Atlas of
HUMAN
ANATOMY

A **Slide Atlas of Human Anatomy** based on the material in this book is available. In the slide atlas format each of the seven chapters in the book is presented in a vinyl binder together with labelled and numbered 35mm colour transparencies of each illustration. Each slide atlas volume also contains a list of abbreviated slide captions for easy reference when using the slides. The complete set of seven slide atlas volumes is contained in a durable presentation slip case. The complete slide atlas contains 506 slides.

Volume 1	Basic Anatomical Concepts	32 slides
Volume 2	Thorax	60 slides
Volume 3	Upper Limb	96 slides
Volume 4	Abdomen	98 slides
Volume 5	Pelvis and Perineum	40 slides
Volume 6	Lower Limb	92 slides
Volume 7	Head and Neck	88 slides

Further information may be obtainted from:
Gower Medical Publishing,
101 Fifth Avenue
New York, New York 10003
USA

Atlas of HUMAN ANATOMY
with integrated text

from Manchester University Department of Anatomy:

J.A. Gosling MD, MB ChB
Professor of Anatomy

P.F. Harris MD, MB ChB, MSc
Professor of Anatomy and Director of the
Anatomical Laboratories

J.R. Humpherson MB ChB
Senior Lecturer in Anatomy

I. Whitmore MD, MB BS, LRCP, MRCS
Lecturer in Anatomy

P.L.T. Willan MB ChB, FRCS
Senior Lecturer in Anatomy

Photography by:

A.L. Bentley ABIPP, AIMBI, MBKS
Medical photographer

J.L. Hargreaves BA(Hons)
Medical photographer

Department of Anatomy
University of Manchester
Manchester, UK

J.B. Lippincott Company · Philadelphia

Gower Medical Publishing London · New York

Distributed in the USA and Canada by:
  J.B. Lippincott Company,
  East Washington Square,
  Philadelphia, PA. 19105, USA

Distributed in Japan by:
  Nankodo Co. Ltd.,
  Tokyo International P.O. Box 5272,
  42-6, Hongo 3-chome,
  Bunkyo-ku, Tokyo 113, Japan.

Distributed in all countries except USA, Canada and Japan by:
  Churchill Livingstone,
  Robert Stevenson House,
  1–3 Baxter's Place,
  Leith Walk,
  Edinburgh EH1 3AF

ISBN: 0-906923-27-1 (Gower)
ISBN: 0-397-58284-6 (Lippincott)

Library of Congress Catalog Card Number: 85-50212

Library Cataloging in Publication Data is available.

Printed in Hong Kong by Mandarin Offset International Ltd.

Project Editor: Sharyn Wong

Design: Mehmet Hussein

Illustration: Robin Nicholl
               Lynda Payne
               Chris Furey
               Maurizia Olanrewaju

Preface

Despite the many anatomical atlases and textbooks currently available, there appeared to be a need for a book which combined the advantages of each of these forms of presentation. This book was conceived with the intention of filling that need. With a unique combination of photographs of dissections, accompanying diagrams and concise text, this volume aims to provide the student with a better understanding of human anatomy.

The basis of this work is the cadaver as seen in the dissecting room; therefore, reference to surface and radiological anatomy is minimal. Likewise, comments on the clinical and functional significance of selected anatomical structures are brief. However, comparison is made where appropriate between the anatomy of the living and that of the cadaver.

Each dissection was specially prepared and photographed to display only a few important features. However, since photographs of dissections are inherently difficult to interpret, each is accompanied by a guide in the form of a drawing. Each drawing is coloured and labelled to highlight the salient features of the dissection and is accompanied by axes to indicate the orientation of the specimen. Adjacent photographs often depict different stages of the same dissection to help the student construct a three-dimensional image.

The first chapter introduces anatomical terminology, provides general information about the basic tissues of the body, and includes overall views of selected systems. Because the six subsequent chapters describe anatomy primarily through dissection, a regional approach has been employed. Features of bones are described only when considering their related structures, especially muscles and joints; osteology is not considered in its own right. The internal structure of the ear and eye are beyond the scope of this book since the study of these topics requires microscopy; the anatomy of the brain and spinal cord are also excluded as they are usually taught in special courses.

The level of detail contained in this book is appropriate for current courses in topographical anatomy for medical and dental undergraduates. In addition, it will be of value to postgraduates and to students entering those professions allied to medicine in which anatomy is part of the curriculum.

The terminology employed is that which is most frequently used in clinical practice. Where appropriate, alternatives (such as those recommended in *Nomina Anatomica*) are appended in brackets.

Preparation of the dissections and the text has occupied the authors for nearly five years. Our objective was to create a high quality and visually attractive anatomical work and we hope that the time and effort spent in its preparation is reflected in the finished product.

Acknowledgements

The authors are indebted to the mortuary technician of the Anatomy Department, Mr. J. Davis, who embalmed the cadavers and helped in cutting the sections. The secretarial staff have assisted greatly in typing various drafts of text, usually trying to meet a deadline already passed.

Other members of the Department of Anatomy have provided valuable comment and have graciously tolerated seemingly endless conversations on the quality of this or that dissection or portion of text.

Our families deserve a special mention, as without their untiring support and patience this volume would certainly not have come to fruition.

The staff at Gower Medical Publishing have worked extremely hard in drawing all the diagrams and executing the page layouts. Sharyn Wong, project editor, has been a stalwart communicator, providing guidance in publishing matters and correcting our English.

We thank them all.

J.A.G., P.F.H., J.R.H., I.W. & P.L.T.W.
Manchester, 1985

User Guide

ORGANIZATION

This book begins with a chapter on basic anatomical concepts which is followed by six chapters, each dealing with one of the anatomical regions. Within each chapter the information is presented usually in a dissectional order suitable for teaching, progressing from the surface to deeper structures. The limbs are described from proximal to distal with the joints considered at the ends of the appropriate chapters.

The numbering of the pages and illustrations is sequential within each chapter; thus 'page 1.24' means the twenty-fourth page in Chapter 1 and 'Fig. 1.24' refers to the twenty-fourth picture in Chapter 1.

TEXT AND PHOTOGRAPHS

Usually each topic is presented on self-contained spreads, the photographs being accompanied by the relevant text. Within the text, cross-references are given to other relevant text and illustrations.

ACCOMPANYING DIAGRAMS

The line diagrams augment the photographs and each diagram uses a colour code to focus the attention of the reader on structures of particular importance in the dissection.

LABELS AND LEADER LINES

On each diagram only the structures of interest have been labelled. In many instances the leader line from a label is branched. If only one structure is named, the leader line and any branch(es) it may have indicates different parts of that structure. However, when more than one stucture is named, the first structure is indicated by the main leader line and the subsequent structures are indicated by branches given off the main leader line at progressively shorter distances from the label. A leader line ending with an arrowhead indicates a space or cavity (see below).

ORIENTATION GUIDES

Each diagram is accompanied by a set of axes which indicates the orientation of the specimen. The abbreviations used in these axes are:

L	Left	I	Inferior	l	lateral
R	Right	P	Posterior	m	medial
S	Superior	A	Anterior	d	distal
				p	proximal

These axes show the direction in the plane of the page in relation to the anatomical position. Thus, when looking at the whole body the axes appear as follows:

$$R \leftarrow\!\!\!\overset{\textstyle S}{\underset{\textstyle I}{+}}\!\!\!\rightarrow L$$
(from in front)

$$L \leftarrow\!\!\!\overset{\textstyle S}{\underset{\textstyle I}{+}}\!\!\!\rightarrow R$$
(from behind)

$$L \leftarrow\!\!\!\overset{\textstyle A}{\underset{\textstyle P}{+}}\!\!\!\rightarrow R$$
(from above)

When views are oblique, the axis which emerges from the plane of the page towards the reader is shown with a large arrowhead and long shaft. Conversely, the axis which passes into the page away from the reader is shown with a small arrowhead and short shaft. Thus, the axes below indicate a left anterolateral view (as seen in Fig. 1.1).

$$A \leftarrow\!\!\!\overset{\textstyle S}{\underset{\textstyle I}{+}}\!\!\!\rightarrow P$$

TERMINOLOGY

The terminology is that used most frequently in clinical practice. Where appropriate, alternative names (including those recommended in *Nomina Anatomica*) are appended in brackets.

SELF ASSESSMENT

The photographs are unfettered by labels, leader lines and other superimposed markings; thus, the reader can readily use this book to test his knowledge by either masking the whole of the accompanying diagram and studying the photograph alone or covering only the labels around the diagram.

Contents

1
BASIC ANATOMICAL CONCEPTS

TERMS OF POSITION AND MOVEMENT

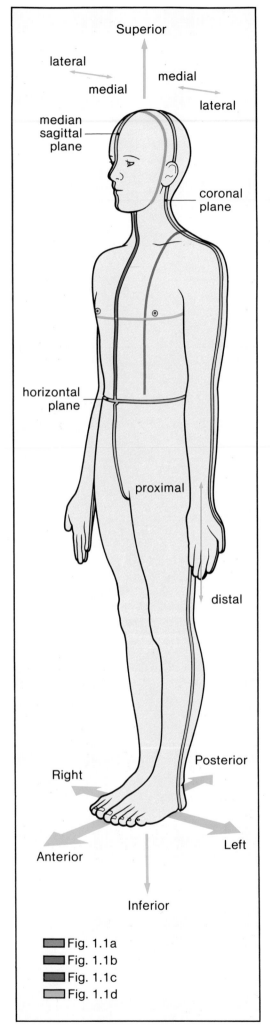

Superior

lateral

medial

medial

lateral

median sagittal plane

coronal plane

horizontal plane

proximal

distal

Posterior

Right

Left

Anterior

Inferior

Fig. 1.1a
Fig. 1.1b
Fig. 1.1c
Fig. 1.1d

Fig. 1.1 *Basic terms conventionally used in anatomical description.*

To avoid ambiguity and confusion, anatomical terms of position and movement are defined according to an internationally accepted convention. This convention defines the 'anatomical position' as one in which the human body stands erect with the feet together and the face, eyes and palms of the hands directed forwards (Fig. 1.1).

Fig. 1.1a *Coronal section through the head.*

S

R — L

I

brain

ramus of mandible   oral cavity

S

A — P

I

heart   lung

diaphragm   stomach   kidney   liver

Fig. 1.1b *Sagittal section through the trunk. This section lies to the left of the median sagittal plane.*

With the subject in the anatomical position, three sets of planes, mutually at right angles, can be defined. **Horizontal** (or **transverse**) **planes** transect the body from side to side and front to back.

Vertical (or longitudinal) planes are termed either **coronal** or **sagittal**. **Coronal planes** pass from one side to the other while **sagittal planes** pass from front to back. One particular sagittal plane, the **median sagittal plane**, lies in the midline and divides the body into right and left halves (Fig. 1.1c).

A transverse section may be cut at right angles to the long axis of any organ or part of the body, and a longitudinal section along its long axis.

The terms **medial** and **lateral** are used to indicate the position of structures relative to the median sagittal plane. For example, the ring finger lies lateral to the little finger but medial to the thumb. The front and back of the body are usually termed the **anterior** (or ventral) and **posterior** (or dorsal) surfaces respectively. Thus, one structure is described as anterior to another because it is placed further forwards (Fig. 1.1).

Superior and **inferior** are terms used to indicate the relative head/tail positions of structures (Fig. 1.1). Those lying towards the head (or cranial) end of the body are described as superior to others which are inferior (or caudal). Thus, the heart lies superior to the diaphragm; the diaphragm is inferior to the heart. In the limbs the terms **proximal** and **distal** have comparable meanings. For example, the elbow joint is proximal to the wrist but distal to the shoulder.

The terms **superficial** and **deep** indicate the location of structures in relation to the body surface. Thus, the ribs lie superficial to the lungs but deep to the skin of the chest wall (Fig. 1.1d).

Fig. 1.1c *Median sagittal section through the trunk.*

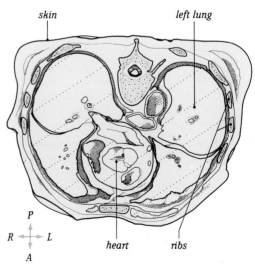

Fig. 1.1d *Transverse section through the thorax at the level of vertebra T6.*

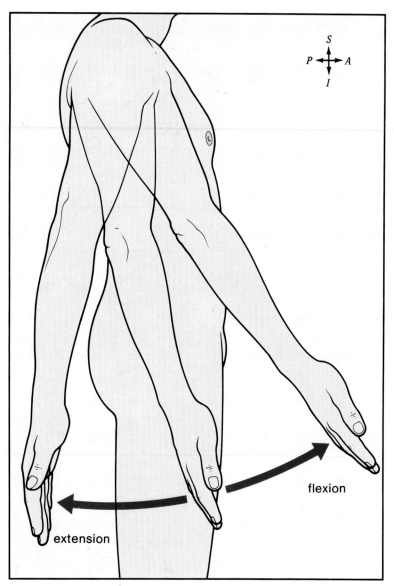

Fig. 1.2 *Movements of flexion and extension of the shoulder joint.*

Fig. 1.3 *Movements of abduction and adduction. In adduction, flexion of the shoulder joint allows the limb to be carried anterior to the trunk.*

Movements at joints are also described by specific terms. From the anatomical position, forward movement of one part in relation to the rest of the body is called **flexion**. **Extension** carries the same part posteriorly (Fig. 1.2). However, because in the fetus the developing upper and lower limbs rotate in different directions, the movements of flexion and extension in all joints from the knee downwards occur in opposite directions when compared with the equivalent joints in the upper limb. In **abduction** the stucture moves away from the median sagittal plane in a lateral direction whereas **adduction** returns it towards the midline (Fig. 1.3). For the fingers and toes, the terms abduction and adduction are used in reference to a longitudinal plane passing along the middle finger or the second toe respectively. Movement around the longitudinal axis of part of the body is called rotation. In **medial** (or internal) **rotation** the anterior surface of a limb rotates medially whilst **lateral** (or external) **rotation** turns the anterior surface laterally (Fig. 1.4). Movements which combine flexion, extension, abduction, adduction, and medial and lateral rotation (for instance, 'windmilling' action seen at the shoulder joint) are known as **circumduction**.

Fig. 1.4 *Movement of the forearm indicates medial and lateral rotation at the shoulder joint. The elbow is flexed.*

1. Skin

Skin (Fig. 1.5) is a protective covering for the surface of the body and comprises a superficial layer called the epidermis, and a deeper layer, the dermis. The epidermis is an epithelium consisting of a surface layer of dead cells which are continually shed and replaced by cells from the deeper germinal layer. The dermis is a layer of connective tissue containing blood vessels, lymphatics and nerves. In most areas of the body the skin is thin and mobile over the underlying structures. Specializations of the skin include finger- and toenails, hair follicles and sweat glands. On the palms of the hands and soles of the feet (and corresponding surfaces of the digits), hair follicles are absent and the epidermis is relatively thick. Also, the skin in these regions is firmly anchored to underlying structures, reducing its mobility during gripping and standing. Lines of tension occur within skin and are of importance to surgeons. Scars following surgical incisions made along these lines tend to be narrower than those made across the lines of tension.

Skin is usually well vascularized and receives blood from numerous subcutaneous vessels. Knowledge of this vascular supply is important when operations are undertaken which involve the use of skin flaps.
Skin has a rich nerve supply, responding to touch, pressure, heat, cold, vibration and pain. In certain areas such as the fingertips, the skin is especially sensitive to touch and pressure. Skin is innervated by superficial (cutaneous) branches of spinal or cranial nerves. The area of skin supplied by each cranial or spinal nerve is remarkably constant and is known as a dermatome (see Fig. 1.24).

2. Superficial fascia

Immediately deep to the skin is a layer of loose connective tissue, the superficial fascia (Fig. 1.5), which contains networks of superficial veins and lymphatics and is traversed by cutaneous nerves and arteries. It also contains fat, which varies considerably in thickness from region to region and between individuals. For example, over the buttock the fat is particularly thick whilst on the back of the hand it is relatively thin.

Fig. 1.5 *Multilevel 'step dissection' through the right midcalf to show layers of skin, fascia and intermuscular septa.*

3. Deep fascia

The deep fascia (Fig. 1.5) consists of a layer of dense connective tissue immediately beneath the superficial fascia. Although thin over the thorax and abdomen, it forms a substantial layer in the limbs (for example, fascia lata; see page 6.3) and neck (for example, investing fascia; see page 7.2). Near the wrist and ankle joints, the deep fascia is thickened to form retinacula which maintain the tendons in position as they cross the joints. Deep fascia also provides attachment for muscles and gives anchorage to intermuscular septa which separate the muscles into compartments.

external
oblique

apo-
neurosis

external
oblique
(cut)

costal
cartilages

S
R ← → L
I

S
R ← → L
I

1.6   **Fig. 1.6a** *External oblique is a flat muscle with an extensive aponeurosis.*   **Fig. 1.6b** *External oblique cut to show its thickness.*

Fig. 1.6c *Subscapularis is a multipennate muscle.*

Fig. 1.6d *Flexor pollicis longus is a unipennate muscle.*

4. Muscle

Muscle is a tissue in which active contraction either shortens its component cells or generates tension along their length. There are three basic types: smooth muscle; cardiac striated muscle; and voluntary striated muscle. 'Striated' and 'smooth' describe the microscopic appearance of the muscle.

Smooth muscle is present in the organs of the alimentary, genitourinary and respiratory systems and in the walls of blood vessels. Capable of slow sustained contraction, smooth muscle is usually controlled by the autonomic nervous system (see page 1.18) and, in some organs, by endocrine secretions (hormones).

Cardiac striated muscle (myocardium) is confined to the wall of the heart and is able to contract spontaneously and rhythmically. Its cyclical activity is coordinated by the specialized conducting tissue of the heart and can be modified by the autonomic nervous system.

Voluntary striated muscle (often called skeletal) is the basic component of those muscles which produce movements at joints. These actions are controlled by the somatic nervous system (see page 1.17) and may be voluntary or reflex. Each muscle cell (fibre) has its own motor nerve ending which initiates contraction of the fibre. Muscles may be attached to the periosteum of bones either directly or by fibrous connective tissue in the form of deep fascia, intermuscular septa or tendons. Direct fleshy attachment can be extensive but tendons are usually attached to small areas of bone. Muscles with similar actions tend to be grouped together; and in limbs these groups form compartments (for instance, extensor compartment of forearm).

Usually each end of a muscle has an attachment to bone. The attachment that remains relatively fixed when the muscle performs its prime action is known as the origin whereas the insertion is the more mobile attachment. However, in some movements the origin moves more than the insertion; therefore these terms are only of limited significance.

The muscle fibres within voluntary muscle are arranged in differing patterns which reflect the function of the muscle (Figs. 1.6a–1.6e). Sometimes they are found as thin flat sheets (as is external oblique). Strap muscles (such as sartorius) have long fibres which reach without interruption from one end of the muscle to the other. Pennate muscles are characterized by fibres that run obliquely. Unipennate muscles (for example, flexor pollicis longus) have fibres running from their origin to attach along only one side of the tendon of insertion. In bipennate muscles (such as rectus femoris), the fibres are anchored to both sides of the tendon of insertion.

Multipennate muscles (for example, subscapularis) have several tendons of origin and insertion with muscle fibres passing obliquely between them. Some muscles, for instance digastric, have two fleshy parts (bellies) connected by an intermediate tendon.

Most tendons are thick and round or flattened in cross-section, although some form thin sheets called aponeuroses (Fig. 1.6a). When tendons cross projections or traverse confined spaces they are often enveloped in a double layer of synovial membrane (see page 1.12) to minimize friction. Where they cross joints, tendons are often held in place by bands of thick fibrous tissue which prevent 'bowstringing' when the joints are moved. Examples include the retinacula at the wrist and ankle joints, and tendon sheaths in the fingers and toes (Figs. 1.7 & 1.8).

The nerve supply to a skeletal muscle contains both motor and sensory fibres which usually enter the fleshy part of the muscle. Groups of muscles with similar actions tend to be supplied by nerve fibres derived from the same spinal cord segments.

As metabolically very active tissue, muscle has a rich arterial blood supply usually carried by several separate vessels. The contraction and relaxation of muscles in the limbs compresses the veins in each compartment. As the veins contain unidirectional valves, this 'muscle pump' action assists the return of venous blood from the limbs to the trunk.

5. Cartilage

Cartilage is a variety of hard connective tissue which gains its nutrition by diffusion from blood vessels in the surrounding tissues. It is classified by its histological structure into hyaline cartilage, fibrocartilage and elastic cartiliage.

Hyaline cartilage occurs in costal cartilages (Fig. 1.6b), the cartilages of the larynx and trachea, and in developing bones. In synovial joints (see Fig. 1.13) it forms the glassy smooth articular surfaces which reduce friction during movement. Articular cartilage is partly nourished by diffusion from the synovial fluid in the joint cavity.

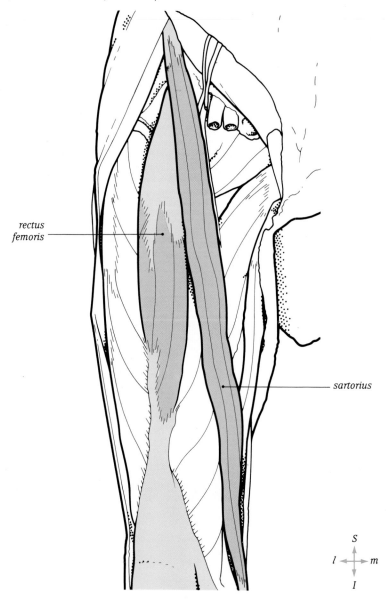

rectus femoris

sartorius

Fig. 1.6e *Rectus femoris is a bipennate muscle and sartorius is a strap muscle.*

The inclusion of tough inelastic collagen fibres in the matrix constitutes fibrocartilage, which is stronger and more flexible than the hyaline type. Fibrocartilage is found in intervertebral discs (see Fig. 1.12), the pubic symphysis, the manubriosternal joint, and as articular discs in some synovial joints (for example, knee and temporomandibular).

Elastic cartilage, which occurs in the external ear and epiglottis, is the most flexible form of cartilage. It contains predominantly elastic fibres and has a yellowish appearance.

Cartilage may become calcified in old age, becoming harder and more rigid.

Fig. 1.7 *Anterior view of the left hand dissected to reveal its fibrous sheaths and tendons.*

Fig. 1.8 *Posterior view of the left hand dissected to show the extensor retinaculum at the wrist.*

1.9

6. Bone

Bone forms the basis of the skeleton and is characterized by a hard calcified matrix which gives rigidity. In most bones two zones are visible. Near the surface the outer cortical layer of bone appears solid and is called compact bone whereas centrally the bone appears spongy and is known as cancellous bone. Many bones contain a cavity (medulla) occupied by the bone marrow, a potential site of blood cell production (Fig. 1.9).

The numerous bones comprising the human skeleton vary considerably in shape and size and are classified into long bones (for example, femur), short bones (bones of the carpus), flat bones (parietal bone of skull), irregular bones (maxilla of skull) and sesamoid bones (patella). Sesamoid bones develop in tendons, generally where the tendon passes over a joint or bony projection. Some bones are described as pneumatized because of their air-filled cavities (for instance, ethmoid).

Bone is enveloped by a thin layer of fibrous tissue called periosteum (see Fig.1.5) which provides anchorage for muscles, tendons and ligaments. Periosteum is a source of cells for bone growth and repair and is richly innervated and exquisitely sensitive to pain.

Bone has a profuse blood supply which is provided partly via the periosteal vessels and partly by nutrient arteries, which enter bones via nutrient foramina and also supply the marrow. Fractured bones often bleed profusely from damaged medullary and periosteal vessels.

Several names are given to the different parts of a long bone in relation to its development (Fig. 1.10). The shaft (or diaphysis) ossifies first and is separated by growth plates from the secondary centres of ossification (or epiphyses) which usually lie at the extremities of the bone. The part of a diaphysis next to a growth plate is called a metaphysis and has a particularly rich blood supply. When increase in bone length ceases, the growth plates disappear and the epiphyses fuse with the diaphysis.

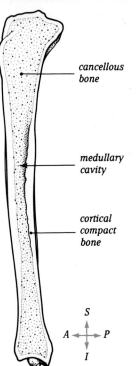

cancellous bone

medullary cavity

cortical compact bone

S

A ←→ P

I

7. Joints

Joints are classified according to their structure into fibrous, cartilaginous and synovial types. In fibrous joints (Fig. 1.11) which are relatively immobile, the two bones are joined by fibrous tissue (for example, sutures seen between the bones of the skull).

Cartilage is interposed between bone ends in cartilaginous joints. Primary cartilaginous joints contain hyaline cartilage, are usually capable of only limited movement, and occur between the ribs and sternum. In secondary cartilaginous joints (Fig. 1.12), fibrocartilage unites the bone ends. These joints, which generally allow more movement than those of the primary type, all lie in the midline. Examples include the intervertebral discs, the manubriosternal joint and the pubic symphysis.

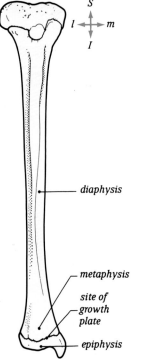

S

l ←→ m

I

diaphysis

metaphysis

site of growth plate

epiphysis

1.10   **Fig. 1.9** *Longitudinal section of an adult tibia.*   **Fig. 1.10** *Anterior view of a child's tibia.*

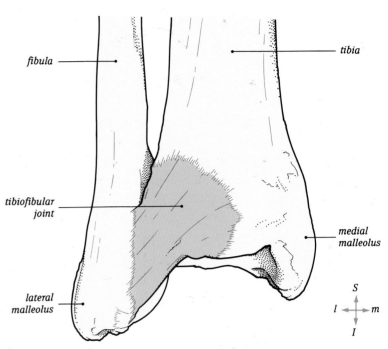

Fig. 1.11 *The inferior tibiofibular joint is an example of a fibrous joint.*

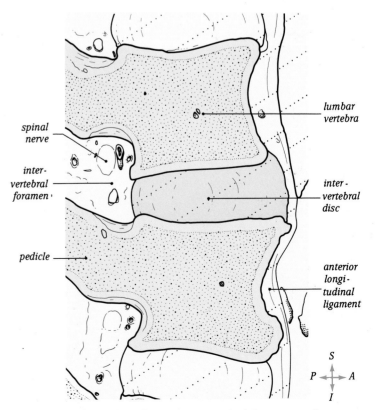

Fig. 1.12 *Sagittal section to show an intervertebral disc, a secondary cartilaginous joint.*

1.11

BASIC TISSUES AND STRUCTURES

SYNOVIAL JOINTS

The most common type of joint is the synovial joint, which is complex and usually highly mobile. They are classified according to the shape of the joint surfaces (such as plane, saddle, ball-and-socket) or the type of movement they permit (such as sliding, pivot, hinge). In a typical synovial joint (Fig. 1.13) the articulating surfaces are coated with hyaline cartilage and the bones are joined by a fibrous capsule, a tubular sleeve which is attached around the periphery of the areas of articular cartilage. In every synovial joint all of the interior (except for intra-articular cartilage) is lined with synovial membrane. This thin vascular membrane secretes synovial fluid into the joint space, providing nutrition for the cartilage and lubrication for the joint.

The capsule is usually thickened to form strengthening bands known as capsular ligaments (for example, the pubofemoral ligament). In addition, fibrous bands, discrete from the capsule, may form extracapsular ligaments (such as the costoclavicular ligament). In some joints there are intracapsular

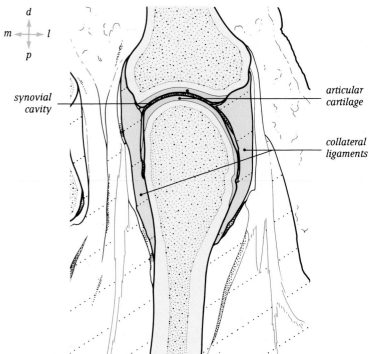

Fig. 1.13 *Coronal section through a metacarpophalangeal joint, a typical synovial joint. The collateral ligaments are thickenings of the joint capsule.*

Fig. 1.14 *Removal of part of the shoulder joint capsule reveals the intracapsular but extrasynovial tendon of the long head of biceps brachii.*

ligaments (for instance, the ligament of the head of the femur) which are covered by synovial membrane. Tendons sometimes fuse with the capsule (as in the rotator cuff) or they may run within the joint, covered by synovial membrane, before gaining their bony attachment (for example, biceps brachii at the shoulder joint; Fig. 1.14).

Fluid containing sacs of synovial membrane called bursae (Fig. 1.15) separate some tendons and muscles from other structures. Bursae which lie close to

joints may communicate with the cavity of the joint through a small opening in the capsule (as does the subscapularis bursa).

In some joints (for example, the knee joint) a disc of cartilage (Fig. 1.16) is interposed between the articular cartilage covering the bone ends. This provides a matched shape for each bone end, thus allowing freer movement without compromising stability. In addition, different types of movement are permitted in each half of the joint.

Fig. 1.15 *Sagittal section through the elbow joint. The olecranon bursa does not communicate with the joint cavity.*

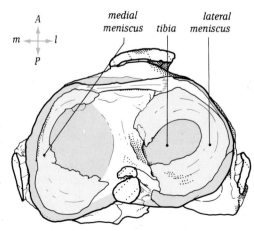

Fig. 1.16 *Disarticulated knee joint to show the menisci.*

Stability varies considerably from one synovial joint to another, as several factors limit excessive movement and contribute to the stability of the joint. These include the shape of the articulating surfaces, the strength of the capsule and associated ligaments, the tone of the surrounding muscles and, where present, intra-articular discs and ligaments. At the hip joint the ligaments and the shape of the bones provide its main stability whereas the tone of the surrounding muscles stabilize the shoulder joint.

Joints, particularly their capsules, receive a rich sensory innervation derived from the nerves supplying the muscles that act on the joint. For instance, the axillary nerve supplies the shoulder joint and deltoid.

Blood vessels around joints frequently take part in rich anastomoses, which allow alternative pathways for blood flow when the joint has moved to a different position and ensure an adequate supply to the synovial membrane (such as in knee joint; Fig. 1.17).

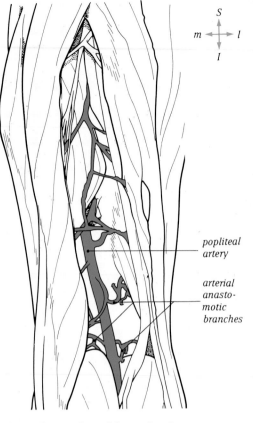

popliteal artery

arterial anasto- motic branches

Fig. 1.17 *Branches of the popliteal artery anastomose around the knee joint.*

8. Skeleton

The skeleton is composed of bones and cartilages held together by joints, and gives rigidity and support to the body. It has axial and appendicular components. The axial component includes the skull, vertebral column, ribs, costal cartilages and sternum. The appendicular skeleton comprises the bones of the upper and lower limbs and their associated girdles. In this book individual bones are described in the appropriate regions. However, since the vertebral column spans the neck and trunk, a brief outline of some of its salient features is given here.

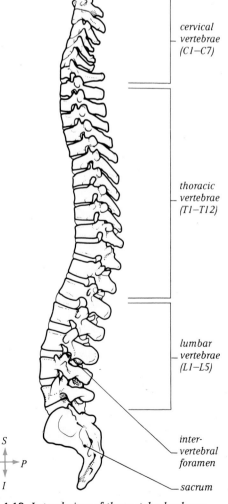

cervical vertebrae (C1–C7)

thoracic vertebrae (T1–T12)

lumbar vertebrae (L1–L5)

inter- vertebral foramen

sacrum

VERTEBRAL COLUMN

The vertebral column (Fig. 1.18) has five regions, each with a characteristic number of vertebrae. There are usually seven cervical, twelve thoracic, five lumbar, five sacral and between one and four coccygeal vertebrae. The sacrum is formed by the fusion of the five sacral vertebrae. In the anatomical position the vertebral column has a series of gentle curves with the cervical and lumbar vertebrae forming curves which are convex anteriorly (lordosis) and the thoracic and sacral vertebrae curved in the opposite direction.

A typical vertebra possesses a body from which arise two posteriorly projecting processes, the pedicles. Each pedicle carries a transverse process, and superior and inferior articular processes. The neural arch is completed posteriorly by two laminae which fuse and give rise to the spinous process (Fig. 1.19). The neural arches and bodies of the vertebrae enclose the vertebral canal which contains the spinal cord, spinal nerves and their associated membranes. Individual spinal nerves emerge from this canal via intervertebral foramina between adjacent vertebrae (see Fig. 1.12).

Fig. 1.18 *Lateral view of the vertebral column.*

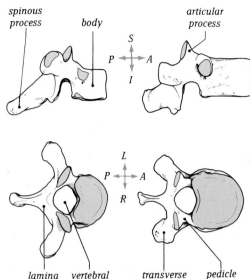

spinous process   body   articular process

S
P ← → A
I

lamina   vertebral foramen   transverse process   pedicle

L
P ← → A
R

Fig. 1.19 *Lateral and superior views of typical thoracic vertebrae.*

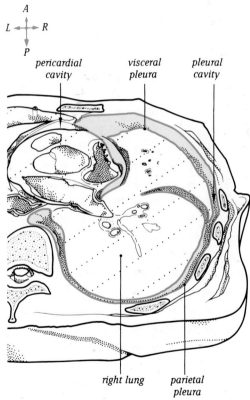

A
L ← → R
P

pericardial cavity   visceral pleura   pleural cavity

right lung   parietal pleura

Fig. 1.20 *Transverse section through the thorax at the level of T5 showing the right pleural cavity.*

Vertebrae articulate with each other at two types of joint. Between the bodies lie the fibrocartilaginous intervertebral discs, forming secondary cartilaginous joints. Between the articular processes are synovial joints at which the inferior facet of one vertebrae articulates with the superior facet of the vertebra below. Movement in the vertebral column is limited by posterior and anterior longitudinal ligaments applied to the respective surfaces of the vertebral bodies, and by intertransverse, interspinous and supraspinous ligaments. The shapes and orientations of the articular processes allow different movements in the various regions of the column. Thus the thoracic spine is much less mobile than the cervical spine.

9. Serous membranes and cavities

Pericardium, pleura and peritoneum comprise the serous membranes lining the cavities that separate the heart, lungs and abdominal viscera respectively from their surrounding structures. Where the membrane lines the outer wall of the cavity it is called parietal, and where it covers the appropriate organ it is called visceral. The parietal and visceral parts are in continuity around the root of the viscus and are separated from each other by a cavity which normally contains only a thin film of serous fluid. Although the membranes are in close contact, they are lubricated by the intervening fluid which permits movement between the viscus and its surroundings (Fig. 1.20).

1.15

10. Blood vessels

Blood vessels convey blood around the body and are classified into three main types, namely arteries, capillaries and veins.

Arteries are relatively thick-walled vessels which convey blood in a branching system of decreasing calibre away from the heart. Some arteries are named after the region through which they pass (such as the femoral artery) while others are named according to the structures they supply (for instance, the renal artery). The largest vessels, such as the aorta, have elastic walls and therefore are called elastic arteries. They give rise to arteries whose walls are more muscular (muscular arteries), such as the radial artery in the forearm. A particularly thick smooth muscle coat is also a feature of the walls of the microscopic arterioles. The tone of arteriolar smooth muscle is under the control of the autonomic nervous system and hormones and is an important factor in the maintenance of pressure in the arterial system. In general, there are few alternative pathways for arterial blood to reach its destination. However, in some regions (for example, joints and at the base of the brain), arterial supply is provided by more than one vessel (see Fig. 1.17). Such arteries may communicate directly with each other at sites known as arterial anastomoses.

Capillaries link the smallest arteries and the smallest veins and convey blood at low pressure through the tissues. Collectively these thin-walled microscopic vessels have a very extensive surface area, facilitating gaseous and metabolic exchange between the blood and tissues.

Veins carry blood at low pressure from the capillary bed back to the heart. They may be deep (accompanying arteries) or superficial (lying in the superficial fascia) (Fig. 1.21) and are usually linked by venous anastomoses. Veins accompanying arteries are often arranged as several interconnecting vessels called venae comitantes. In the limbs the deep veins can be compressed by local muscular action, thus assisting venous return. Many veins (excluding the venae cavae and those draining viscera and within the cranium) contain unidirectional valves which direct the flow of blood towards the heart (Fig. 1.22). The venous pattern is often variable, and numerous anastomotic connections provide alternate pathways for venous return. In some regions, numerous intercommunicating veins form meshworks called plexuses (such as the pelvic venous plexus). In the cranial cavity, venous blood is carried in special vessels formed by the dura mater lining the interior of the skull. These dural sinuses receive the venous return from the brain.

11. Lymphatic vessels and nodes

Tissue fluid is collected by microscopic open-ended channels called lymphatics. From a particular region or organ these valved lymphatic vessels drain into aggregations of lymphoid tissue called lymph nodes which filter lymph. Groups of lymph nodes are often found close to an organ (for example, hilar nodes) or at the root of a limb (for example, axillary lymph nodes). Ultimately, lymph drains into the venous system in the root of the neck through larger lymph channels called the thoracic duct and the right lymphatic trunk.

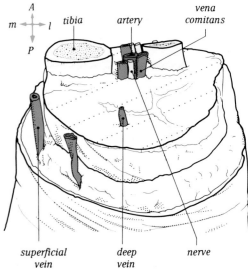

Fig. 1.21 *Multilevel 'step dissection' through the right midcalf showing the vascular supply.*

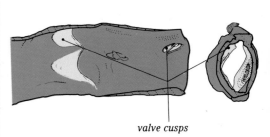

Fig. 1.22 *Portion of saphenous vein seen in cross-section and opened longitudinally.*

Since they filter the fluid passing through them, lymph nodes may become involved in the spread of infection or malignancy (for example, cancer). Thus, the surgeon removing a cancerous organ may also excise the lymph nodes which drain that organ.

12. Nervous tissue

Nervous tissue contains two types of cell, neurones and neuroglia. The neurone is the functional unit responsible for the conduction of nerve impulses. It consists of a cell body and its associated processes. One type of process, of which there is only one per neurone, is the axon. This may be relatively short but sometimes is very long, as in peripheral nerves where axons comprise the individual nerve fibres. The neuroglia undertake supporting roles and include Schwann cells, which provide the myelin sheaths around axons. These sheaths insulate the axons, thus increasing their speeds of conduction.

The nervous system consists of central and peripheral parts. The brain and spinal cord comprise the central nervous system and are not considered in this book.

The peripheral nervous system consists of spinal, cranial and autonomic nerves, and their associated ganglia. Bundles of nerve cell processes and their supporting Schwann cells form peripheral nerves. Several nerve processes, bound together by connective tissue, form a nerve bundle; and numerous bundles, surrounded by a fibrous sheath (epineurium), constitute the complete peripheral nerve. Nerve cell bodies also form part of the peripheral nervous system and are usually grouped together into ganglia. The peripheral nervous system is subdivided into somatic and autonomic parts.

SOMATIC NERVES

In general, the somatic nerves innervate skeletal muscle and transmit sensation from all parts of the body except the viscera. Twelve pairs of cranial nerves are attached to the brain and are named: olfactory (I); optic (II); oculomotor (III); trochlear (IV); trigeminal (V); abducens (VI); facial (VII); vestibulocochlear (VIII); glossopharyngeal (IX); vagus (X); accessory (XI); and hypoglossal (XII). The majority of these nerves supply structures in the head and neck, but the vagus nerve also supplies thoracic and abdominal viscera.

Spinal nerves are also in pairs and each is attached to a specific segment of the spinal cord by anterior and posterior roots. There are eight cervical (C1–C8), twelve thoracic (T1–T12), five lumbar (L1–L5), five sacral (S1–S5), and one or two coccygeal (Co) spinal nerves. Thoracic spinal nerves illustrate the typical segmental pattern of distribution to the body wall (Fig. 1.23). The area of skin supplied by one spinal (or cranial) nerve is called a dermatome. In the trunk the dermatome pattern involves substantial overlap between adjacent areas (Fig. 1.24). Similarly, all the muscles supplied by a single spinal (or cranial) nerve comprise a myotome.

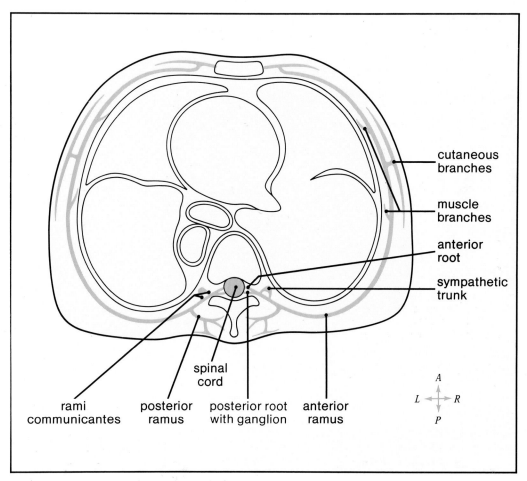

Fig. 1.23 *Course and distribution of a typical thoracic spinal nerve.*

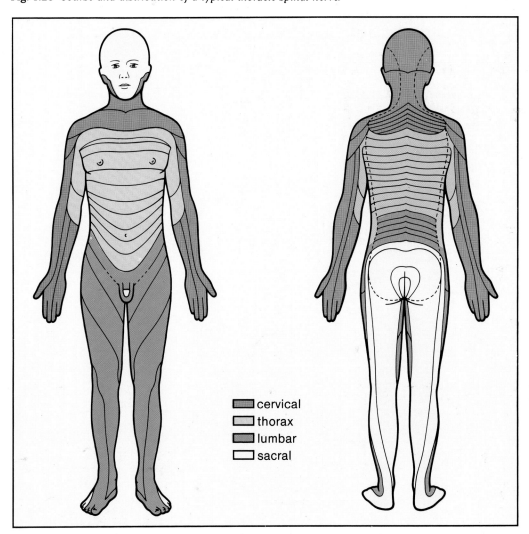

Fig. 1.24 *Dermatomes of the trunk and limbs. The area within the broken line (right) is innervated by the posterior rami.*

1.17

The regular pattern of innervation in the trunk is modified in the limbs, each being supplied by several spinal nerves through a complex network, a plexus (such as the brachial plexus of the upper limb; Fig. 1.25). Plexus formation modifies the pattern of myotomes so that spinal cord segments innervate muscles according to their prime actions. For example, flexors of the elbow joint are supplied by the spinal cord segments C5 and C6. Sensory cell bodies are located in ganglia on peripheral nerves near the central nervous system (for instance, trigeminal ganglion, posterior root ganglia). However, the cell bodies of somatic motor nerves are located in the central nervous system.

Fig. 1.25 *The axilla has been dissected to show the brachial plexus.*

AUTONOMIC NERVES

The autonomic nervous system innervates smooth and cardiac muscle, and also glands. It is divided into two parts, sympathetic and parasympathetic, whose effects for the most part are antagonistic (for example, sympathetic stimulation increases while parasympathetic stimulation reduces heart rate). In both sympathetic and parasympathetic components, preganglionic myelinated axons leave the central nervous system and synapse on neurones in peripheral ganglia distributed throughout the body. The postganglionic axons which pass to the effector organs are non-myelinated. Autonomic sensory fibres accompany autonomic efferent fibres in peripheral nerves but their cell bodies are located in the posterior root ganglia in company with somatic sensory neurones.

The parts of the central nervous system from which the autonomic nerves emerge differ for the sympathetic and parasympathetic components (Fig. 1.26).

SYMPATHETIC NERVES

Preganglionic sympathetic fibres leave the central nervous system only in the spinal nerves of all the thoracic and the upper two lumbar segments (thoracolumbar outflow) and enter the ganglionated sympathetic trunks via white rami communicantes. The two sympathetic trunks lie on either side of the vertebral column and extend throughout most of its length. Each trunk consists of sympathetic ganglia and interconnecting nerve trunks.

Unmyelinated postganglionic axons destined for the blood vessels and sweat glands of the body wall, including the limbs, leave the ganglia by grey rami communicantes and are distributed by the spinal nerves. Special visceral branches pass directly from the trunks to reach the appropriate organ. Postganglionic sympathetic nerve fibres are often conveyed to their destinations as intimate plexuses on the walls of arteries.

PARASYMPATHETIC NERVES

In the parasympathetic system, myelinated preganglionic fibres leave the central nervous system as part of cranial nerves III, VII, IX and X and as part of sacral spinal nerves S2, S3 and S4 to form the craniosacral autonomic outflow. These preganglionic fibres synapse in ganglia lying close to or in the wall of the target organ. Relatively short non-myelinated postganglionic axons emerge from these ganglia to innervate the appropriate tissue. In the head there are four paired ganglia (ciliary, pterygopalatine, submandibular and otic) that receive preganglionic parasympathetic fibres from cranial nerves III, VII and IX. The postganglionic fibres from these ganglia supply the eye, and lacrimal, nasal and salivary glands. Preganglionic fibres from the vagus (X) nerve synapse with postganglionic neurones which innervate cervical, thoracic and abdominal viscera. Those from the sacral nerves (nervi erigentes) supply the pelvic organs. The parasympathetic ganglia associated with the vagus and sacral nerves usually comprise small clusters of cells in the walls of the innervated organs (Fig. 1.26).

Fig. 1.26 *Pattern of innervation in the parasympathetic and sympathetic autonomic nervous systems.*

BODY SYSTEMS

There are several systems which span more than one region of the body but each of the subsequent chapters covers only one region. Therefore, overall views of selected systems are here included. Figs. 1.27 to 1.32 depict the skeleton, the vascular system (including lymphatics), the spinal nerves and the digestive tract.

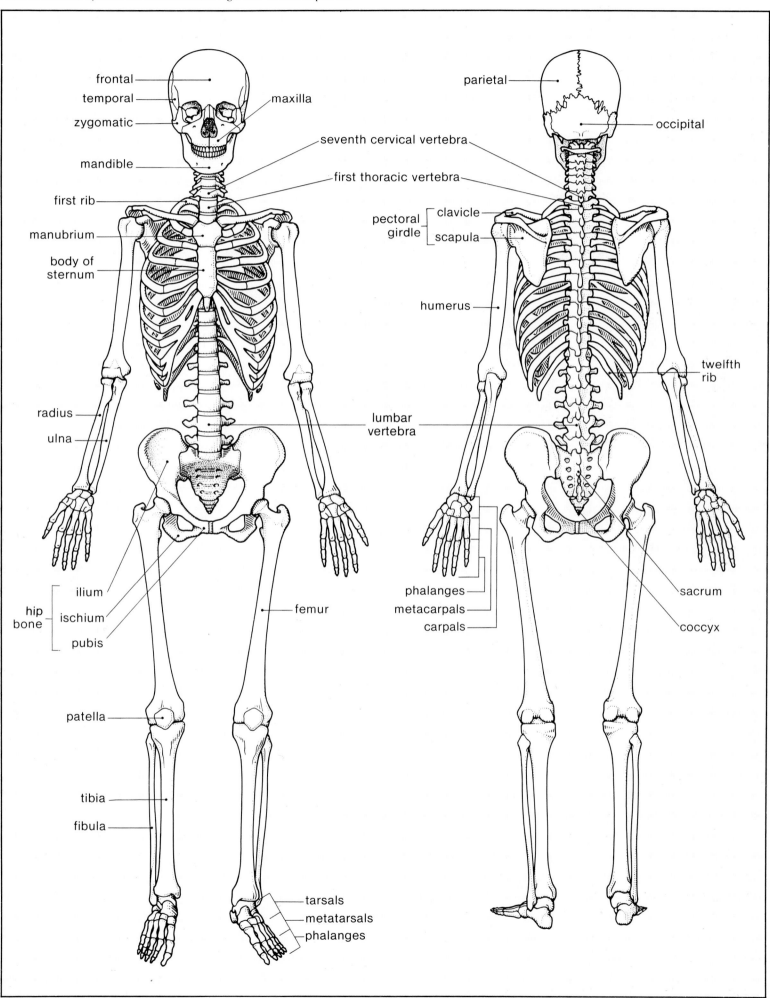

Fig. 1.27 *Anterior and posterior views of the bones of the skeleton.*

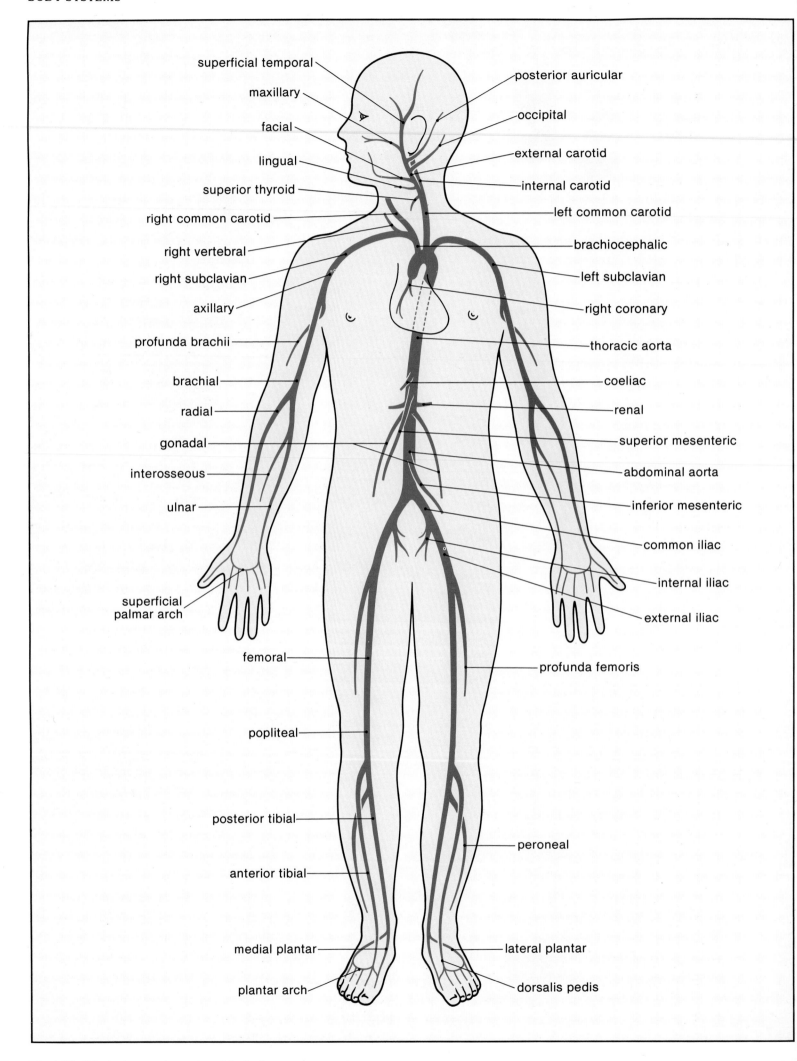

superficial temporal

maxillary

facial

lingual

superior thyroid

right common carotid

right vertebral

right subclavian

axillary

profunda brachii

brachial

radial

gonadal

interosseous

ulnar

superficial
palmar arch

femoral

popliteal

posterior tibial

anterior tibial

medial plantar

plantar arch

posterior auricular

occipital

external carotid

internal carotid

left common carotid

brachiocephalic

left subclavian

right coronary

thoracic aorta

coeliac

renal

superior mesenteric

abdominal aorta

inferior mesenteric

common iliac

internal iliac

external iliac

profunda femoris

peroneal

lateral plantar

dorsalis pedis

Fig. 1.28 *Principal systemic arteries of the body.*

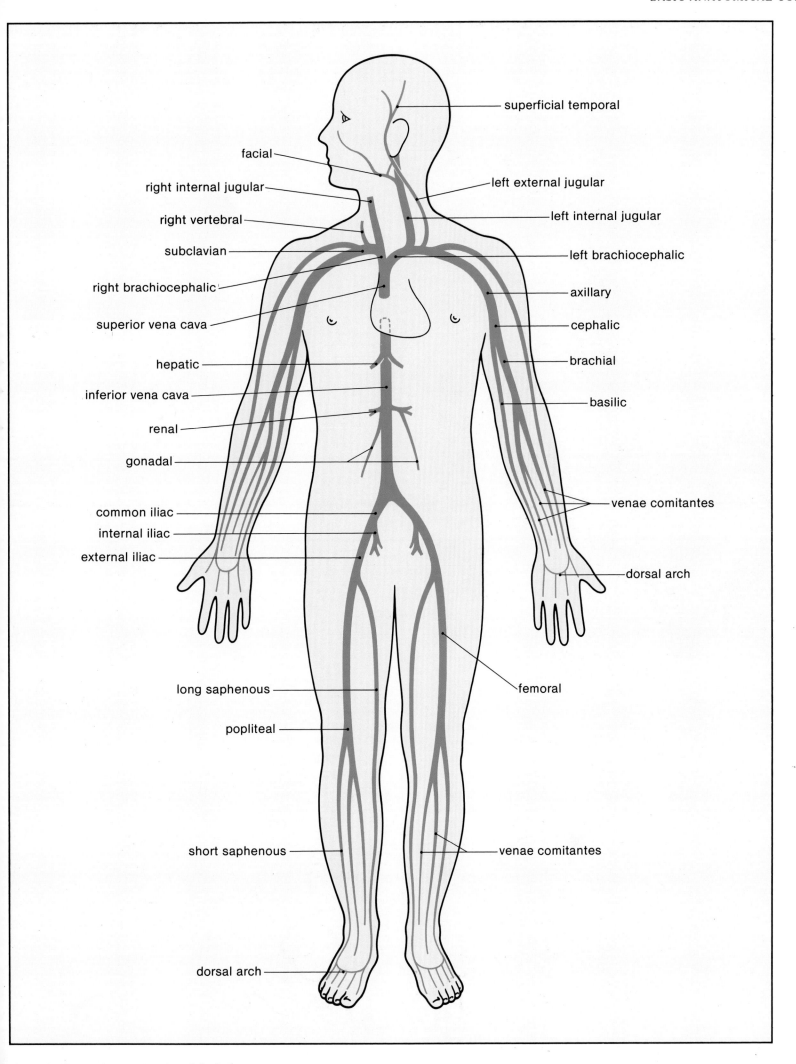

superficial temporal

facial

right internal jugular

right vertebral

subclavian

right brachiocephalic

superior vena cava

hepatic

inferior vena cava

renal

gonadal

common iliac

internal iliac

external iliac

long saphenous

popliteal

short saphenous

dorsal arch

left external jugular

left internal jugular

left brachiocephalic

axillary

cephalic

brachial

basilic

venae comitantes

dorsal arch

femoral

venae comitantes

Fig. 1.29 *Principal systemic veins of the body.*

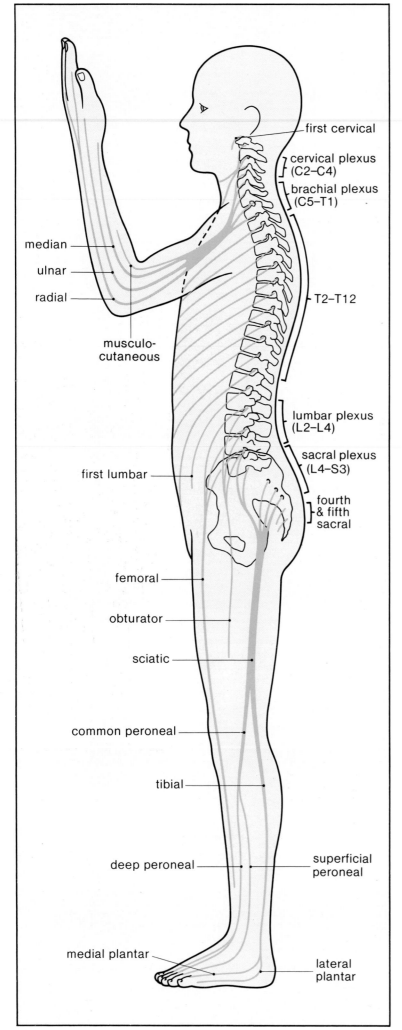

median

ulnar

radial

musculo-
cutaneous

first cervical

cervical plexus
(C2–C4)

brachial plexus
(C5–T1)

T2–T12

lumbar plexus
(L2–L4)

sacral plexus
(L4–S3)

first lumbar

fourth
& fifth
sacral

femoral

obturator

sciatic

common peroneal

tibial

deep peroneal

superficial
peroneal

medial plantar

lateral
plantar

Fig. 1.30 *Lateral view of the distribution of the anterior rami of the spinal nerves.*

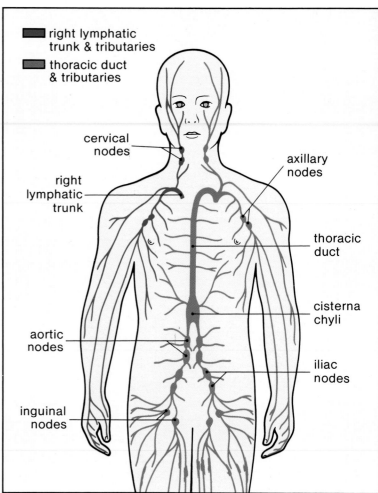

right lymphatic
trunk & tributaries

thoracic duct
& tributaries

cervical
nodes

right
lymphatic
trunk

aortic
nodes

inguinal
nodes

axillary
nodes

thoracic
duct

cisterna
chyli

iliac
nodes

Fig. 1.31 *The main lymphatic nodes and vessels of the body.*

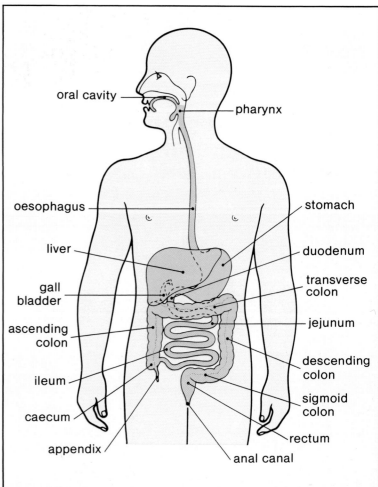

oral cavity

oesophagus

liver

gall
bladder

ascending
colon

ileum

caecum

appendix

pharynx

stomach

duodenum

transverse
colon

jejunum

descending
colon

sigmoid
colon

rectum

anal canal

Fig. 1.32 *Principal organs of the alimentary tract. The pancreas has been omitted for clarity.*

2

THORAX

SKELETON OF THORAX

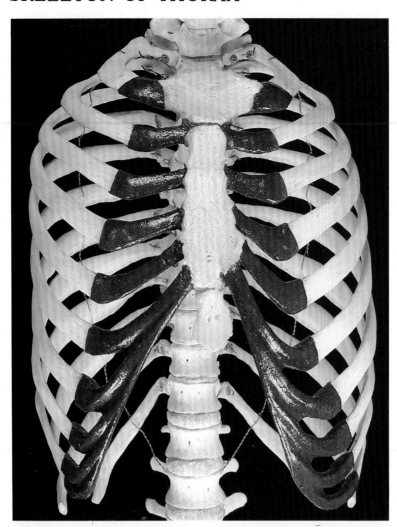

The skeleton of the thorax consists of twelve thoracic vertebrae, the twelve pairs of ribs and their costal cartilages, and the sternum (Fig. 2.1). Structures in continuity between the root of the neck and the upper part of the thoracic cavity pass through the thoracic inlet which is bounded by the first thoracic vertebral body, the first pair of ribs and costal cartilages and the upper border of the sternum. The thoracic outlet through which structures pass between the thoracic and abdominal cavities is formed by the twelfth thoracic vertebral body, the twelfth and eleventh ribs and the costal margin (the fused costal cartilages of the seventh to tenth ribs inclusive).

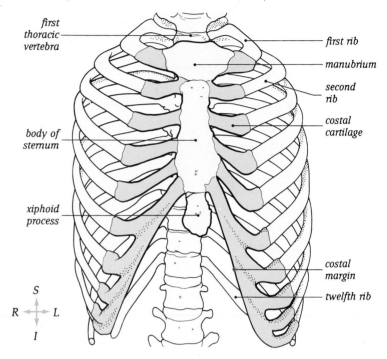

Fig. 2.1 *Articulated bones of the thorax showing the relationships between the vertebral column, ribs, costal cartilages and sternum.*

Fig. 2.2 *Right lateral and superior views of the (left) second and (right) tenth thoracic vertebrae.*

THORACIC VERTEBRAE

Each thoracic vertebra possesses a body anteriorly and a neural arch (paired pedicles and laminae) posteriorly (Fig. 2.2). The bodies gradually increase in size from above downwards. Posteriorly adjacent to the attachment of the pedicles the vertebral body is characterized by at least one small depression, the costal facet. These facets form synovial joints with the vertebral ends (heads) of the ribs. Typically, a vertebral body possesses one pair of facets on each side. The upper facet receives the rib whose number is the same as that of the thoracic vertebra; the lower facet articulates with the head of the rib below. The first, tenth, eleventh and twelfth vertebrae possess only one pair of facets which are for their own ribs.

From each pedicle a superior articular process projects upwards (to form a synovial joint with the inferior articular process of the vertebra above) and an inferior process extends downwards (for the vertebra below). At the union of the pedicle and lamina on each side, a transverse process projects backwards and laterally and near its tip carries an articular facet for the tubercle of the corresponding rib. From the junction of each pedicle and transverse process the lamina slopes downwards and medially to unite in the midline with its fellow and complete the neural arch enclosing the vertebral foramen. In the midline posteriorly the spinous process projects downwards and backwards from the junction of the laminae.

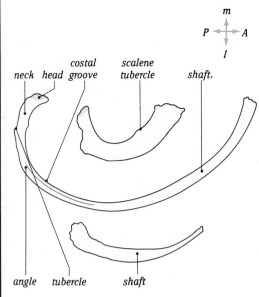

Fig. 2.3 *Superior view of, in descending order, the first, seventh and twelfth ribs showing their surface features and relative sizes.*

RIBS

Although the ribs differ in size and shape, the majority (3-9 inclusive) have features in common and are described as 'typical ribs' (Fig. 2.3). Each typical rib consists of a head, neck, tubercle, shaft, upper and lower borders and inner and outer surfaces. The heads of the ribs are those parts which articulate with the thoracic vertebral bodies. The lower part of the head forms a synovial joint with its own vertebral body whilst the upper part articulates with the vertebra above. The intermediate part of the head lies against the intervertebral disc. The neck of the rib connects the head and the tubercle and lies in front of the transverse process. The tubercle of the rib faces posteriorly and the medial part of its surface forms a synovial joint with the articular facet on the transverse process of the corresponding vertebra. The shaft forms the remainder of the rib and ends anteriorly at a shallow depression which receives the costal cartilage. Passing laterally from the tubercle, the shaft slopes downwards and backwards before turning forwards and outwards to form the angle. Lateral to the angle the shaft possesses a sharp lower border which bounds a prominent costal groove.

The first rib is atypical. Its head possesses an articular facet solely for its own vertebral body. The shaft is short and broad and has superior and inferior surfaces. In addition, its superior surface carries a ridge which forms a projection on the inner border of the rib, the scalene tubercle, to which is attached scalenus anterior. Two grooves lie across the shaft, one in front of the ridge (for the subclavian vein) and the other behind (for the subclavian artery and lowest trunk of the brachial plexus). The tenth, eleventh and twelfth ribs are atypical in that each head possesses a single facet and the rib is usually devoid of a tubercle and an angle.

Costal cartilages

All ribs possess costal cartilages and those of the upper seven pairs (true ribs) articulate with the sides of the sternum. Pairs eight, nine and ten (false ribs) fall short of the sternum and articulate with the cartilage immediately above. Pairs eleven and twelve (floating ribs) are pointed and end freely in the muscle of the abdominal wall.

STERNUM

The sternum is a flat bone and consists of the manubrium, the body (Fig. 2.4) and the xiphoid process. The manubrium articulates with the medial end of each clavicle at the sternoclavicular joint and with the first costal cartilage. Its upper margin is broad and forms part of the thoracic inlet. A palpable secondary cartilaginous joint (the manubriosternal joint) unites the manubrium and body and forms a useful guide to the second costal cartilage which abuts the sternum at the lateral margin of the joint. The lateral margins of the body of the sternum are indented by the medial ends of the second to the seventh costal cartilages. The xiphoid process lies in the subcostal angle and projects downwards and backwards from the body of the sternum.

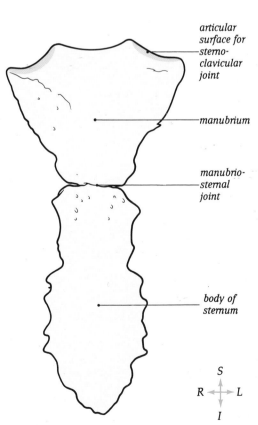

Fig. 2.4 *The manubrium and the body of the sternum. The xiphoid process is absent.*

THORACIC WALL

BREAST

The breast (Fig. 2.5) consists of glandular tissue and a quantity of fat embedded in the superficial fascia of the anterior chest wall. In the male and immature female the gland is rudimentary. Although the size and shape of the breast in the adult female are variable, the base (the part lying on the deep fascia covering pectoralis major, serratus anterior and rectus abdominis) is constant in position. In the adult female the base is roughly circular and extends between the second and sixth ribs. Medially the gland overlies the lateral border of the sternum. Part of the breast extends upwards and laterally and reaches the anterior fold of the axilla. This is the axillary tail and is the only part of the breast to penetrate beneath the deep fascia.

The glandular elements consist of fifteen to twenty lobes arranged radially, each draining into a lactiferous duct. These ducts open independently onto the surface of the nipple. The skin of the nipple is surrounded by an area of pink skin, the areola, which may develop brown pigmentation during pregnancy.

The gland is traversed by fibrous septa (Fig. 2.5) which subdivide the lobes and loosely attach the skin of the breast to the deep fascia covering the chest wall. Normally the breast is freely mobile over the underlying muscles.

Blood supply
The fat and glandular elements of the breast receive blood from arteries which also supply the deeper structures of the chest wall. These vessels include perforating branches from the internal thoracic artery and the second, third and fourth intercostal arteries. The lateral thoracic and thoracoacromial arteries arising from the axillary artery also supply the breast. The gland is drained by veins which accompany the arteries.

Lymph drainage
Within the substance of the breast the lymphatic vessels form a system of interconnecting channels which collect lymph from all parts of the organ. The superior and lateral aspects of the breast usually drain into central and apical axillary nodes via infraclavicular and pectoral nodes. The medial and inferior parts of the breast drain deeply into glands along the internal thoracic vessels and thence via the bronchomediastinal lymph trunk into the confluence of lymphatic vessels in the root of the neck (see page 7.8). Lymphatics may also cross the midline to communicate with vessels in the opposite breast.

Fig. 2.5 *Sagittal section through the right breast and underlying chest wall. In this dissection, the glandular structure of the breast cannot be distinguished.*

MUSCLES

The outer surfaces of the ribs, costal cartilages and sternum give attachment to muscles involved in movements of the upper limb and the scapula, namely pectoralis major, pectoralis minor and serratus anterior. In addition, the external surfaces of the lower ribs provide attachment for rectus abdominis and the external oblique muscles of the anterior abdominal wall (see pages 4.4 & 4.5).

Pectoralis major

This large fan-shaped muscle (Fig. 2.6) attaches to the clavicle, sternum and upper costal cartilages and forms the bulk of the anterior wall of the axilla. The clavicular head is attached to the anterior surface of the medial half of the clavicle. The sternocostal head is anchored to the manubrium and body of the sternum, and the upper six costal cartilages. Laterally both parts of the muscle attach to the humerus along the lateral lip of the intertubercular sulcus (see page 00).

Pectoralis major is supplied by the medial and lateral pectoral nerves from the brachial plexus. Functionally it is a powerful adductor and flexor of the arm at the shoulder joint and also produces medial rotation of the humerus. When the upper limb is fixed the sternocostal part may act as an accessory muscle of inspiration by elevating the ribs.

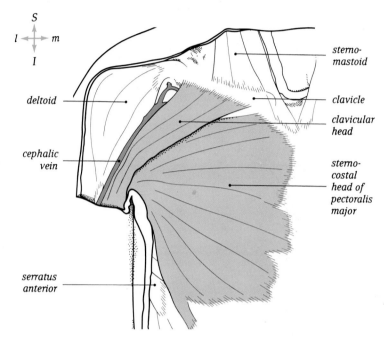

Fig. 2.6 *Pectoralis major revealed by removal of the skin and superficial fascia.*

Pectoralis minor

This small muscle (Fig. 2.7) lies deep to pectoralis major and is usually attached to the third, fourth and fifth ribs. The muscle converges on the medial border of the coracoid process of the scapula. Pectoralis minor is supplied by the medial and lateral pectoral nerves and assists in movements of protraction and rotation of the scapula (see page 3.40).

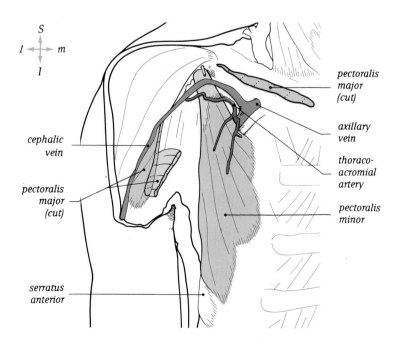

Fig. 2.7 *Pectoralis minor exposed by removal of pectoralis major.*

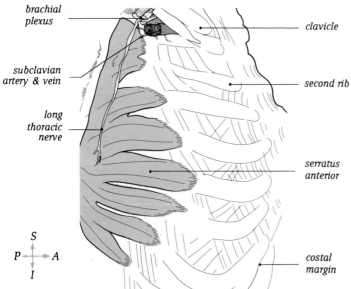

Fig. 2.8 *Serratus anterior seen after removal of the pectoral muscles and displacement of the scapula backwards.*

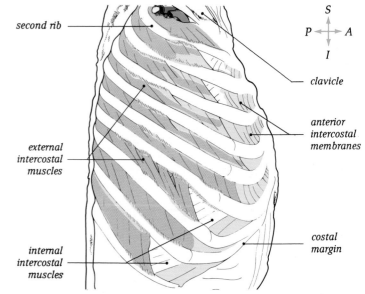

Fig. 2.9 *External intercostal muscles exposed by removal of the upper limb and serratus anterior.*

Serratus anterior

This large muscle lies between the scapula and chest wall and attaches to the lateral aspects of the upper eight ribs (Fig. 2.8) forming part of the medial wall of the axilla. The muscle fibres from the upper four ribs attach to the superior angle and to the costal surface of the medial border of the scapula. The fibres from ribs five to eight converge on the costal surface of the inferior angle of the scapula.

Innervation is provided by the long thoracic nerve arising in the neck from the upper three roots (C5, C6 & C7) of the brachial plexus. The muscle is a powerful protractor of the scapula and assists trapezius in producing scapular rotation during abduction of the upper limb. In addition, the muscle helps to stabilize the scapula during movements of the upper limb.

INTERCOSTAL SPACES

The interval between two adjacent ribs is called an intercostal space. On each side of the thorax there are eleven such spaces, numbered from above and occupied by muscles, membranes, nerves and vessels. The number given to each intercostal space and its neurovascular structures corresponds to that of the rib which limits the space superiorly. The nerves and vessels immediately inferior to the twelfth ribs are termed the subcostal nerves and vessels. The intercostal nerves and vessels supply the intercostal muscles and the parietal pleura deep to each space. Branches from these vessels also supply the overlying muscles of the body wall, the superficial fascia and skin. Most intercostal nerves have cutaneous branches which supply the skin covering the chest and abdominal walls.

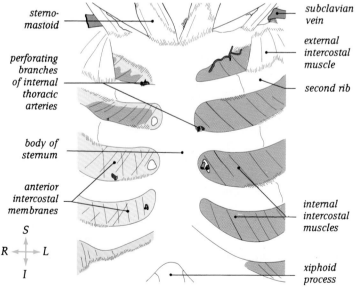

Fig. 2.10 *Anterior intercostal membranes and the anterior fibres of the internal intercostal muscles.*

Fig. 2.11 *Internal intercostal muscles exposed by removal of the anterior parts of the external intercostal muscles.*

INTERCOSTAL MUSCLES

There are three layers of intercostal muscles which lie superficial, intermediate and deep, and these are named the external, the internal and the innermost intercostal muscles.

External intercostal muscles

The fibres of the external intercostal muscles slope downwards and forwards from the lower border of one rib to the upper border of the subjacent rib (Fig. 2.9). The muscle extends from the tubercle of the rib posteriorly to the junction of the rib and its costal cartilage anteriorly. Between costal cartilages the muscle fibres are replaced by a thin fascial sheet called the anterior intercostal membrane which reaches the lateral border of the sternum (Fig. 2.10).

Internal intercostal muscles

The internal intercostal muscles (Fig. 2.11) lie immediately deep to the external intercostal muscles. The fibres of the two muscles are mutually at right angles, those of the internal intercostal muscles running downwards and backwards from the lower border of one rib to the upper border of the subjacent rib. Anteriorly each muscle continues between the costal cartilages to reach the lateral border of the sternum (Fig. 2.10). Posteriorly each muscle extends only to the angles of the ribs where it is replaced by the posterior intercostal membrane which continues as far as the tubercles of the ribs.

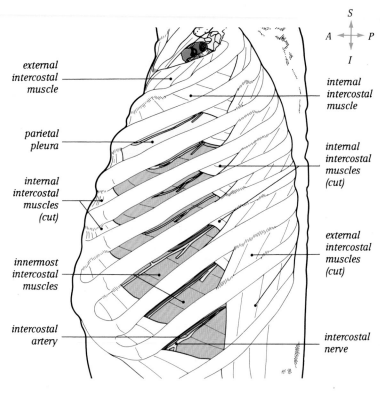

Fig. 2.12 *Innermost intercostal muscles and intercostal nerves exposed after removing parts of the internal intercostal muscles. In the third intercostal space the innermost intercostal muscle has been removed to expose the parietal pleura.*

Innermost intercostal muscles

These muscles lie on a plane deep to that of the internal intercostal muscles (Fig. 2.12). They form the lateral part of an incomplete layer of muscle called the transversus thoracis, which includes sternocostalis anteriorly and subcostalis posteriorly. Each innermost intercostal muscle connects the inner surface of one rib to that of its neighbours.

Nerve supply

All the intercostal muscles in a particular intercostal space are supplied by the corresponding intercostal nerve.

Actions

Although the main role of the intercostal muscles is in ventilation of the lungs, it must be emphasized that during normal quiet breathing the muscles of the thoracic wall make only a small contribution. Inspiration is usually brought about mainly by the diaphragm whose movements increase the vertical capacity of the chest. The transverse and anteroposterior diameters of the thorax are increased, especially in deep inspiration, by the external intercostal muscles which incline the ribs outwards, upwards and forwards so that the intercostal spaces are widened. During quiet breathing, expiration is largely due to the 'elastic' recoil of the lungs and thoracic wall and involves minimal activity by the intercostal muscles. Even when expiration is 'forced', for example, during vigorous physical exertion or when coughing, the main muscular effort is provided by the muscles of the abdominal wall rather than the chest wall. However, the internal intercostal muscles contribute to forced expiration by drawing the ribs downwards and inwards, thereby narrowing the intercostal spaces.

INTERCOSTAL VESSELS AND NERVES

Each intercostal space has a principal artery, vein and nerve which collectively form the neurovascular bundle (Fig. 2.12). This bundle lies in the neurovascular plane between the internal and innermost intercostal muscles and runs along the upper border of the intercostal space occupying the subcostal groove of the rib. Usually the vein lies superiorly and the nerve inferiorly in the bundle. A collateral nerve and collateral vessels arise posteriorly from the neurovascular bundle and run forwards along the lower border of the intercostal space to supply the intercostal muscles.

Intercostal arteries

Intercostal arteries enter from both anterior and posterior ends of the intercostal space. Anteriorly the internal thoracic arteries (Fig. 2.13) arising from the subclavian arteries in the root of the neck (see page 7.8) provide branches which run laterally to supply the upper six pairs of intercostal spaces. On each side the lower five spaces receive anterior intercostal arteries from the musculophrenic artery, one of the terminal branches of the internal thoracic artery. These anterior arteries anastomose end-to-end with the posterior intercostal arteries.

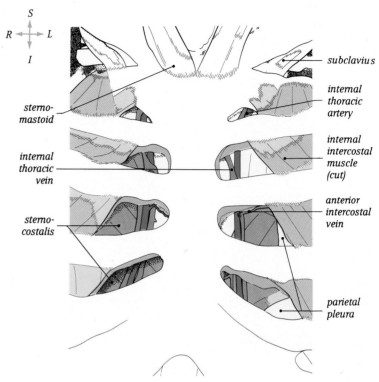

Fig. 2.13 *Internal thoracic vessels revealed by removal of the anterior parts of the intercostal muscles.*

Posterior intercostal arteries to the lower nine intercostal spaces arise as direct branches from the descending thoracic aorta (see Fig. 2.59). For the first and second spaces the posterior intercostal arteries are derived from the superior intercostal branch of the costocervical trunk. This trunk arises from the subclavian artery (see page 7.9) and its superior intercostal branch enters the thorax by crossing the neck of the first rib. The anastomoses between anterior and posterior intercostal arteries and between the scapular arteries and posterior intercostals are important because they enable blood to reach the descending aorta when the aortic arch is abnormally narrowed (coarctation of the aorta).

Intercostal veins
Anteriorly the intercostal veins from the lower five intercostal spaces drain into the musculophrenic veins. The upper six intercostal veins and the musculophrenic veins drain into the internal thoracic veins, which themselves are tributaries of the brachiocephalic veins in the root of the neck. Posteriorly the intercostal veins drain into the azygos venous system. On the right, those in the lower eight spaces terminate directly in the azygos vein (see Fig. 2.59). The veins from the second and third spaces combine into a single vessel, the right superior intercostal vein, which drains into the arch of the azygos vein. The first posterior intercostal vein leaves the thorax to terminate in the root of the neck, usually in the right vertebral vein.

On the left, the lower eight posterior intercostal veins enter either the hemiazygos or accessory hemiazygos veins (see Fig. 2.60). The left superior intercostal vein drains the second and third spaces and crosses the left side of the arch of the aorta to terminate in the left brachiocephalic vein. As on the right, the first posterior intercostal vein leaves the thorax to terminate usually in the vertebral, but occasionally in the brachiocephalic, vein.

Intercostal nerves
The intercostal nerves comprise the ventral rami of the thoracic spinal nerves. Each intercostal nerve enters the neurovascular plane posteriorly (see Fig. 2.60) and gives a collateral branch which supplies the intercostal muscles of the space. Except for the first, each intercostal nerve gives off a lateral cutaneous branch near the midaxillary line which pierces the overlying muscle. This cutaneous nerve divides into anterior and posterior branches which supply the adjacent skin. The intercostal nerves of the second to the sixth spaces enter the superficial fascia near the lateral border of the sternum and divide into medial and lateral cutaneous branches.

Most of the fibres of the ventral ramus of the first thoracic spinal nerve join the brachial plexus for distribution to the upper limb (see page 3.8). The small first intercostal nerve is the collateral branch and supplies only the muscles of the intercostal space, not the overlying skin.

The intercostal nerves of the lower five spaces continue in the neurovascular plane beyond the costal margin to supply the muscles and skin of the abdominal wall (see page 4.6).

PLEURA

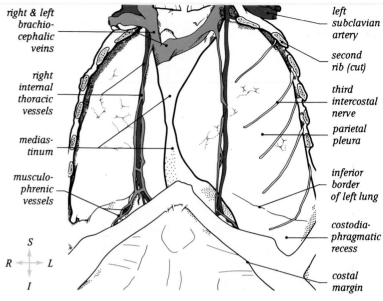

Fig. 2.14 *Removal of the anterior chest wall has exposed the internal thoracic vessels and costal part of the parietal pleura, through which the lungs are visible.*

Fig. 2.15 *Transverse section through the thorax at the level of the tracheal bifurcation and the fourth thoracic vertebra.*

The thoracic cavity lies within the walls of the thorax and is separated from the abdominal cavity by the diaphragm. The cavity contains the right and left lungs, each surrounded by a serous membrane called the pleura. Between the lungs is a central partition, the mediastinum, which includes the heart and great vessels, the trachea and the oesophagus. Superiorly, numerous mediastinal structures enter or leave the root of the neck through the thoracic inlet (see pages 7.8 & 7.9). Inferiorly, important structures including the aorta, inferior vena cava and oesophagus pass between the mediastinum and the abdomen through openings in the diaphragm (see page 4.56).

The pleura surrounds the lungs and lines the walls of the thoracic cavity and is subdivided into visceral and parietal parts. The visceral layer covers the surface of the lung and is continuous with the parietal layer around the mediastinal attachment of the lung at the lung root. The parietal layer covers the lateral aspect of the mediastinum, the upper surface of the diaphragm and the inner aspect of the chest wall (Fig. 2.14). Although the parietal and visceral layers are normally in contact, a space, the pleural cavity (Fig. 2.15), exists between them and contains a thin film of serous fluid. The fluid ensures close apposition of the two pleural surfaces and reduces friction during respiratory movements. Injury or disease may produce an accumulation of gas (pneumothorax) or fluid (pleural effusion) within the pleural cavity, causing the lung to collapse.

PARIETAL PLEURA

The parietal pleura is named according to the surfaces it covers. Thus, the mediastinal pleura conforms to the contours of the structures forming the lateral surface of the mediastinum and is innervated by sensory branches of the phrenic nerve. Inferiorly the diaphragmatic pleura clothes the upper surface of the diaphragm. The central portion receives sensory branches from each phrenic nerve whilst the periphery is innervated by lower intercostal nerves. The pleura covering the inner surface of the thoracic wall is called the costal pleura and is innervated segmentally by the intercostal nerves (Fig. 2.14).

The periphery of the diaphragm slopes steeply downwards towards it attachment to the thoracic wall, creating a narrow gutter, the costo-diaphragmatic recess. Within this recess, which is particularly deep laterally and posteriorly, the costal and diaphragmatic parts of the parietal pleura lie in mutual contact.

The parietal pleura extending into the root of the neck is called the cervical pleura. It is applied to the undersurface of a firm fascial layer, the suprapleural membrane, which prevents upward movement of the apex of the lung and pleura during ventilation. The cervical pleura covering the apex of the lung is innervated by the first intercostal nerve.

Surface markings of the parietal pleura

Because the parietal pleura is reflected from the thoracic wall onto both the mediastinum and the diaphragm, a line of pleural reflection can be mapped out on the body surface. Traced from its upper limit, approximately 2.5 cm above the medial third of the clavicle, this line descends behind the sternoclavicular joint and approaches the midline at the level of the manubriosternal joint. On the right the pleural reflection descends vertically to the level of the sixth costal cartilage while on the left the heart displaces the pleura laterally (Fig. 2.14) so that from the fourth to the sixth costal cartilages the line of reflection lies just lateral to the edge of the sternum. This displacement exposes part of the pericardium underlying the medial ends of the fourth and fifth intercostal spaces. Traced laterally from the sixth costal cartilage the surface marking is the same on each side, crossing the eighth rib in the midclavicular line and the tenth rib in the midaxillary line.

Posteriorly the parietal pleura continues horizontally, crosses the twelfth rib 5 cm from the midline and continues medially for a further 2.5 cm. Thus, a small area of parietal pleura lies below the level of the twelfth rib.

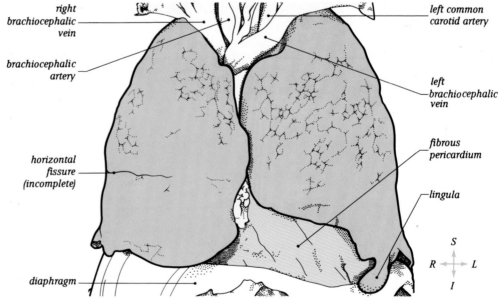

Fig. 2.16 *Lungs, after removal of the anterolateral thoracic wall and parietal pleura. The lungs cover more of the mediastinum in this specimen than is usual.*

VISCERAL PLEURA

The visceral pleura (Fig. 2.15) is continuous with the mediastinal parietal pleura around the root of the lung. Structures entering or leaving the lung occupy the upper part of this pleural sleeve, the lower part consisting of an empty fold of pleura called the pulmonary ligament. The visceral pleura firmly adheres to the surface of the lung and extends into the depths of the fissures. Unlike the parietal layer, visceral pleura does not have a somatic innervation.

Surface markings of the visceral pleura

Since the visceral pleura covers the surface of the lung, its surface markings coincide with those of the lung (see page 2.15).

LUNGS

The two lungs lie in the thoracic cavity and are separated by the structures in the mediastinum (Fig. 2.16). Although the lungs of infants are pink, those of older individuals may have a mottled appearance due to deposits of inhaled carbon. Living lungs are elastic, enabling their volumes to change during ventilation, in contrast to embalmed lungs, which are rigid and often bear the imprints of adjacent structures. Each lung is covered in visceral pleura and is cone-shaped with the base or diaphragmatic surface directed downwards and the apex upwards. The costal surface is smoothly convex while the mediastinal surface is irregular and bears the hilum of the organ. Fissures are usually present which divide each lung into lobes (usually three lobes on the right and two on the left). Most of the lung consists of the peripheral part of the respiratory tract and the associated pulmonary vascular system. Having entered the lung, the bronchi and pulmonary vessels subdivide extensively.

Fig. 2.17 *Costal surface of the right lung showing oblique and horizontal fissures, and the upper, middle and lower lobes.*

Fig. 2.18 *Costal surface of the left lung showing the single oblique fissure and upper and lower lobes.*

FISSURES

Although variations occur, each lung is usually divided into upper and lower lobes by an oblique fissure. On the right the upper lobe is further subdivided by the horizontal fissure (Fig. 2.17) which runs from the anterior border of the lung into the oblique fissure and demarcates the middle lobe. On the left the horizontal fissure is usually absent and the middle lobe represented by the lingula (Fig. 2.18).

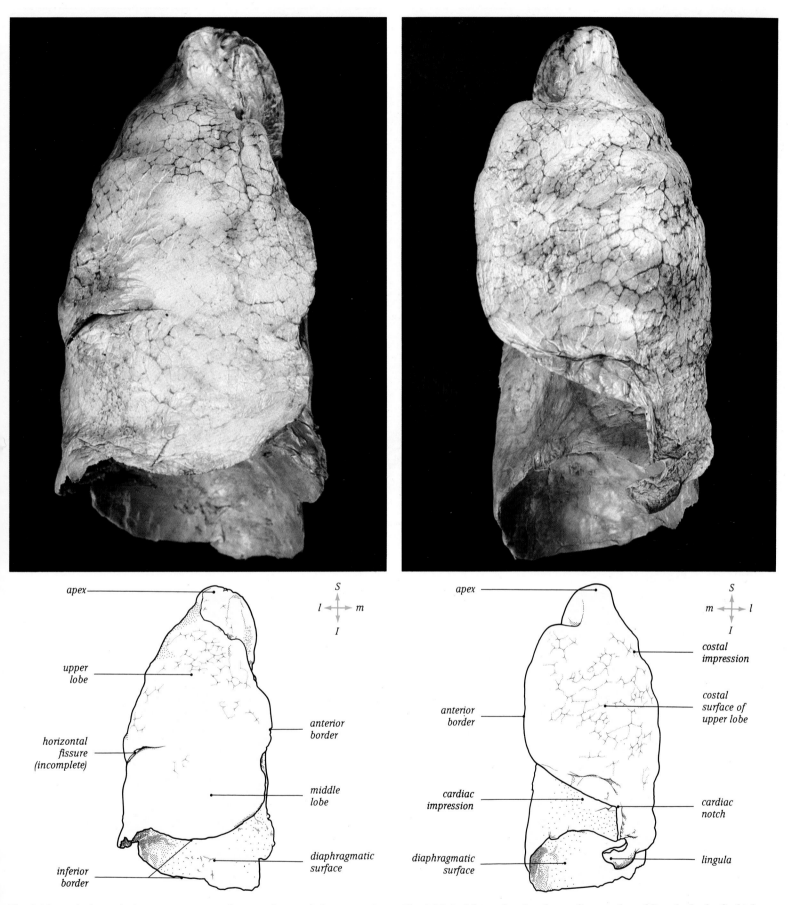

Fig. 2.19 *Right lung showing its concave inferior surface and sharp anterior and inferior borders.*

Fig. 2.20 *Left lung showing the cardiac notch and lingula, both of which are particularly marked in this specimen.*

SURFACES, BORDERS AND RELATIONS

The costal surface is convex and extends upwards into the cervical part of the pleura to form the apex of the lung which is closely related to the corresponding subclavian artery and vein. The inferior surface (base) is markedly concave (Figs. 2.19 & 2.20), conforming to the upward convexity of the dome of the diaphragm. The costal and diaphragmatic surfaces meet at the sharp inferior border. The anterior border is also sharp and is formed where the costal and mediastinal surfaces are in continuity. In contrast, the posterior border is rounded and rather indistinct.

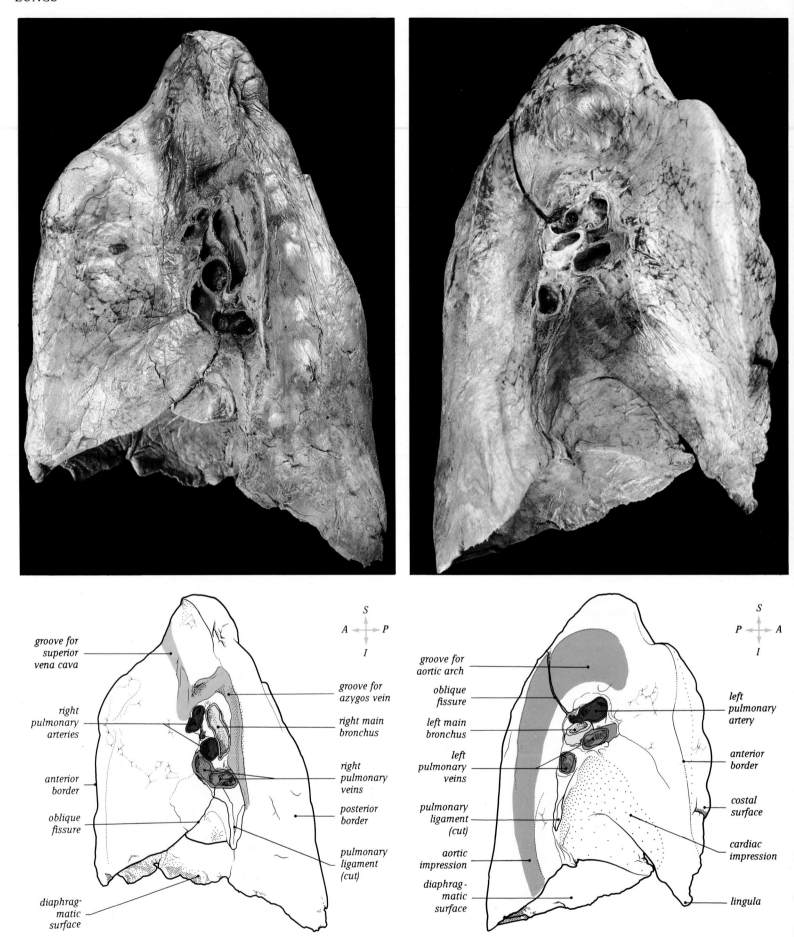

Fig. 2.21 *Mediastinal surface of the right lung showing the hilum lying relatively close to the rounded posterior border.*

Fig. 2.22 *Mediastinal surface of the left lung shows clearly the impressions of the heart and aorta.*

Each lung is attached to the mediastinum by the lung root, the principal components of which are the pulmonary vessels and the bronchi. These structures, accompanied by bronchial vessels, lymphatics and autonomic nerves, enter or leave the lung through the hilum. Usually, two pulmonary veins emerge from each lung, the inferior vein being the lowest structure in the hilum (Figs. 2.21 & 2.22). The bronchi and pulmonary arteries are adjacent

as they pass through the hilum and on the left the main bronchus lies anterior to the pulmonary artery. However, on the right the main bronchus frequently divides into two branches, the upper and lower lobe bronchi, before reaching the lung and each bronchus is accompanied by a branch of the pulmonary artery. The hila of both lungs often contain lymph nodes which are recognizable by their acquired dark coloration (Fig. 2.23).

Each lung has its own medial relations. The anterior part of the mediastinal surface of the right lung is related to the right brachiocephalic vein, the superior vena cava and the pericardium covering the right atrium of the heart. Between these structures and the mediastinal pleura is the intervening right phrenic nerve which descends in front of the hilum to reach the diaphragm. The upper part of the hilum is related to the azygos vein (Fig. 2.21) which arches forwards to terminate in the superior vena cava. The trachea and accompanying right vagus nerve are related to the right upper lobe.

On the mediastinal surface of the left lung are distinct impressions produced by the fibrous pericardium and the heart (Fig. 2.22). The left phrenic nerve is related to the mediastinal pleura and passes in front of the hilum as it descends across the pericardium. The aorta creates an obvious groove (Fig. 2.22) where it arches over the lung root and descends behind the hilum as the descending thoracic aorta.

Surface markings

The apex of each lung rises above the medial third of the clavicle. From here the anterior border of the lung follows the reflection of the parietal pleura, passing behind the sternoclavicular and manubriosternal joints. On the right the border descends vertically close to the midline from the level of the second to the fifth costal cartilages. On the left the heart displaces the lung and parietal pleura so that the pericardium is exposed behind the medial ends of the fourth and fifth intercostal spaces. On both sides the inferior border of the lung crosses the sixth rib in the midclavicular line, the eighth rib in the midaxillary line and the tenth rib 5cm from the midline posteriorly. The lower border of the lung lies at a higher level than the line of pleural reflection; this part of the pleural cavity not occupied by lung is called the costodiaphragmatic recess.

BRONCHI

The bifurcation of the trachea in the mediastinum gives rise to the right and left main (principal) bronchi. The right main bronchus (Fig. 2.23) is wider and more steeply inclined than the left. The main bronchi give rise to lobar (secondary) bronchi which are confined to their respective lobes. On the right the upper lobe bronchus arises outside the hilum in the lung root, whereas on the left the lobar bronchi arise entirely within the lung. In each lobe, further subdivision occurs into segmental (tertiary) bronchi which are constant in position and supply specific portions of lung called bronchopulmonary segments. Each lobe consists of a definite number of these segments. Within individual segments the bronchi further subdivide into bronchioles, then respiratory bronchioles, which in turn lead into the alveolar ducts and alveoli. Bronchial arteries derived from the descending thoracic aorta accompany and supply the major bronchi. Venous return from the bronchi is through bronchial veins which termi-nate in the azygos venous system (see page 2.35).

Fig. 2.23 *Transverse section through the thorax at the level of the fifth thoracic vertebra.*

PULMONARY VESSELS

The right and left pulmonary arteries divide into branches which correspond to and accompany the subdivisions of the bronchi within the lungs. The bronchi and pulmonary arteries lie centrally in the bronchopulmonary segments. The arteries ultimately give rise to pulmonary capillaries in the alveolar walls. Oxygenated blood drains from these capillaries into tributaries of the pulmonary veins which occupy intersegmental positions. These vessels empty into two pulmonary veins which usually emerge separately through each hilum (Figs. 2.21 & 2.22) and drain into the left atrium.

AUTONOMIC NERVES

The pulmonary plexus, most of which lies behind the lung root, contains both sympathetic and parasympathetic fibres which accompany the bronchi into the lung. Sympathetic nerves originate in the upper thoracic ganglia of the sympathetic chain and supply smooth muscle in the walls of the bronchi and pulmonary blood vessels. The parasympathetic fibres are derived from the vagus nerves and supply bronchial smooth muscle and mucous glands.

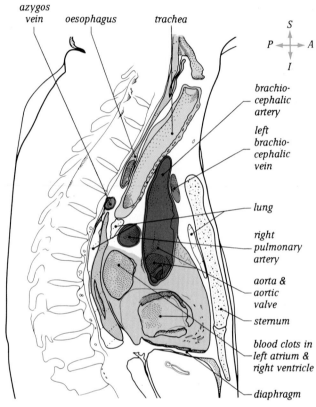

Fig. 2.24 *Near midline sagittal section through the thorax showing some mediastinal structures.*

Labels in Fig. 2.24:
- azygos vein
- oesophagus
- trachea
- brachio-cephalic artery
- left brachio-cephalic vein
- lung
- right pulmonary artery
- aorta & aortic valve
- sternum
- blood clots in left atrium & right ventricle
- diaphragm

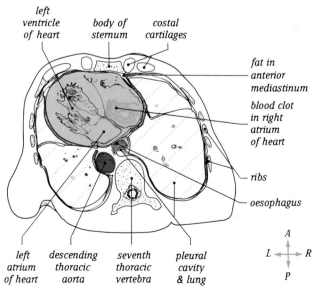

Fig. 2.25 *Transverse section at the level of the seventh thoracic vertebra. The heart is abnormally large.*

Labels in Fig. 2.25:
- left ventricle of heart
- body of sternum
- costal cartilages
- fat in anterior mediastinum
- blood clot in right atrium of heart
- ribs
- oesophagus
- left atrium of heart
- descending thoracic aorta
- seventh thoracic vertebra
- pleural cavity & lung

The central part of the thorax between the two pleural cavities contains a group of structures collectively termed the mediastinum. These include the heart and great vessels, the trachea and the oesophagus. The mediastinum extends from the thoracic inlet above to the diaphragm below and from the sternum in front to the thoracic vertebral bodies behind (Figs. 2.24 & 2.25). By convention the mediastinum is divided into superior and inferior parts by an imaginary horizontal plane passing through the manubriosternal joint and the lower part of the fourth thoracic vertebra. The superior mediastinum lies between this plane and the thoracic inlet and contains the superior vena cava and its tributaries, the arch of the aorta and its branches, and the trachea. Also passing through this region are the oesophagus, the thoracic duct and the right and left vagus and phrenic nerves.

The inferior mediastinum lies between the imaginary plane and the diaphragm and consists of three compartments. The largest of these is the middle mediastinum composed of the heart and its covering of fibrous pericardium. In front of the middle mediastinum lies the anterior mediastinum consisting of a small amount of fat and the remnants of the thymus gland. Behind the fibrous pericardium lies the posterior mediastinum, traversed by the descending thoracic aorta, the oesophagus and the thoracic duct.

FIBROUS PERICARDIUM

The fibrous pericardium is a sac of dense connective tissue surrounding the heart. In addition to the heart, it contains the roots of the great arteries and veins and is covered on its inner surface by serous pericardium (see below). The broad base of the fibrous pericardium is attached to the central tendon of the diaphragm (Fig. 2.26) and is pierced by the inferior vena cava. Superiorly the sac fuses with the adventitial layers of the aorta, pulmonary trunk and superior vena cava. On each side, the posterior part of the sac blends with the walls of the pulmonary vessels.

The anterior aspect of the fibrous pericardium is related to the anterior parts of the two lungs and the anterior reflections of the pleura. Between the pleural reflections the pericardium lies close to the body of the sternum and to the medial ends of the adjacent fourth and fifth left costal cartilages and associated intercostal structures. During infancy and childhood the thymus (most of which lies in the superior mediastinum) is related to the anterior surface of the pericardium, but after puberty the thymus regresses and is gradually replaced by fat.

Laterally, the pericardium is covered by mediastinal pleura and is crossed by the right and left phrenic nerves as they descend to the diaphragm. These nerves supply sensory fibres to the fibrous pericardium and the mediastinal pleura. Most of the blood supply to the fibrous pericardium is provided by the internal thoracic arteries and veins via pericardiophrenic vessels that accompany the phrenic nerves.

Behind the fibrous pericardium lie the oesophagus, the descending thoracic aorta and the thoracic duct (see page 2.34).

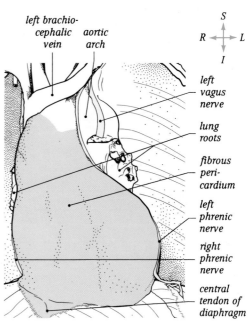

Fig. 2.26 *The fibrous pericardium is firmly attached to the diaphragm and to the adventitia of the great vessels.*

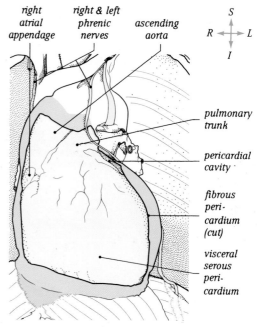

Fig. 2.27 *The fibrous pericardium has been opened to expose the visceral pericardium covering the anterior surface of the heart.*

SEROUS PERICARDIUM

Deep to the fibrous pericardium lies the serous pericardium consisting of parietal and visceral layers. Between the two layers is the pericardial cavity, a narrow space containing a thin film of serous fluid. The parietal layer lines the inner surface of the fibrous pericardium, to which it is firmly attached. The visceral layer covers the outer surface of the heart and the roots of the great vessels (Fig. 2.27). The two layers slide freely against each other and are in continuity where the great vessels pierce the fibrous pericardium. The reflections between the parietal and visceral layers

form two sleeves. One sleeve surrounds the ascending aorta and pulmonary trunk; the second is more extensive and surrounds the superior and inferior venae cavae and pulmonary veins. The two pericardial sleeves lie adjacent to each other and the narrow intervening channel is called the transverse pericardial sinus. A second sinus lies behind the left atrium of the heart. This is the oblique pericardial sinus which is limited superiorly by the pericardial reflection around the pulmonary veins and superior vena cava (see Fig. 2.31).

HEART

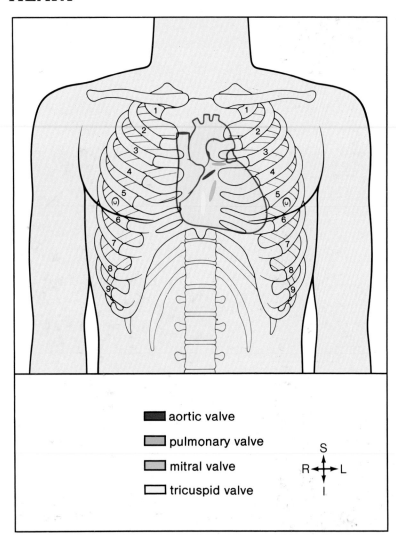

aortic valve
pulmonary valve
mitral valve
tricuspid valve

S
R ←—→ L
I

Fig. 2.28 *Borders and valves of the heart and their relationships to the anterior chest wall.*

EXTERNAL FEATURES

The heart, enclosed in pericardium, occupies the middle mediastinum. It is roughly cone-shaped and lies behind the sternum with its base facing posteriorly and its apex projecting inferiorly and to the left, producing the cardiac impression in the left lung.

The heart consists of four chambers, namely the right and left atria and the right and left ventricles. A fat-filled groove, the atrioventricular sulcus, separates the surfaces of the atria from the ventricles and carries the right and left coronary arteries and the coronary sinus. The right atrium receives the superior and inferior venae cavae and the coronary sinus. The left atrium drains the right and left pulmonary veins. The right ventricle is continuous with the pulmonary trunk while the left ventricle opens into the ascending aorta.

Borders

It is useful in clinical practice to represent the outline of the heart as a projection onto the anterior chest wall. When represented in this way the heart has right, inferior and left borders (Fig. 2.28). The right border is formed by the right atrium and runs between the third and sixth right costal cartilages approximately 3cm from the midline. The inferior border is formed mainly by the right atrium and right ventricle. At its left extremity, the border is completed by that part of the left ventricle which forms the apex of the heart. The inferior border runs from the sixth right costal cartilage approximately 3cm from the midline to the apex, which usually lies behind the fifth left intercostal space 6cm from the midline. In the living, the apex usually produces an impulse (apex beat) palpable on the anterior chest wall. The left ventricle together with the left atrial appendage form the left border of the heart, which slopes upwards and medially from the apex to the second left intercostal space approximately 3cm from the midline.

Surfaces

The majority of the anterior surface of the heart consists of the right atrium and right ventricle (Fig. 2.29). The left ventricle contributes a narrow strip adjacent to the left border of the heart. The anterior surface is completed by the right and left atrial appendages. The atrioventricular sulcus descends more or less vertically across the anterior surface and contains the right coronary artery surrounded by fat. The anterior surfaces of the right and left ventricles are separated by the anterior interventricular artery (Fig. 2.29).

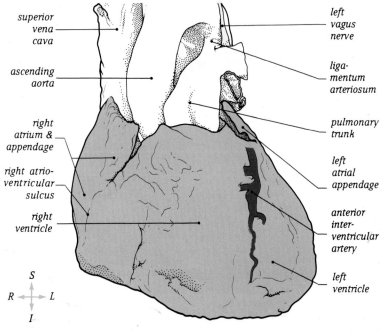

superior vena cava
ascending aorta
right atrium & appendage
right atrio-ventricular sulcus
right ventricle

left vagus nerve
liga-mentum arteriosum
pulmonary trunk
left atrial appendage
anterior inter-ventricular artery
left ventricle

S
R ←—→ L
I

Fig. 2.29 *Anterior surface of the heart. The fibrous pericardium has been removed.*

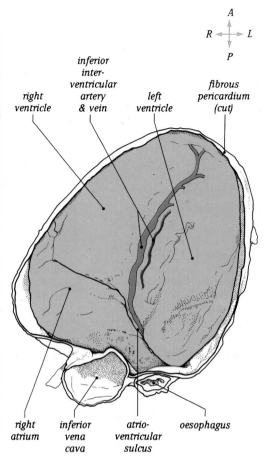

Fig. 2.30 *Inferior surface of the heart. The inferior part of the fibrous pericardium has been removed with the diaphragm.*

Most of the inferior (diaphragmatic) surface of the heart (Fig. 2.30) consists of the two ventricles, the left usually contributing the greater area. The inferior interventricular vessels mark the junction between these two chambers. The surface is completed by a small portion of the right atrium adjacent to the termination of the inferior vena cava.

The posterior surface or base of the heart (Fig. 2.31) consists mostly of the left atrium together with a small part of the right atrium.

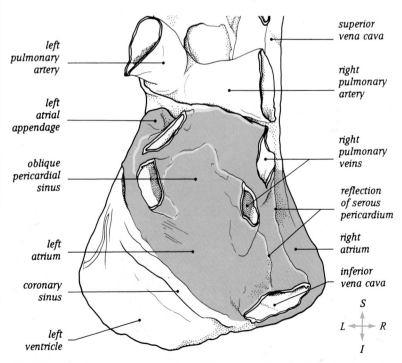

Fig. 2.31 *The base (posterior surface) of the heart showing the reflection of the serous pericardium and the site of the oblique pericardial sinus.*

CHAMBERS AND VALVES

The cavities of the right and left atria are continuous with those of their respective ventricles through the atrioventricular orifices. Each orifice possesses an atrioventricular valve which prevents backflow of blood from the ventricle into the atrium. The myocardium of the atria is separated from that of the ventricles by connective tissue which forms a complete fibrous ring around each atrioventricular orifice. Interatrial and interventricular septa separate the cavities of the atria and ventricles. Valves, each with three semilunar cusps, guard the orifices between the right ventricle and pulmonary trunk (pulmonary valve) and the left ventricle and ascending aorta (aortic valve).

Right atrium

The right atrium receives blood from the superior and inferior venae cavae and from the coronary sinus and cardiac veins which drain the myocardium. The superior vena cava enters the upper part of the chamber. Adjacent to its termination is a broad triangular prolongation of the atrium, the atrial appendage, which overlaps the ascending aorta (Fig. 2.32).

Internally the anterior wall of the right atrium possesses a vertical ridge, the crista terminalis (Fig. 2.32). From the crista, muscular ridges (musculi pectinati) run to the left and extend into the appendage. The posterior (septal) wall is relatively smooth but possesses a well-defined ridge surrounding a shallow depression named the fossa ovalis. This fossa is the site of the foramen ovale which, in the fetus, allowed blood to pass directly from the right to left atrium. The coronary sinus empties into the chamber close to the atrioventricular orifice. Inferiorly the right atrium receives the inferior vena cava immediately after the vessel has pierced the central tendon of the diaphragm. A fold called the valve of the inferior vena cava (Fig. 2.32) projects into the chamber and is the remnant of a fetal structure which directed the flow of blood across the right atrium towards the foramen ovale.

Tricuspid valve

From the right atrium, blood flows into the right ventricle through the right atrioventricular orifice which is guarded by the tricuspid valve (Fig. 2.33). The valve possesses three cusps, the bases of which attach to the margins of the atrioventricular orifice, while their free borders project into the cavity of the right ventricle (Fig. 2.34) where they are anchored by fibrous strands (chordae tendineae) to the papillary muscles of the ventricle. During ventricular contraction (systole) the papillary muscles pull on the chordae, preventing eversion of the valve cusps and reflux of blood into the atrium. The valve lies in the midline behind the lower part of the body of the sternum and its sounds are heard best by auscultation over the xiphisternum.

Right ventricle

The right ventricle has the right atrium on its right and the left ventricle both behind and to its left. The chamber forms parts of the anterior and inferior surfaces of the heart and narrows superiorly at the infundibulum, which leads into the pulmonary trunk (Fig. 2.34). The walls of the right ventricle are thicker than those of the right atrium and internally possess numerous muscular ridges called trabeculae carneae (see Fig. 2.39). One of these, the moderator band (see Fig. 2.50), often bridges the cavity of the chamber, connecting the interventricular septum to the anterior ventricular wall. When present, it carries the right branch of the atrioventricular bundle of conducting tissue (see page. 2.35). Projecting from the ventricular walls into the interior of the chamber are processes of myocardium, the papillary muscles, each attached at its apex to several chordae tendineae.

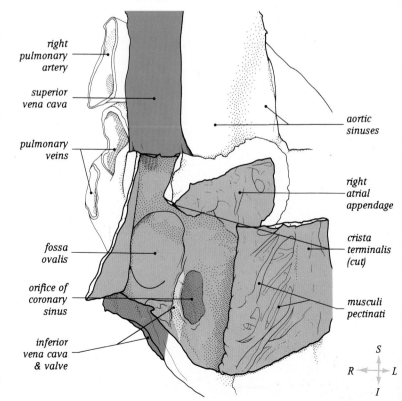

Fig. 2.32 *Interior of the right atrium and atrial appendage exposed by reflection and excision of part of the anterior atrial wall.*

right pulmonary artery

superior vena cava

pulmonary veins

fossa ovalis

orifice of coronary sinus

inferior vena cava & valve

aortic sinuses

right atrial appendage

crista terminalis (cut)

musculi pectinati

S
R ← → L
I

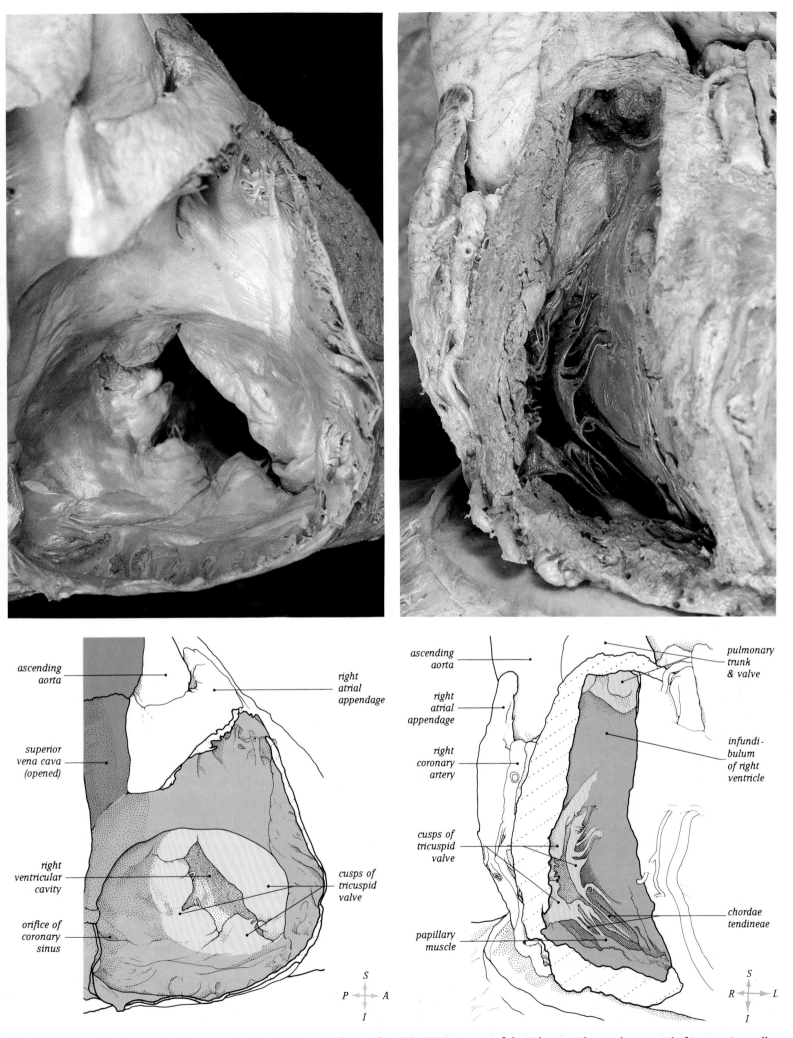

Fig. 2.33 *Tricuspid valve revealed by removal of the lateral wall of the right atrium.*

Fig. 2.34 *Interior of the right ventricle seen by removal of its anterior wall.*

2.21

Pulmonary valve

The pulmonary orifice lies between the infundibulum and the pulmonary trunk and is guarded by the pulmonary valve (Figs. 2.35 & 2.36) which consists of three semilunar cusps. The valve closes during ventricular relaxation (diastole), preventing backflow of blood from the pulmonary trunk into the right ventricle. The valve lies behind the left border of the sternum at the level of the third costal cartilage. Sounds generated by this valve are loudest over the anterior end of the second left intercostal space.

Left atrium

The left atrium lies behind the right atrium and forms the base of the heart. It possesses a hook-like appendage which projects forwards to the left of the pulmonary trunk and infundibulum. The chamber receives superior and inferior pulmonary veins from each lung (see Fig. 2.31). The four pulmonary veins, together with the two venae cavae, are all enclosed in a sleeve of serous pericardium, forming the superior limit of the oblique pericardial

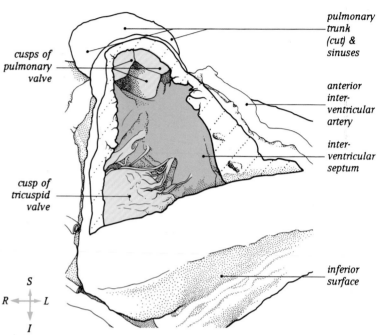

Fig. 2.35 *Ventricular surfaces of the cusps of the pulmonary valve seen after removal of part of the anterior wall of the right ventricle.*

Fig. 2.36 *Pulmonary and aortic valves seen from above.*

sinus. The left atrium forms the anterior wall of this sinus which separates the chamber from the fibrous pericardium and oesophagus. Most of the inner surface of the left atrium is smooth (Fig. 2.37), although musculi pectinati are present in the appendage.

Mitral (bicuspid) valve

The left atrium communicates anteroinferiorly with the left ventricle through the left atrioventricular orifice which is guarded by the mitral (bicuspid) valve. This valve possesses two cusps whose bases attach to the margins of the atrioventricular orifice (Fig. 2.37) while their free borders and cusps are anchored by chordae tendineae to the papillary muscles within the left ventricle (Fig. 2.38). The valve prevents reflux during ventricular contraction. Although it lies in the midline at the level of the fourth costal cartilages, the sounds of the mitral valve are best heard over the apex of the heart.

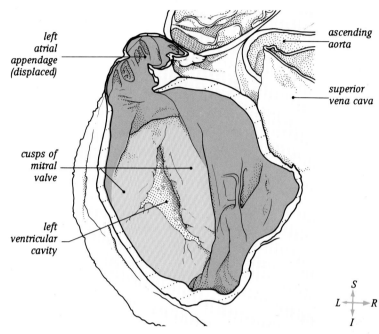

Fig. 2.37 *Mitral valve and interior of the left atrium and appendage seen by removal of the posterior wall of the chamber.*

Fig. 2.38 *Interior of the left ventricle seen after removal of part of its wall.*

Left ventricle

From the left atrioventricular orifice the left ventricle extends forwards and to the left as far as the apex. The thickness of the wall of the chamber is normally three times that of the right ventricle (Fig. 2.39). Internally there are prominent trabeculae carneae and papillary muscles (Fig. 2.42). The chamber narrows as it passes upwards and to the right behind the infundibulum to form the aortic vestibule (Fig. 2.40), the part of the ventricle which communicates with the ascending aorta through the aortic orifice.

Aortic valve

The aortic valve consists of three semilunar cusps (Figs. 2.41) which prevent backflow of blood from the ascending aorta during ventricular diastole. The valve lies behind the sternum to the left of the midline at the level of the anterior end of the third left intercostal space. However, its sounds are best heard over the medial ends of the first and second right intercostal spaces.

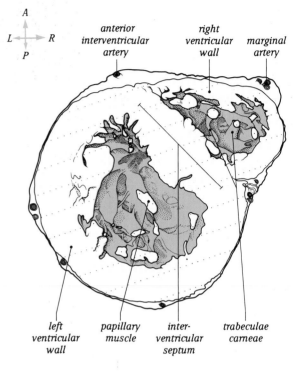

Fig. 2.39 *Section through the heart shows the apical portions of the left and right ventricles.*

Fig. 2.40 *Mitral valve and aortic vestibule exposed by removal of part of the left ventricular wall.*

monary trunk and ascending aorta

pulmonary trunk and the ascending aorta lie within the fibrous
icardium, enclosed together in a sleeve of serous pericardium anterior to
transverse pericardial sinus. The pulmonary trunk extends upwards and
ckwards while the ascending aorta initially lies behind it and passes
vards and forwards, overlapped by the right atrial appendage. At the origin
each vessel are three dilatations or sinuses (Fig. 2.41), one immediately
ve each of the cusps of the pulmonary and aortic valves. When ventricular
traction ceases, blood flows into the sinuses, thus pushing against the
ps and closing the valves. Two of the aortic sinuses give rise to the right
left coronary arteries.

The pulmonary trunk emerges from the pericardium and divides into right
and left pulmonary arteries in the concavity of the aortic arch, anterior to the
bifurcation of the trachea at the level of the fourth thoracic vertebra. As the
ascending aorta pierces the fibrous pericardium it turns backwards and to the
left, becoming the arch of the aorta.

Connecting the aortic arch to the pulmonary trunk (or to the commencement
of the left pulmonary artery) is the ligamentum arteriosum (Fig. 2.42), the
remnant of the fetal ductus arteriosus which conveyed blood from the
pulmonary trunk to the aorta, bypassing the pulmonary circulation.
Occasionally the ductus remains patent after birth, giving rise to serious
circulatory abnormalities.

Fig. 2.41 *Aortic and pulmonary valves viewed obliquely from above.*

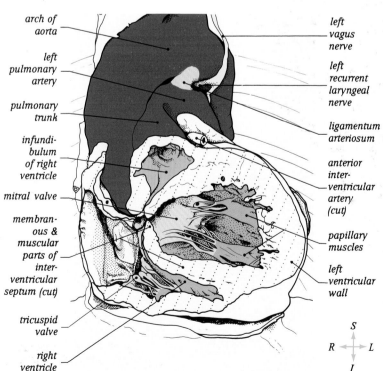

Fig. 2.42 *Anterior view of the aorta, pulmonary trunk and ligamentum
arteriosum. Most of the muscular part of the interventricular septum has been
removed to show the interior of the left ventricle.*

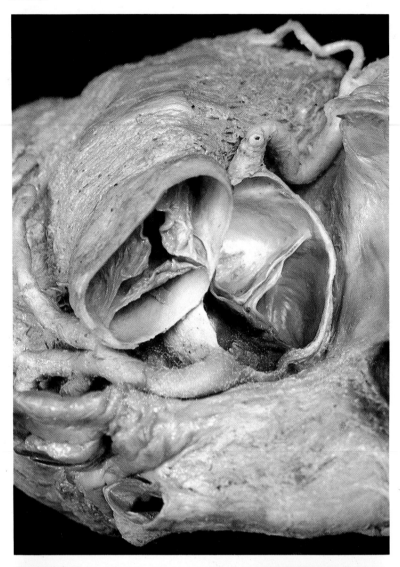

BLOOD VESSELS

The arterial supply to the heart is provided by the right and left coronary arteries which arise from the ascending aorta just above the aortic valve (Fig. 2.43). They supply the myocardium, including the papillary muscles and conducting tissue. The principal venous return is via the coronary sinus and the cardiac veins.

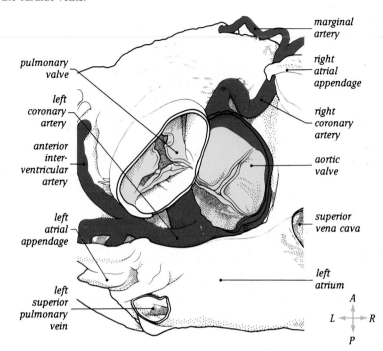

Fig. 2.43 *Origins of the right and left coronary arteries from the root of the ascending aorta seen from above.*

Right coronary artery

This vessel arises from the anterior aspect of the root of the aorta and descends in the anterior atrioventricular groove (Figs. 2.43 & 2.44). At the inferior border it gives off a marginal branch which runs to the left towards the apex of the heart. The right coronary artery continues on the inferior surface in the atrioventricular groove (Fig. 2.45) and terminates by anastomosing with the left coronary artery. On the inferior surface, the inferior interventricular artery arises from the right coronary artery (occasionally the left coronary artery) and runs in the inferior interventricular groove towards the apex. The right coronary artery and its branches supply the anterior surface of the right atrium, the lower part of the left atrium, most of the right ventricle, and parts of the left ventricle and interventricular septum. In addition, branches from this artery usually supply most of the conducting tissue of the heart (see page 2.35).

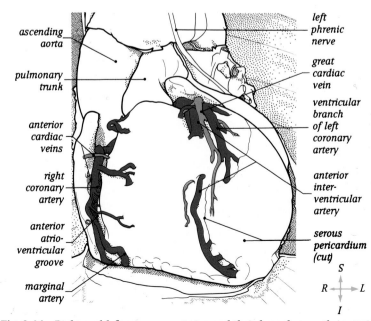

Fig. 2.44 *Right and left coronary arteries and their branches on the anterior surface of the heart.*

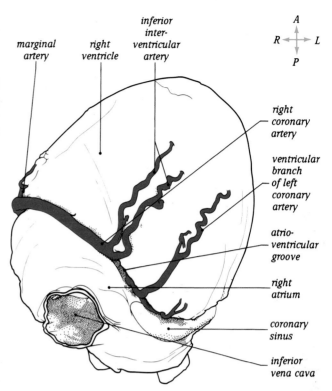

marginal artery · right ventricle · inferior inter-ventricular artery

A · R · L · P

right coronary artery

ventricular branch of left coronary artery

atrio-ventricular groove

right atrium

coronary sinus

inferior vena cava

Fig. 2.45 *Right and left coronary arteries and their branches on the inferior surface of the heart. The inferior interventricular artery is duplicated in this specimen.*

Left coronary artery

This artery takes origin from the posterior aspect of the root of the ascending aorta and runs to the left behind the pulmonary trunk where its major branch, the anterior interventricular artery, arises (Figs. 2.43 & 2.46). The latter vessel descends in the anterior interventricular groove towards the apex of the heart. The left coronary artery continues as the circumflex artery in the posterior part of the atrioventricular groove and terminates by anastomosing with the right coronary artery. The vessel supplies the posterior wall of the left atrium and appendage, most of the left ventricle, and parts of the right ventricle and interventricular septum.

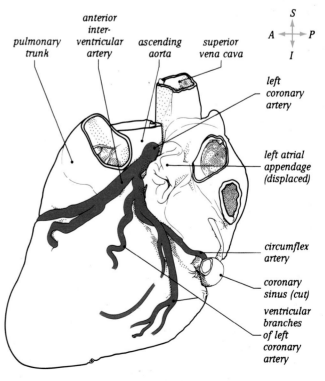

pulmonary trunk · anterior inter-ventricular artery · ascending aorta · superior vena cava

S · A · P · I

left coronary artery

left atrial appendage (displaced)

circumflex artery

coronary sinus (cut)

ventricular branches of left coronary artery

Fig. 2.46 *Left coronary artery and its branches viewed from the left.*

Coronary sinus and cardiac veins

Most of the venous return from the heart is carried by the coronary sinus, which runs along the posterior part of the atrioventricular groove and terminates in the right atrium. The coronary sinus is formed near the left border of the heart by the union of the posterior vein of the left ventricle and the great cardiac vein (Fig. 2.47), which accompanies the anterior interventricular artery. Other veins enter the coronary sinus, including the middle cardiac vein (Fig. 2.48) which accompanies the inferior interventricular artery. Some cardiac veins enter the right atrium independently.

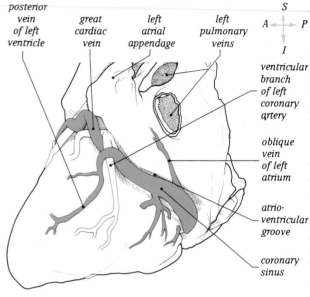

Fig. 2.47 *Oblique view of the coronary sinus lying in the atrioventricular groove.*

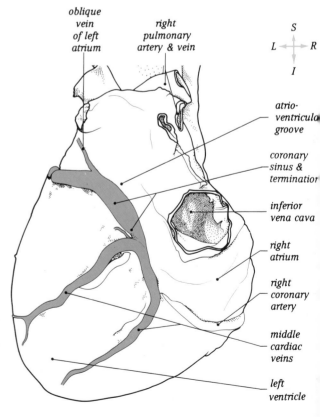

Fig. 2.48 *Posteroinferior view of the termination of the coronary sinus in the right atrium.*

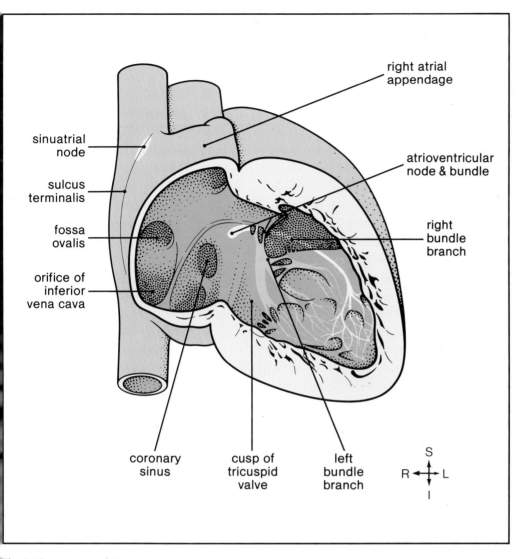

right atrial
appendage

atrioventricular
node & bundle

right
bundle
branch

sinuatrial
node

sulcus
terminalis

fossa
ovalis

orifice of
inferior
vena cava

coronary
sinus

cusp of
tricuspid
valve

left
bundle
branch

Fig. 2.49 *Location of the conducting tissue in the walls of the chambers.*

CONDUCTING SYSTEM

Coordinated contraction of the myocardium is controlled by specialized conducting tissues, consisting of the sinuatrial (SA) node, the atrioventricular (AV) node, the atrioventricular bundle (of His) and its right and left branches (Fig. 2.49).

The sinuatrial node lies in the anterior wall of the right atrium close to the termination of the superior vena cava. It occupies part of the root of the atrial appendage and the upper end of the sulcus terminalis. Numerous autonomic nerves supply the node and modify its rate of discharge. The SA node usually receives blood from an atrial branch of either the right or left coronary artery. From the SA node the cardiac excitation wave passes through the atrial myocardium to reach the AV node.

The atrioventricular node lies in the interatrial septum anterosuperior to the termination of the coronary sinus. It is continuous with the atrioventricular bundle which passes through the fibrous ring separating the atria and ventricles. The bundle gains the upper part of the interventricular septum and promptly divides into right and left branches. The AV node and bundle are supplied by branches of the inferior interventricular artery.

Lying beneath the endocardium the right branch of the atrioventricular bundle descends in the interventricular septum and often passes in the moderator band (Fig. 2.50) to ramify within the anterior wall of the right ventricle. The left branch runs on the left side of the interventricular septum. Both branches divide repeatedly at the ventricular apices and spread out into the myocardium of the respective ventricles.

ascending
aorta
& right
coronary
artery

infundi-
bulum

right
ventricular
wall (cut)

inter-
ventricular
septum

cusp of
tricuspid
valve

chordae
tendineae

moderator
band

Fig. 2.50 *Moderator band seen through a window cut in the anterior wall of the right ventricle.*

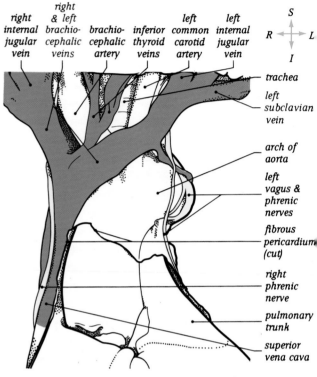

Fig. 2.51 *Relationships of the brachiocephalic veins to the great arteries arising from the aortic arch.*

Labels on figure: right internal jugular vein; right & left brachiocephalic veins; brachiocephalic artery; inferior thyroid veins; left common carotid artery; left internal jugular vein; trachea; left subclavian vein; arch of aorta; left vagus & phrenic nerves; fibrous pericardium (cut); right phrenic nerve; pulmonary trunk; superior vena cava

BRACHIOCEPHALIC VEINS

On each side the brachiocephalic vein is formed in the root of the neck by the union of the internal jugular and subclavian veins. At its origin the vein lies behind the sternoclavicular joint and in front of the first part of the subclavian artery.

The right brachiocephalic vein runs a short vertical course in the superior mediastinum to unite with the left brachiocephalic vein (Fig. 2.51) behind the medial end of the first right intercostal space. It receives the right vertebral and internal thoracic veins, together with the right jugular and subclavian lymph trunks and the right lymph duct. The vessel is accompanied by the right phrenic nerve.

The left brachiocephalic vein enters the thorax and runs obliquely to the right passing behind the manubrium. The vessel lies in front of the origin from the arch of the aorta of the left common carotid artery and the brachiocephalic artery. At its commencement the vein is joined by the termination of the thoracic duct and, along its course, receives the left vertebral, internal thoracic and superior intercostal veins and, usually, the inferior thyroid veins.

SUPERIOR VENA CAVA

Formed by the union of the two brachiocephalic veins, this large vessel descends vertically (Fig. 2.51) and terminates in the right atrium of the heart. It lies to the right of the ascending aorta and to the left of the right phrenic nerve, and receives the azygos vein before piercing the fibrous pericardium.

ARCH OF AORTA AND BRANCHES

The arch of the aorta lies within the superior mediastinum in continuity with the ascending aorta. The vessel curves backwards and to the left to reach the left side of the fourth thoracic vertebral body where it becomes the descending aorta. The arch possesses a concavity inferiorly, left and right sides, and a superior convexity.

The concavity is related to the bifurcation of the pulmonary trunk and the left main bronchus. The ligamentum arteriosum attaches the pulmonary trunk (or left pulmonary artery) to the concavity of the aortic arch and is closely related to the left recurrent laryngeal nerve (see Fig. 2.42).

The left side of the aortic arch is crossed by the left phrenic and vagus nerves (Fig. 2.52) and covered by mediastinal pleura. The phrenic nerve lies in front of the vagus and passes onto the fibrous pericardium in front of the lung root. The vagus nerve inclines backwards to pass behind the lung root, having given off the left recurrent laryngeal nerve. The left superior intercostal vein passes forwards across the arch and usually terminates in the left brachiocephalic vein.

The right side of the arch is related, from in front backwards, to the superior vena cava, trachea, left recurrent laryngeal nerve, oesophagus and thoracic duct. These structures lie between the aorta and the right mediastinal pleura.

The convexity of the arch gives rise to the brachiocephalic, left common carotid and left subclavian arteries (Fig. 2.53) which ascend into the root of the neck. The brachiocephalic artery is the first branch of the arch of the aorta and arises behind the left brachiocephalic vein. The artery slopes upwards and to the right across the anterior surface of the trachea, leaving the thorax to the right of the trachea to divide in the root of the neck into the right subclavian and right common carotid arteries.

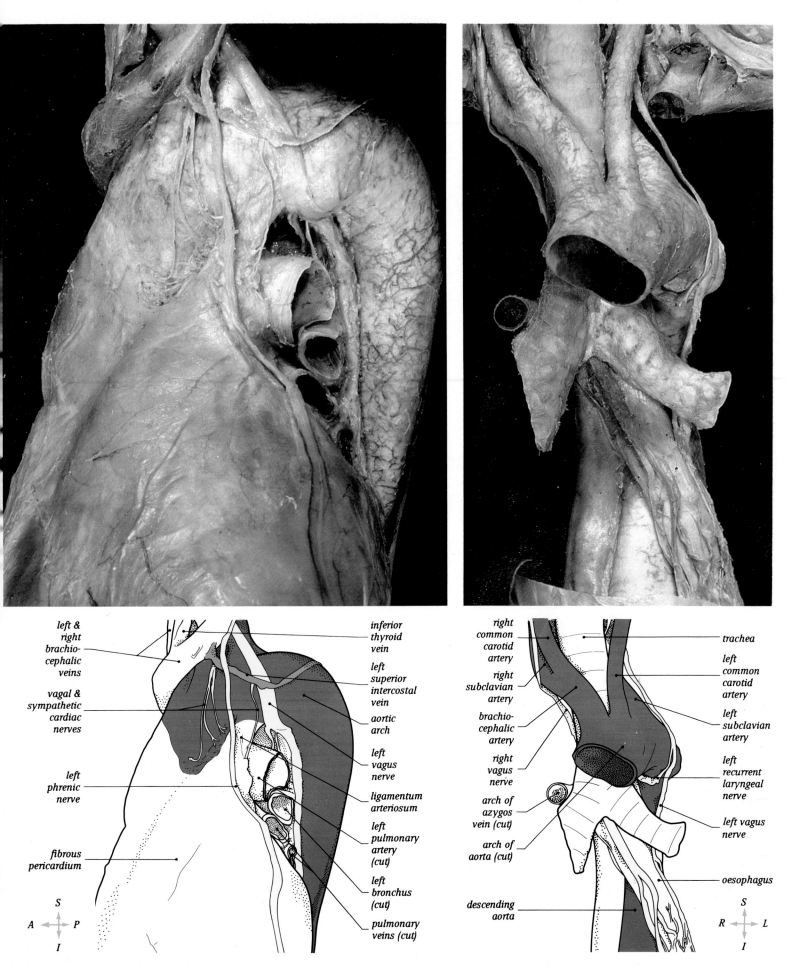

Fig. 2.52 *Oblique view of the arch of the aorta showing the courses of the left vagus and phrenic nerves.*

Fig. 2.53 *Arch of the aorta and its branches viewed anteriorly.*

Labels for Fig. 2.52:
left & right brachio-cephalic veins
vagal & sympathetic cardiac nerves
left phrenic nerve
fibrous pericardium
inferior thyroid vein
left superior intercostal vein
aortic arch
left vagus nerve
ligamentum arteriosum
left pulmonary artery (cut)
left bronchus (cut)
pulmonary veins (cut)

Labels for Fig. 2.53:
right common carotid artery
right subclavian artery
brachio-cephalic artery
right vagus nerve
arch of azygos vein (cut)
arch of aorta (cut)
descending aorta
trachea
left common carotid artery
left subclavian artery
left recurrent laryngeal nerve
left vagus nerve
oesophagus

The left common carotid artery arises behind the brachiocephalic artery and ascends, in company with the left phrenic and vagus nerves, through the superior mediastinum on the left of the trachea into the root of the neck.

The left subclavian artery is the most posterior artery arising from the aortic arch and lies immediately behind the left common carotid artery. It runs upwards and laterally, closely related to the pleura covering the apex of the left lung, entering the root of the neck behind the sternoclavicular joint.

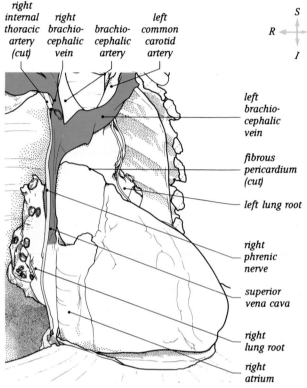

Fig. 2.54 *Oblique view of the course of the right phrenic nerve in the thorax.*

PHRENIC NERVES

The right and left phrenic nerves (C3, C4 & C5) pass through the thoracic inlet behind the respective subclavian veins. Due to the asymmetry of the mediastinal organs, the intrathoracic courses of the two nerves differ. The right phrenic nerve, covered by mediastinal pleura, accompanies the right brachiocephalic vein and the superior vena cava in front of the root of the right lung (Fig. 2.54). It descends vertically across the fibrous pericardium covering the right atrium and pierces the diaphragm alongside the inferior vena cava.

The left phrenic nerve, also covered by mediastinal pleura, lies lateral to the left common carotid artery and crosses the left side of the aortic arch to gain the fibrous pericardium in front of the left lung root (Fig. 2.55). The nerve then descends across the pericardium as far as the apex of the heart where it pierces the diaphragm.

The phrenic nerves supply the muscle of the diaphragm, excluding the crura. They give sensory fibres to the fibrous pericardium and the mediastinal and diaphragmatic pleura, and sensory branches to the peritoneum covering the inferior surface of the diaphragm.

TRACHEA

The trachea descends through the neck, where normally it is palpable, and enters the thorax in the midline, immediately behind the upper border of the manubrium. It runs vertically through the superior mediastinum and, at the level of the aortic arch, divides into right and left main bronchi (Fig. 2.56). The right main bronchus is wider than the left and inclines steeply downwards to enter the right lung root. The right upper lobar bronchus often arises outside the hilum of the lung. The left main bronchus runs obliquely to the left within the concavity of the arch of the aorta, passing behind the left pulmonary artery to gain the left lung root.

The thoracic part of the trachea is crossed anteriorly by the brachiocephalic artery and the left brachiocephalic vein. In addition, the trachea is overlapped by the anterior margins of the pleura and lungs and the thymus (or its remnants). The trachea is related on the left to the arch of the aorta and left common carotid and subclavian arteries, on the right to the superior vena cava, the termination of the azygos vein, the right vagus nerve and the mediastinal pleura, and posteriorly to the oesophagus and the left recurrent laryngeal nerve. (The right recurrent laryngeal nerve does not enter the thorax but passes around the right subclavian artery in the root of the neck; see page 7.9).

The vascular supply of the trachea is from the inferior thyroid artery and vein. The recurrent laryngeal nerves supply sensory and parasympathetic secretomotor fibres to the mucous membrane and motor fibres to the smooth muscle (trachealis).

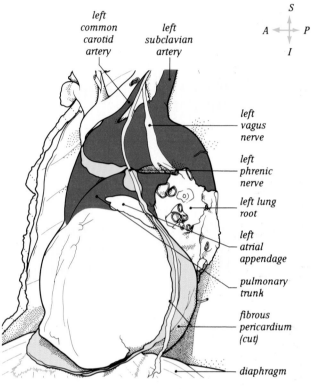

Fig. 2.55 *Oblique view of the intrathoracic course of the left phrenic nerve.*

Labels (Fig. 2.55):
- left common carotid artery
- left subclavian artery
- S / A – P / I
- left vagus nerve
- left phrenic nerve
- left lung root
- left atrial appendage
- pulmonary trunk
- fibrous pericardium (cut)
- diaphragm

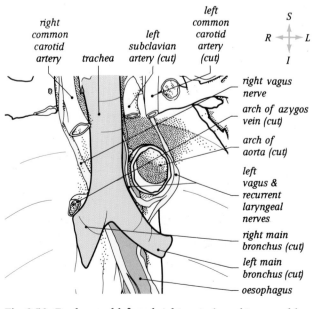

Fig. 2.56 *Trachea and left and right main bronchi exposed by removal of the anterior part of the aortic arch.*

Labels (Fig. 2.56):
- right common carotid artery
- trachea
- left subclavian artery (cut)
- left common carotid artery (cut)
- S / R – L / I
- right vagus nerve
- arch of azygos vein (cut)
- arch of aorta (cut)
- left vagus & recurrent laryngeal nerves
- right main bronchus (cut)
- left main bronchus (cut)
- oesophagus

MEDIASTINAL STRUCTURES

OESOPHAGUS

The oesophagus descends through the root of the neck and traverses the thoracic inlet behind the trachea. In the superior mediastinum the oesophagus lies in front of the upper four thoracic vertebral bodies and behind the trachea, the left main bronchus and left recurrent laryngeal nerve. The aortic arch and the thoracic duct are on its left while the azygos vein arches forwards on its right (Fig. 2.57).

The oesophagus continues into the posterior mediastinum in front of the fifth thoracic vertebra accompanied by the right and left vagus nerves. It descends behind the fibrous pericardium and inclines to the left to cross in front of the descending aorta. On its right side the oesophagus is covered by mediastinal pleura. On the left, once anterior to the descending aorta, it is related to pleura as far as the diaphragm. Accompanied by branches of the vagus nerves (see below), the oesophagus passes through the diaphragm at the level of the tenth thoracic vertebra.

The oesophagus is supplied by branches from the inferior thyroid arteries and from the descending thoracic aorta. Its lower part receives branches from the left gastric artery which ascend through the oesophageal opening in the diaphragm. Radicles of the left gastric vein (a tributary of the portal vein) anastomose with veins which drain venous blood from the oesophagus into the azygos system. The upper part of the oesophagus is drained by the brachiocephalic veins. Sensory and parasympathetic motor fibres to the oesophagus are provided by the vagi and their recurrent laryngeal branches.

VAGUS (X) NERVES

In the superior mediastinum the relationships of the right and left vagi differ. The right vagus nerve enters the thorax behind the bifurcation of the brachiocephalic artery and on the right of the trachea. The nerve, covered by mediastinal pleura, inclines backwards and passes behind the right lung root to gain the oesophagus. The left vagus nerve descends behind the left common carotid artery to cross the left side of the aortic arch, gives off the left recurrent laryngeal nerve, and continues behind the left lung root to reach the oesophagus.

The left recurrent laryngeal nerve (Fig. 2.57) passes around the arch of the aorta adjacent to the ligamentum arteriosum and ascends in the interval between the trachea and oesophagus. In the posterior mediastinum the right and left vagus nerves divide on the surface of the oesophagus to form a network, the oesophageal plexus. The terminal branches of the plexus (the anterior and posterior vagal trunks) enter the abdomen with the oesophagus (see page 4.50).

DESCENDING THORACIC AORTA AND BRANCHES

The descending aorta (Fig. 2.58) is continuous with the aortic arch and initially lies to the left of the fifth thoracic vertebral body. As it traverses the posterior mediastinum it inclines forwards and to the right, gaining the midline anterior to the twelfth thoracic vertebra. On the right, the upper part of the descending aorta is related to the thoracic vertebral bodies and the oesophagus. The lower part and all of its left side are covered by mediastinal pleura. The thoracic duct and the azygos vein lie to the right of the aorta and anteriorly it is crossed by the oesophagus sloping obliquely from the midline to the left. The descending aorta leaves the thorax in front of the twelfth thoracic vertebra and behind the median arcuate ligament of the diaphragm with the thoracic duct and azygos vein.

Posterior intercostal arteries from the descending aorta supply the third to the eleventh intercostal spaces on both sides. They anastomose with the anterior intercostal arteries derived from either the internal thoracic or the musculophrenic arteries. Other branches from the aorta supply the right and left bronchi and the oesophagus.

THORACIC DUCT

Arising from the upper part of the cisterna chyli (see page 4.49), the thoracic duct passes into the thorax lying between the azygos vein and descending aorta and with these structures (Figs. 2.58 & 2.59) ascends through the

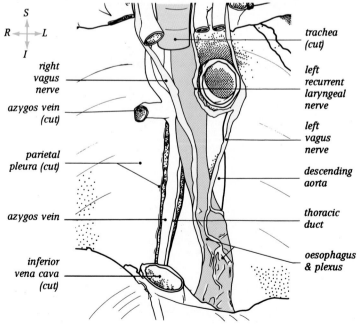

Fig. 2.57 *Intrathoracic part of the oesophagus and accompanying vagus nerves after removal of the bifurcation of the trachea*

posterior mediastinum to gain the superior mediastinum on the left of the oesophagus. The duct then curves forwards and to the left, crossing the apex of the left lung to enter the root of the neck where it terminates in the confluence of the left internal jugular and subclavian veins.

Fig. 2.58 *Descending aorta and thoracic duct exposed by removal of the thoracic part of the oesophagus.*

Fig. 2.59 *Azygos vein, right intercostal nerves and posterior intercostal vessels exposed by removal of the parietal pleura.*

AZYGOS VENOUS SYSTEM

This system of veins drains blood from most of the posterior thoracic wall and from the bronchi, the pericardium and part of the intrathoracic oesophagus. The azygos vein enters the thorax through the aortic opening and receives posterior intercostal veins from the lower eight spaces on the right (Fig. 2.59). Veins from the second and third spaces drain into the right superior intercostal vein which terminates in the azygos vein as it arches over the right lung root to join the superior vena cava (see Fig. 2.21). The venous return from the first space drains into the right brachiocephalic vein. The azygos also receives one or more branches from the hemiazygos veins.

2.35

The hemiazygos and accessory hemiazygos veins drain the lower eight posterior intercostal spaces on the left side. The lowermost four spaces usually empty into the hemiazygos vein, which crosses the midline to terminate in the azygos vein (see Fig. 2.60). Veins from the next four intercostal spaces usually join to form the accessory hemiazygos vein, which also crosses to end in the azygos. Sometimes, the hemiazygos and accessory

hemiazygos veins drain into the azygos vein by a single vessel. The second and third spaces on the left are drained by the left superior intercostal vein (see Fig. 2.52) which crosses the aortic arch to end in the left brachiocephalic vein. The first left intercostal space drains into the corresponding brachiocephalic vein.

THORACIC SYMPATHETIC TRUNK

The thoracic part of the sympathetic trunk (chain) runs along the lateral aspects of the thoracic vertebral bodies (Figs. 2.60 & 2.61). In continuity with the cervical and abdominal parts, the thoracic sympathetic trunk consists of a series of interconnected enlargements (ganglia) occurring at intervals along its length. Usually, each thoracic spinal nerve is connected to its own ganglion by two branches, a white (preganglionic) and a grey (postganglionic) ramus communicans. Not infrequently, adjacent ganglia fuse together and, most often, the inferior cervical and first thoracic ganglia fuse to form the stellate ganglion.

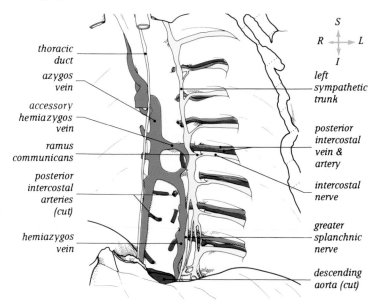

Fig. 2.60 *Oblique view of left sympathetic trunk, hemiazygos vein, intercostal nerves and posterior intercostal vessels after removal of the descending aorta and parietal pleura on the left side of midline.*

Branches

Fine nerve filaments running from the sympathetic trunk contribute to the autonomic prevertebral plexuses supplying the thoracic organs, including the heart (cardiac plexuses), lungs (pulmonary plexuses) and the oesophagus (oesophageal plexus). The lower thoracic ganglia give rise to a collection of autonomic fibres which form the greater (Fig. 2.61), lesser and least splanchnic nerves, which are destined to supply intra-abdominal structures which are gained by piercing the crura of the diaphragm. All thoracic spinal nerves receive from the grey rami communicantes sympathetic postganglionic fibres which are distributed to various structures of the body wall (for example, blood vessels, hair follicles and sweat glands) by the segmental spinal nerves.

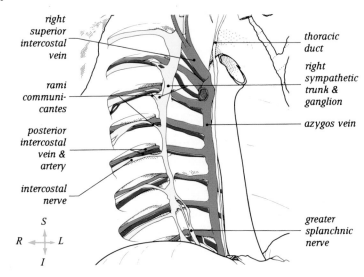

Fig. 2.61 *Oblique view of right sympathetic trunk and posterior intercostal vessels and intercostal nerves after removal of the parietal pleura.*

3
UPPER LIMB

INTRODUCTION

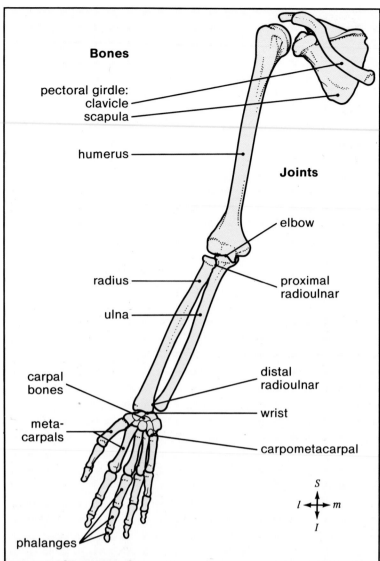

Bones

pectoral girdle:
clavicle
scapula

humerus

Joints

elbow

radius

proximal
radioulnar

ulna

carpal
bones

distal
radioulnar

meta-
carpals

wrist

carpometacarpal

phalanges

Fig. 3.1 *Bones and joints of the upper limb.*

scapular region

axilla

compartments of arm:
posterior
anterior

cubital fossa

compartments
of forearm:
posterior
anterior

carpal
region

dorsum
of hand

palm
of hand

Fig. 3.2 *Parts of the upper limb.*

The upper limb (extremity) comprises several bones and their joints (Fig. 3.1), clothed by soft tissues. For descriptive purposes the limb is divided into regions (Fig. 3.2), each enveloped by fascia and containing muscles with nerve and vascular supplies. The scapula with its associated muscles and soft tissues constitute the scapular region while the muscles attaching between the front of the chest wall and the upper limb (together with the overlying fascia, breast and skin) constitute the pectoral region. The scapula and the clavicle, which together form the pectoral girdle, articulate at the acromioclavicular joint. Also, the clavicle articulates with the trunk at the sternoclavicular joint and the scapula with the humerus at the shoulder (glenohumeral) joint.

Between the proximal part of the limb and the chest wall is the axilla, a region traversed by the principal nerves and vessels passing between the upper limb and the root of the neck.

The arm is that part of the upper limb between the shoulder and the elbow. The muscles of the arm are disposed in anterior (flexor) and posterior

(extensor) compartments, separated by the humerus and the medial and lateral intermuscular septa (Fig. 3.3). In front of the elbow joint (at which the humerus, radius and ulna articulate) lies the cubital fossa, a region traversed by vessels and nerves passing between the arm and the forearm.

The forearm lies between the elbow and the wrist, and its muscles are arranged in anterior (flexor) and posterior (extensor) compartments, separated by the radius, ulna, and interosseous membrane (Fig. 3.4). Rotation at the joints between the bones of the forearm (proximal and distal radioulnar joints) permits the hand to function either in the supinated (palm facing up) or pronated (palm facing down) position.

The forearm articulates with the carpus at the wrist (radiocarpal) joint. Together with the flexor retinaculum, the bones of the carpus form the carpal tunnel which links the anterior compartment of the forearm and the hand. Anterior to the metacarpals are the structures of the palm while posteriorly is the dorsum of the hand. The digits are named, from lateral to medial, the thumb and the index, middle, ring and little fingers.

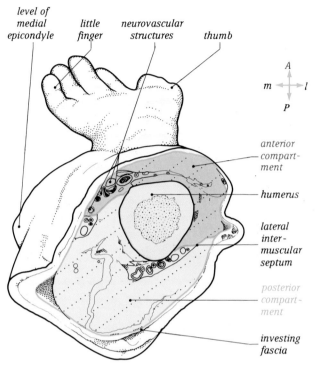

level of medial epicondyle   *little finger*   *neurovascular structures*   *thumb*

A
m — l
P

anterior compartment

humerus

lateral intermuscular septum

posterior compartment

investing fascia

Fig. 3.3 *Transverse section midway between shoulder and elbow joints to show the compartments of the arm.*

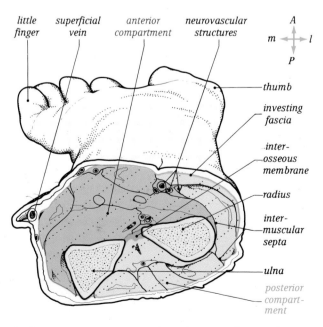

little finger   *superficial vein*   *anterior compartment*   *neurovascular structures*

A
m — l
P

thumb

investing fascia

interosseous membrane

radius

intermuscular septa

ulna

posterior compartment

Fig. 3.4 *Transverse section midway between elbow and wrist joints to show the compartments of the forearm.*

DELTOID

Deltoid is a large multipennate muscle responsible for the rounded contour of the shoulder region (Fig. 3.5). The muscle overlies the shoulder joint and the attachments of the short scapular muscles to the upper end of the humerus (Fig. 3.6). Proximally it has a continuous attachment to the lateral third of the clavicle and to the acromion and spine of the scapula. The distal attachment is to a roughened area, the deltoid tuberosity, midway down the lateral surface of the shaft of the humerus. Deltoid acts only on the shoulder joint where it is the main abductor. During this movement, produced by the acromial fibres, the joint is stabilized by the clavicular fibres and those from the scapular spine. Acting alone the anterior fibres produce flexion whereas the posterior fibres extend the shoulder joint. Deltoid is supplied by the axillary nerve, a terminal branch of the posterior cord of the brachial plexus (see page 3.8).

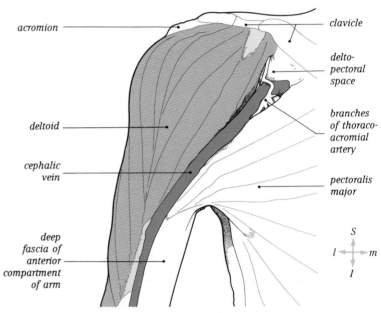

Fig. 3.5 *Anterior view of deltoid. The cephalic vein lies in the deltopectoral groove. Deformity of the clavicle is due to a healed fracture.*

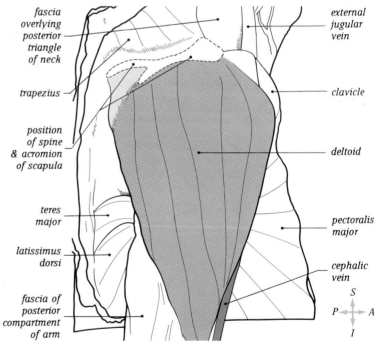

Fig. 3.6 *Lateral view. Deltoid has a continuous proximal attachment to the spine and acromion of the scapula and the lateral part of the clavicle.*

AXILLARY NERVE

The axillary nerve leaves the axilla through the quadrilateral space (see Fig. 3.59) accompanied by the posterior circumflex humeral artery. In its course the nerve is closely related to the surgical neck of the humerus and to the capsule of the shoulder joint. It supplies deltoid and teres minor, the shoulder joint and skin overlying the lower part of deltoid. Damage to the nerve may occur during dislocation of the shoulder joint, resulting in weakness of abduction, loss of sensation and, subsequently, in loss of the normal contour of the shoulder as the deltoid muscle becomes wasted.

AXILLA

The axilla is the space between the root of the upper limb and the chest wall. It is traversed by the principal vessels and nerves which pass between the upper limb and the root of the neck. The shape and size of the axilla vary according to the position of the shoulder joint but when the limb is in the anatomical position the axilla is shaped like a truncated pyramid with a narrow apex (inlet) superiorly, a broad base and three walls (Fig. 3.7).

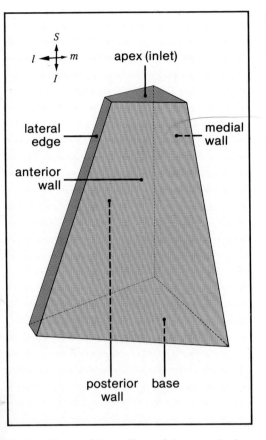

Fig. 3.7 *Shape of the axilla as if the upper limb were in the anatomical position.*

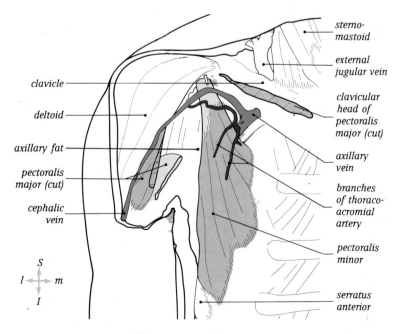

Fig. 3.8 *Axilla from above showing the boundaries of the apex (inlet) and continuity between the root of the neck and the upper limb (arrow).*

WALLS

The upper ribs and intercostal spaces, covered by serratus anterior, form the medial wall (see Fig. 3.10) which is convex laterally. The anterior wall consists of pectoralis major overlying pectoralis minor and subclavius (Fig. 3.9 & see Fig. 3.11) while the posterior wall is formed by subscapularis, teres major and latissimus dorsi. The muscles of the anterior and posterior walls converge on the humerus (see Fig. 3.10) so that the axilla is limited laterally by the narrow bicipital groove of the humerus. The base of the axilla, convex upwards, is formed by fascia passing between the inferior margins of the anterior and posterior walls. The triangular apex of the axilla provides continuity between the root of the neck and the upper limb and is bounded by the clavicle anteriorly, the upper border of the scapula posteriorly and the first rib medially (Fig. 3.8).

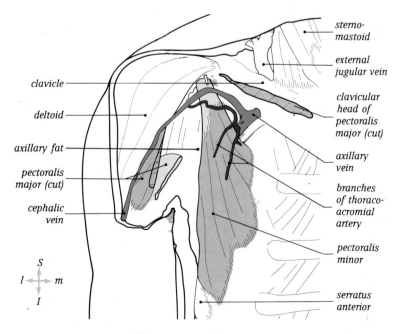

Fig. 3.9 *Structures which pass above pectoralis minor in the anterior wall of the axilla. Pectoralis major and fascia around pectoralis minor have been removed.*

Fig. 3.10 *Transverse section showing (left) the walls and (right) the contents of the axilla. The lung has been removed.*

CONTENTS

The axilla contains the axillary artery and its branches, the axillary vein and its tributaries, the nerves of the brachial plexus and the axillary lymph nodes.

Coracobrachialis and the short and long heads of biceps traverse the axilla. In addition, the tail of the breast may enter the axilla. All these structures are embedded in loose fatty connective tissue (Fig. 3.10).

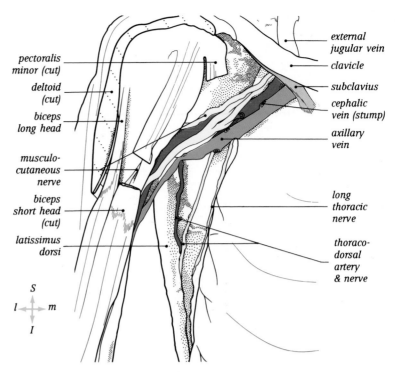

pectoralis minor (cut)

deltoid (cut)

biceps long head

musculo-cutaneous nerve

biceps short head (cut)

latissimus dorsi

external jugular vein

clavicle

subclavius

cephalic vein (stump)

axillary vein

long thoracic nerve

thoraco-dorsal artery & nerve

S
l — m
I

Fig. 3.11 *Axillary neurovascular bundle, exposed by removal of the pectoral muscles and axillary fat.*

Axillary Artery

The subclavian artery continues as the axillary artery beyond the lateral edge of the first rib. Near the inlet the axillary artery lies posterior to the axillary vein (Fig. 3.11), but more distally the artery lies lateral to the vein close to the humerus. The axillary artery and parts of the brachial plexus which surround it are bound together by the axillary sheath. Coracobrachialis and the short head of biceps lie lateral to the artery while pectoralis minor crosses it anteriorly. By convention, the axillary artery may be described in parts which lie above, behind and below pectoralis minor. Distal to the lower border of teres major the vessel continues into the arm as the brachial artery (see Fig. 3.13).

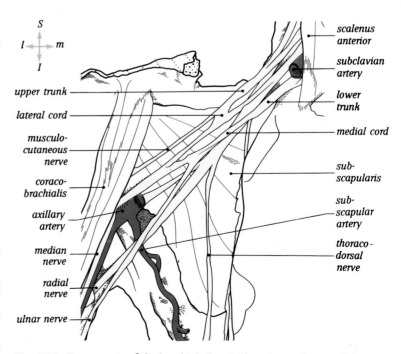

S
l — m
I

upper trunk

lateral cord

musculo-cutaneous nerve

coraco-brachialis

axillary artery

median nerve

radial nerve

ulnar nerve

scalenus anterior

subclavian artery

lower trunk

medial cord

sub-scapularis

sub-scapular artery

thoraco-dorsal nerve

Fig. 3.12 *Components of the brachial plexus. The veins and most of the axillary artery have been removed.*

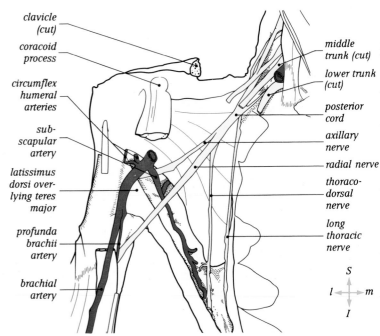

Fig. 3.13 *Some posterior branches of the brachial plexus. The more anterior parts of the plexus have been excised.*

Branches of the axillary artery supply the muscles forming the walls of the axilla and adjacent structures. The thoracoacromial artery (see Fig. 3.9) supplies the anterior wall while the superior thoracic and lateral thoracic arteries supply the medial and anterior walls. The thoracoacromial and lateral thoracic arteries also supply part of the breast. The posterior wall is supplied by the subscapular artery. The anterior and posterior circumflex humeral arteries (Fig. 3.13) pass laterally and encircle the surgical neck of the humerus, supplying the shoulder joint and the upper part of the arm. An important collateral circulation, the scapular anastomosis, is formed by communications between the circumflex scapular branch of the subscapular artery and the suprascapular branch from the thyrocervical trunk, a branch of the subclavian artery.

Axillary vein
The venae comitantes of the brachial artery unite with the basilic vein in the upper part of the arm and continue as the axillary vein above the lower border of teres major. The vein ascends medial to the axillary artery (see Fig. 3.11) passing behind pectoralis minor, and crosses the lateral edge of the first rib to continue as the subclavian vein, lying anterior to its companion artery. A major tributary of the axillary vein is the cephalic vein which ascends in the groove between deltoid and pectoralis major. Just below the clavicle it enters the axilla by piercing the fascia above pectoralis minor (see Fig. 3.9). The progress of a catheter inserted proximally along the cephalic vein may be impeded by the acute angulations often present above pectoralis minor or near its termination in the axillary vein. The axillary vein receives other tributaries which in general correspond to the branches of the axillary artery.

Brachial plexus
The whole plexus will be described here, although only the divisions, cords and certain branches lie within the axilla. The brachial plexus supplies the upper limb and consists of a branching network of nerves derived from the anterior rami of the lower four cervical and the first thoracic spinal nerves. The plexus enables nerve fibres originating in several spinal cord segments to be distributed to each peripheral branch. A knowledge of the segmental arrangement and distribution is necessary for accurate diagnosis in diseases or injuries involving the spinal cord or the brachial plexus. The parts of the plexus are named, from proximal to distal, roots, trunks, divisions and cords (Fig. 3.14). The five roots (anterior rami) give rise to three trunks (upper, middle and lower) which emerge between scalenus medius and scalenus anterior to lie in the floor of the posterior triangle of the neck (see page 7.4). The roots of the plexus lie deep to the prevertebral fascia while the trunks are covered by its lateral extension, the axillary sheath. Each trunk divides into an anterior and a posterior division behind the clavicle, at the apex of the axilla. Within the axilla, the divisions combine to produce the three cords which are named lateral, medial and posterior according to their relationships to the axillary artery. Each cord ends at the lower border of pectoralis minor by dividing into two terminal branches. Other branches of the plexus arise in the neck and axilla directly from the roots, trunks and cords (Fig. 3.15). The anterior divisions form the lateral and medial cords (see Fig. 3.12) whose branches supply the flexor muscles of the arm, forearm and hand and the skin overlying the flexor compartments. The three posterior divisions unite to form the posterior cord (Fig. 3.13) whose branches supply the extensor musculature of the shoulder, arm and forearm and the skin of the posterior surface of the limb.

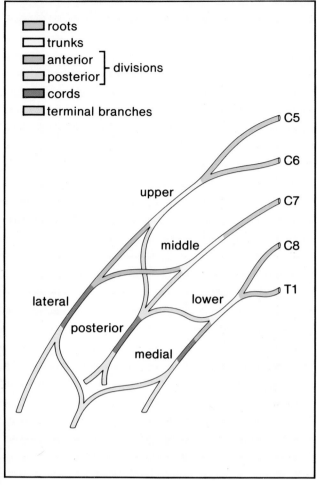

Fig. 3.14 *Main components of the brachial plexus in their usual arrangement.*

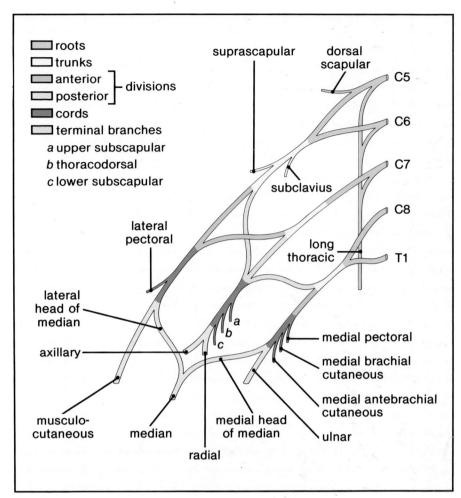

Fig. 3.15 *Branches of the brachial plexus. The arrangement of these nerves may vary considerably.*

Axillary lymph nodes

The axillary lymph nodes receive lymph not only from the upper limb but also from the superficial tissues of the thoracic and abdominal walls above the level of the umbilicus.

The nodes are described in groups according to their positions in the axilla. Anteriorly lies the pectoral group which drains the lateral and anterior aspects of the body wall including the breast. Laterally, along the axillary vessels, is the lateral group of nodes which receives most of the lymph from the upper

limb. Posteriorly the subscapular nodes receive lymph from the dorsal aspect of the body wall. Within the axilla, efferent lymph channels drain centrally and then proximally to apical nodes from which a subclavian lymph trunk arises; this terminates in the root of the neck by joining the right lymphatic duct or the thoracic duct, or by joining the subclavian vein (see page 7.8).

The principal vessels and nerves entering or leaving the axilla are listed in the following table:

Between axilla and root of neck (via inlet of axilla):	Between axilla and arm (lateral to fascia of axillary floor):	Through anterior wall (via interval between clavicle and pectoralis minor):	Through posterior wall (via triangular and quadrilateral intermuscular spaces):
Subclavian/axillary artery Axillary/subclavian vein Trunks/divisions of brachial plexus Subclavian lymph trunk	Axillary/brachial artery Brachial/axillary vein Median nerve Musculocutaneous nerve Ulnar nerve Radial nerve Brachial lymphatics	Thoracoacromial artery Cephalic vein Pectoral nerves Deltopectoral lymphatics	Circumflex branch of subscapular artery Axillary nerve with posterior circumflex humeral artery

The anterior compartment of the arm contains three muscles, namely biceps brachii, coracobrachialis and brachialis, the brachial artery with its venae comitantes, and three nerves, namely the median, ulnar and musculocutaneous nerves.

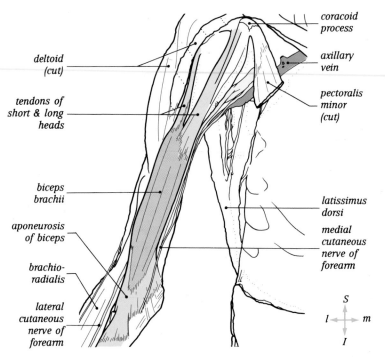

Fig. 3.16 *Anterior view of biceps after removal of deep fascia and anterior fibres of deltoid.*

MUSCLES

The three muscles of the compartment are supplied by the musculocutaneous nerve. The two heads of biceps separate proximally (Fig. 3.16) and have tendinous attachments to the scapula. The short head lies medially and passes distally from the tip of the coracoid process. The tendon of the long head attaches to the supraglenoid tubercle, leaves the shoulder joint deep to the transverse humeral ligament and continues distally in the intertubercular sulcus deep to the tendon of pectoralis major. The muscle bellies fuse and are attached by a tendon (see Fig. 3.22) to the tubercle of the radius and by the bicipital aponeurosis which fuses with deep fascia on the medial side of the forearm. Biceps is a strong flexor of the elbow and supinator of the forearm at the radioulnar joints, and a weak flexor of the shoulder joint.

Coracobrachialis attaches to the coracoid process with the short head of biceps. The muscle attaches distally to the medial side of the shaft of the humerus near its midpoint. Coracobrachialis is pierced by the musculocutaneous nerve (Fig. 3.17) and functions as a weak flexor and adductor of the shoulder joint.

Fig. 3.17 *The musculocutaneous nerve piercing coracobrachialis. The short head of biceps has been divided and the muscle reflected laterally.*

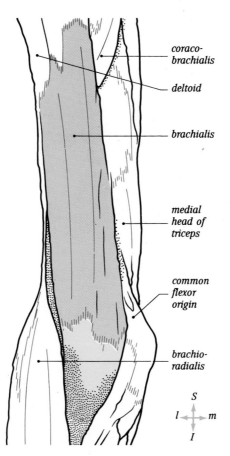

coraco-
brachialis

deltoid

brachialis

medial
head of
triceps

common
flexor
origin

brachio-
radialis

S
l ← → m
I

Fig. 3.18 *Brachialis, revealed by removal of the other components of the anterior compartment. The intermuscular septa have also been excised, exposing triceps.*

Brachialis (Fig. 3.18) lies deeply and has an extensive attachment to the anterior surface of the distal half of the shaft of the humerus and adjacent intermuscular septa. The muscle passes to the coronoid process of the ulna and acts as a powerful flexor of the elbow joint.

VESSELS
The brachial artery is the continuation of the axillary artery distal to teres major. In the upper part of the arm, the brachial artery with its venae comitantes is accompanied by the median and ulnar nerves (Fig. 3.19) and the medial cutaneous nerve of forearm. The artery passes distally and laterally, lying medial to biceps and anterior to coracobrachialis and brachialis. An important branch, the profunda brachii artery (see page 3.30), supplies the posterior compartment of the arm. The division of the brachial artery into its terminal radial and ulnar branches usually occurs in the cubital fossa but may occur at a more proximal level.

Venae comitantes, ascending from the cubital fossa, accompany the brachial artery and are joined by the basilic vein after it has pierced the deep fascia at about the midpoint of the arm. At the lower border of the axilla the venous channels usually combine to form a single axillary vein.

NERVES
The musculocutaneous nerve (Fig. 3.17) is a terminal branch of the lateral cord. It pierces coracobrachialis and lies between biceps and brachialis, supplying each of these muscles. The nerve continues distally as the lateral cutaneous nerve of forearm which pierces the deep fascia between biceps and brachioradialis to lie superficially over the cubital fossa (see Fig. 3.21).

The median and ulnar nerves traverse the entire length of the arm, but neither gives any branches above the elbow joint. The median nerve arises by lateral and medial heads which are terminal branches of the lateral and medial cords. In the upper part of the arm the nerve lies lateral to the brachial artery; but at midarm level it crosses anterior to the vessels and finally lies medial to the artery (Fig. 3.19), a position retained in the cubital fossa. The ulnar nerve is a terminal branch of the medial cord and, together with the medial cutaneous nerve of forearm, initially lies medial to the brachial artery but leaves the artery at midarm level (Fig. 3.19). It then pierces the medial intermuscular septum and enters the posterior compartment to lie between the septum and the medial head of triceps.

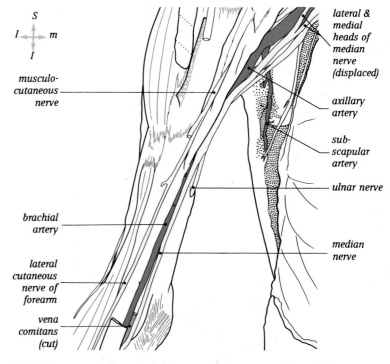

S
l ← → m
I

musculo-
cutaneous
nerve

brachial
artery

lateral
cutaneous
nerve of
forearm

vena
comitans
(cut)

lateral &
medial
heads of
median
nerve
(displaced)

axillary
artery

sub-
scapular
artery

ulnar nerve

median
nerve

Fig. 3.19 *Nerves and artery of the compartment. Biceps, the axillary vein and most venae comitantes of the brachial artery have been excised.*

CUBITAL FOSSA

The cubital fossa is a triangular-shaped space in front of the elbow joint, bounded laterally by brachioradialis and medially by pronator teres (see Fig. 3.23). By convention, the fossa is limited proximally by an imaginary line drawn between the two humeral epicondyles. The roof is formed by deep fascia, reinforced by the aponeurosis of biceps (see Fig. 3.21). The superficial fascia overlying the roof contains branches of the lateral and medial cutaneous nerves of forearm and superficial veins such as the median cubital vein which links the cephalic and basilic veins (Fig. 3.20). The arrangement of these superficial veins may vary considerably between individuals.

Fig. 3.20 *Cutaneous nerves and superficial veins overlying the right cubital fossa. Superficial fascia has been retained medial to the basilic vein.*

Fig. 3.21 *Roof of the cubital fossa after removal of superficial fascia, veins and nerves. A perforating vein communicates with deep veins by passing through the deep fascia.*

Fig. 3.22 *Contents of the cubital fossa. The aponeurosis of biceps and deep fascia have been removed.*

Labels for Fig. 3.20:
- basilic vein
- medial cutaneous nerve of arm
- cephalic vein
- medial cutaneous nerve of forearm
- biceps
- superficial fascia
- median cubital vein
- lateral cutaneous nerve of forearm
- perforating vein

Labels for Fig. 3.21:
- biceps
- basilic vein
- branch of posterior cutaneous nerve of forearm
- tendon & aponeurosis of biceps
- perforating vein
- deep fascia of forearm
- brachio-radialis
- lateral cutaneous nerve of forearm

Labels for Fig. 3.22:
- medial head of triceps
- brachial artery & venae comitantes
- aponeurosis of biceps (cut)
- tendon of biceps
- median nerve
- pronator teres
- radial artery & vena comitans

The fossa is traversed by nerves and vessels passing between the arm and the forearm. Its contents (Figs. 3.22 & 3.24), embedded in fatty connective tissue are, from medial to lateral, the median nerve, the brachial artery and its venae comitantes, the tendon of biceps and the radial nerve. Distally the terminal branches of the radial nerve, the superficial radial and posterior interosseous nerves, and the terminal branches of the brachial artery, namely the radial and ulnar arteries, also lie within the fossa. The floor of the cubital fossa (Fig. 3.24) is formed by supinator and brachialis which overlies the capsule of the elbow joint.

Fig. 3.23 *Boundaries of the cubital fossa after removal of the roof and contents.*

Fig. 3.24 *Brachioradialis and pronator teres have been retracted to reveal the floor of the cubital fossa and expose the radial nerve.*

The anterior compartment of the forearm contains a superficial and a deep group of muscles which include flexors of the wrist, fingers and thumb, and two muscles which act as pronators. The compartment is traversed by the median and ulnar nerves and by the radial and ulnar arteries with their venae comitantes. Investing deep fascia continuous with that on the posterior aspect of the limb encloses the compartment and provides additional attachment for the superficial muscles. In front of the carpus, deep fascia forms the flexor retinaculum (Fig. 3.26) behind which the tendons of the long flexors lie in the carpal tunnel (see page 3.48). Superficial fascia overlying the compartment contains cutaneous nerves and tributaries of the cephalic and basilic veins (Fig. 3.25).

SUPERFICIAL MUSCLES

The superficial muscles are, from lateral to medial, pronator teres, flexor carpi radialis, palmaris longus and flexor carpi ulnaris (Fig. 3.27). Flexor digitorum superficialis is also included in this group but is partly covered by the other muscles.

All the superficial muscles attach proximally to the common flexor origin on the front of the medial epicondyle of the humerus. In addition, pronator teres attaches to the medial side of the coronoid process of the ulna and flexor carpi ulnaris attaches to the medial border of the olecranon and the adjacent part of the subcutaneous border of the ulna. Flexor digitorum superficialis has an additional attachment to the medial collateral ligament of the elbow, the coronoid process and the anterior oblique line of the radius.

Distally pronator teres attaches half-way along the lateral aspect of the shaft of the radius and forms the medial border of the cubital fossa (see page 3.13). The muscle pronates the forearm. Flexor carpi radialis attaches to the bases of the second and third metacarpal bones. It is a flexor and abductor of the wrist joint. Palmaris longus, a vestigial muscle which may be absent, has a long thin tendon which attaches to the palmar aponeurosis. The muscle is a weak flexor of the wrist joint. Flexor carpi ulnaris attaches distally to the pisiform and, via ligaments from the pisiform, to the hook of the hamate and the base of the fifth metacarpal. It is the most medial of the superficial muscles and is a flexor and adductor of the wrist.

Flexor digitorum superficialis (Fig. 3.28) is relatively large and is the deepest of this group of muscles. Distally it gives rise to four tendons, one for each finger, which pass into the hand deep to the flexor retinaculum. In the carpal tunnel the tendons have a characteristic grouping (see Fig. 3.91). Within each finger the tendon forms two slips which pass around the profundus tendon and then partly reunite before attaching to the sides of the middle phalanx (see Fig. 3.36). The muscle flexes the wrist and the metacarpophalangeal and proximal interphalangeal joints of the fingers.

The superficial muscles all pass anterior to the elbow and therefore act as weak flexors of that joint in addition to their roles in the movements of the wrist and hand. Collectively the carpal flexors and extensors stabilize the wrist joint during movements of the fingers and thumb.

All the superficial muscles are innervated by the median nerve except flexor carpi ulnaris, which is supplied by the ulnar nerve.

S
l ⟷ m
I

median
cubital
vein

medial
cutaneous
nerve of
forearm

cephalic
vein

accessory
cephalic
vein

median
vein of
forearm

basilic
vein

Fig. 3.25 *Superficial veins overlying the anterior aspect of the forearm. These vessels are subject to considerable variation.*

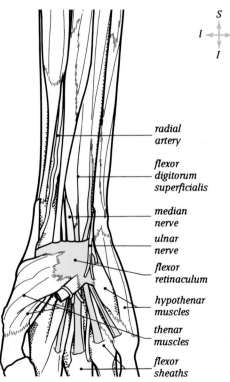

S
l ⟷ m
I

radial
artery

flexor
digitorum
superficialis

median
nerve

ulnar
nerve

flexor
retinaculum

hypothenar
muscles

thenar
muscles

flexor
sheaths

Fig. 3.26 *Flexor retinaculum revealed by removal of superficial and investing layers of fascia. The retinaculum provides attachment for the thenar and hypothenar muscles.*

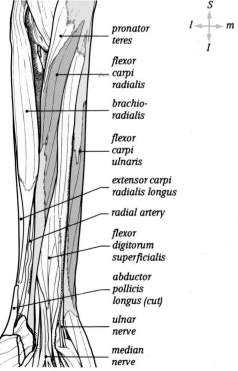

pronator
teres

flexor
carpi
radialis

brachio-
radialis

flexor
carpi
ulnaris

extensor carpi
radialis longus

radial artery

flexor
digitorum
superficialis

abductor
pollicis
longus (cut)

ulnar
nerve

median
nerve

S
l — m
I

Fig. 3.27 *Flexor carpi radialis and flexor carpi ulnaris seen after removal of deep fascia and the flexor retinaculum. This specimen lacks palmaris longus.*

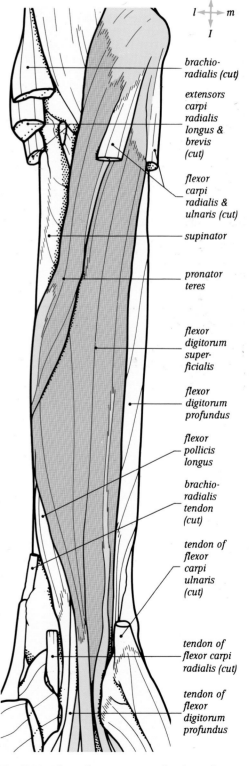

S
l — m
I

brachio-
radialis (cut)

extensors
carpi
radialis
longus &
brevis
(cut)

flexor
carpi
radialis &
ulnaris (cut)

supinator

pronator
teres

flexor
digitorum
super-
ficialis

flexor
digitorum
profundus

flexor
pollicis
longus

brachio-
radialis
tendon
(cut)

tendon of
flexor
carpi
ulnaris
(cut)

tendon of
flexor carpi
radialis (cut)

tendon of
flexor
digitorum
profundus

Fig. 3.28 *Flexor digitorum superficialis and pronator teres revealed by division of flexors carpi ulnaris and radialis, and of brachioradialis.*

DEEP MUSCLES

The deep muscles are flexor pollicis longus, flexor digitorum profundus and pronator quadratus. Their attachments to the radius, ulna and intervening interosseous membrane are illustrated in Fig. 3.29. Distally the flexor pollicis longus tendon (Fig. 3.30) passes through the carpal tunnel and attaches to the base of the distal phalanx of the thumb. The muscle flexes the interphalangeal and metacarpophalangeal joints of the thumb. Flexor digitorum profundus (Fig. 3.30) gives rise to four tendons which traverse the carpal tunnel deep to the tendons of flexor digitorum superficialis (see Fig. 3.34). In the palm the tendons diverge, one entering each finger. Each tendon passes between the slips of the corresponding superficialis tendon, continuing distally to attach to the base of the terminal phalanx. The muscle is a flexor of the fingers and of the wrist joint. Pronator quadratus, a small rectangular muscle lying transversely between the anterior surfaces of the shafts of the radius and ulna (Fig. 3.31), pronates the forearm.

The deep muscles are innervated by the anterior interosseous nerve, except for the medial part of flexor digitorum profundus which is supplied by the ulnar nerve.

VESSELS

In the cubital fossa the brachial artery usually divides into the radial and ulnar arteries (Fig. 3.32). The radial artery passes distally,

under brachioradialis, lying on the flexor muscles. In the lower forearm the vessel is accompanied by the superficial branch of the radial nerve and, near the wrist, is subcutaneous and palpable against the anterior surface of the radius. The artery winds round the lateral aspect of the wrist, traverses the 'anatomical snuff box' and subsequently enters the palm to form the deep palmar arch (see Fig. 3.48). In the forearm the artery gives branches to muscles and contributes to anastomoses around the elbow and wrist joints.

The ulnar artery passes deep to the arch formed by the radial and ulnar attachments of flexor digitorum superficialis and continues between the superficial and deep flexor muscles. In the distal part of the forearm the artery is joined on its medial side by the ulnar nerve. It lies beneath flexor carpi ulnaris but at the wrist emerges to lie lateral to the tendon of this muscle. The ulnar artery crosses superficial to the flexor retinaculum and, as it enters the hand, divides into superficial and deep palmar branches. The ulnar artery gives branches to the muscles of the anterior compartment and to the anastomoses around the elbow and wrist joints. Its largest branch, the common interosseous artery (Fig. 3.32), arises near the origin of the ulnar artery and promptly

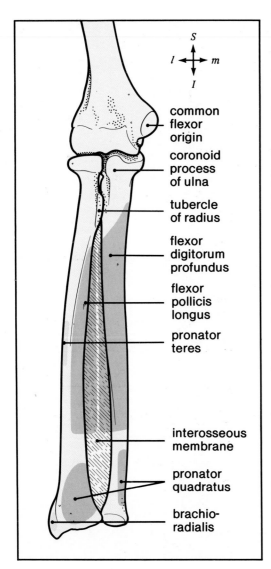

Fig. 3.29 *Attachments of the deep layer of anterior compartment muscles to the radius, ulna and interosseous membrane. The insertions of pronator teres and brachioradialis are also indicated.*

Labels on Fig. 3.29:
- common flexor origin
- coronoid process of ulna
- tubercle of radius
- flexor digitorum profundus
- flexor pollicis longus
- pronator teres
- interosseous membrane
- pronator quadratus
- brachio-radialis

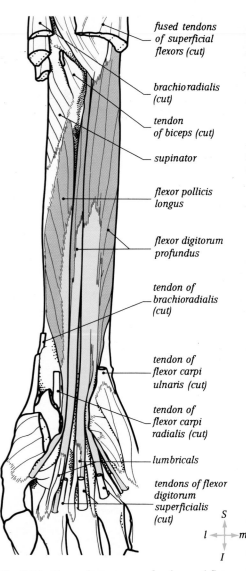

Fig. 3.30 *Flexor digitorum profundus and flexor pollicis longus exposed by removal of the superficial flexors. As in this specimen, the index component of flexor digitorum profundus is often separate from the remainder of the muscle.*

Labels on Fig. 3.30:
- fused tendons of superficial flexors (cut)
- brachioradialis (cut)
- tendon of biceps (cut)
- supinator
- flexor pollicis longus
- flexor digitorum profundus
- tendon of brachioradialis (cut)
- tendon of flexor carpi ulnaris (cut)
- tendon of flexor carpi radialis (cut)
- lumbricals
- tendons of flexor digitorum superficialis (cut)

divides into posterior and anterior interosseous branches. The posterior interosseous artery enters the posterior compartment of the forearm (see Fig. 3.70). The larger anterior interosseous artery passes distally in the anterior compartment, lying on the interosseous membrane, accompanied by the anterior interosseous nerve. The vessel supplies the deep flexor muscles and gives nutrient branches to the radius and ulna. Distally it penetrates the interosseous membrane to assist in the anastomoses around the wrist.

Venae comitantes accompany the arteries of the anterior compartment and drain proximally into veins around the brachial artery.

NERVES

The median nerve enters the forearm from the cubital fossa between the two heads of pronator teres. It crosses anterior to the ulnar artery (Fig. 3.32) and descends between the superficial and deep flexors. At the wrist the median nerve is remarkably superficial, lying medial to the tendon of flexor carpi radialis and just deep to the palmaris longus tendon. The median nerve passes through the carpal tunnel into the hand, where it divides into terminal branches (see Fig. 3.46).

The nerve supplies all the superficial muscles of the anterior compartment except flexor carpi ulnaris. The anterior interosseous branch of the median nerve (Fig. 3.32) supplies all the deep muscles of the compartment except the medial part of flexor digitorum profundus. This branch lies between flexor digitorum profundus and flexor pollicis longus and passes behind pronator quadratus to supply the wrist. In the forearm the median nerve also gives a palmar cutaneous branch which crosses superficial to the flexor retinaculum and supplies skin of the lateral part of the palm.

The ulnar nerve passes behind the medial epicondyle and enters the forearm between the two heads of flexor carpi ulnaris. Lying on flexor digitorum profundus and covered by flexor carpi ulnaris, it traverses the medial side of the anterior compartment, accompanied in the lower part of the forearm by the ulnar artery. Near the wrist the ulnar nerve emerges lateral to the flexor carpi ulnaris tendon and crosses superficial to the flexor retinaculum with the ulnar artery on its lateral side. The nerve terminates in the hand by dividing into superficial and deep branches (see page 3.24). The ulnar nerve supplies the elbow joint and gives branches to flexor carpi ulnaris and the medial part of flexor digitorum profundus. It also provides a palmar cutaneous nerve which supplies skin on the medial aspect of the palm, and dorsal cutaneous branches which innervate the medial part of the dorsum of the hand (see Fig. 3.71).

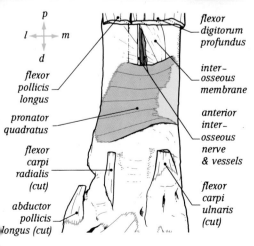

Fig. 3.31 *Pronator quadratus exposed by division of flexor pollicis longus and flexor digitorum profundus.*

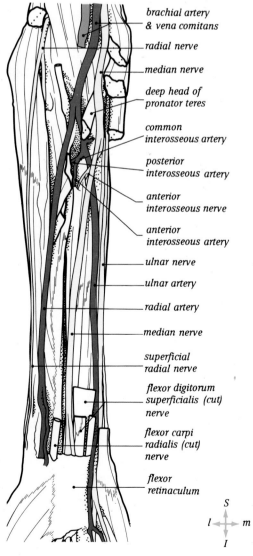

Fig. 3.32 *Vessels and nerves of the anterior compartment of the forearm. The superficial flexor muscles and brachioradialis have been divided, and most of the venae comitantes have been removed.*

PALM AND DIGITS

The palm of the hand contains the palmar aponeurosis, intrinsic muscles, tendons originating from muscles in the anterior compartment of the forearm, and palmar vessels and nerves. The intrinsic muscles comprise the thenar and hypothenar groups, the lumbricals and interossei, and adductor pollicis. The tendons enter the palm through the carpal tunnel (see Fig. 3.91) deep to the flexor retinaculum.

The skin of the anterior surface of the hand is thick, devoid of hair and contains many sweat glands. It is firmly bound to the underlying deep fascia producing characteristic creases.

DEEP FASCIA OF PALM

The deep fascia of the palm is thickened centrally to form the triangular palmar aponeurosis (Fig. 3.33) and is thinner at each side where it covers the thenar and hypothenar muscles. Proximally the palmar aponeurosis attaches to the flexor retinaculum and is continuous with the tendon of palmaris longus. Distally the aponeurosis gives rise to four pairs of digital slips which cross the metacarpophalangeal joints and attach to the proximal phalanges of the fingers via the fibrous flexor sheaths. The aponeurosis covers the superficial palmar arch, the median nerve and the tendons of the long flexors of the digits.

Fig. 3.33 *Palmar aponeurosis exposed by removal of skin and superficial fascia. Investing fascia has been removed proximal to the flexor retinaculum.*

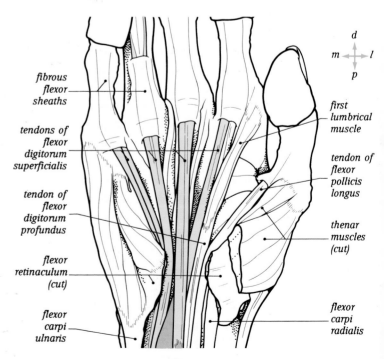

Fig. 3.34 *Tendons of flexor digitorum superficialis in the palm. The palmar aponeurosis, flexor retinaculum and investing fascia, and palmar vessels and nerves have been removed.*

lateral and medial septa pass from the edges of the palmar aponeurosis to the first and fifth metacarpal bones respectively. These septa separate the thenar and hypothenar muscles from a 'central palmar space' which is traversed by the palmar digital vessels and nerves, and by the tendons of the long flexor muscles of the digits.

The superficial fascia of the medial side of the palm usually contains palmaris brevis (Fig. 3.33), a small muscle attaching to the overlying skin and to the palmar aponeurosis.

Fig. 3.35 *Transverse section through the index finger at the level of the proximal phalanx.*

FLEXOR TENDONS IN HAND

The tendons of flexor pollicis longus, flexor digitorum profundus and flexor digitorum superficialis enter the hand deep to the flexor retinaculum (see Fig. 3.92). On reaching the appropriate digit each tendon traverses a tunnel formed by the fibrous flexor sheath and the phalanges (Fig. 3.34). The fibrous sheath is attached to the edges of the anterior surfaces of the phalanges (Fig. 3.35) and continues as far as the distal phalanx (Fig. 3.36). The sheath is thinner and more flexible in front of the interphalangeal joints, allowing flexion of the digit without 'bowstringing' of the tendons and thus facilitating gripping. Within the flexor sheaths the tendons are invested by synovial membrane and receive vincula vasculosa, small folds of synovium which convey blood vessels to the tendons.

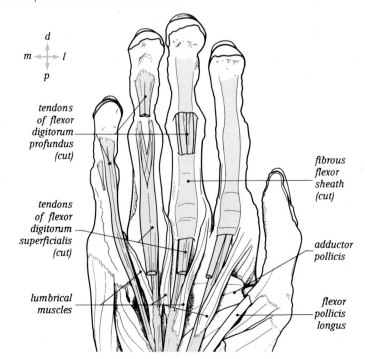

Fig. 3.36 *Digital fibrous flexor sheaths. The partially cut away sheath of the middle finger exposes the tendons of flexor digitorum superficialis and profundus, whose phalangeal attachments are revealed on the ring and little fingers.*

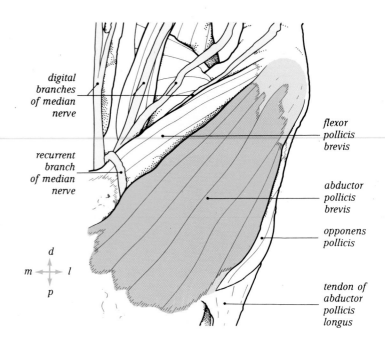

digital
branches
of median
nerve

flexor
pollicis
brevis

recurrent
branch
of median
nerve

abductor
pollicis
brevis

opponens
pollicis

tendon of
abductor
pollicis
longus

Fig. 3.37 *Muscles of the thenar eminence exposed by removal of palmar fascia. Abductor pollicis brevis is superficial to flexor brevis and opponens pollicis.*

THENAR MUSCLES

Abductor pollicis brevis, flexor pollicis brevis and opponens pollicis form the thenar eminence on the lateral side of the palm. They attach proximally to the trapezium and scaphoid and to the lateral part of the flexor retinaculum.

Abductor pollicis brevis (Fig. 3.37) lies superficial to the other thenar muscles and passes from the scaphoid to the base of the proximal phalanx of the thumb. The muscle abducts the thumb, moving the digit anteriorly at right angles to the plane of the palm.

Flexor pollicis brevis, lying deep and medial to the abductor, passes from the trapezium to the proximal phalanx of the thumb. The muscle flexes the carpometacarpal and metacarpophalangeal joints, drawing the thumb across the palm (maintaining the thumbnail at right angles to the palmar plane).

Opponens pollicis (Fig. 3.38), the deepest of the thenar muscles, attaches proximally to the trapezium and distally to the shaft of the first metacarpal. The muscle produces opposition of the thumb, allowing pulp-to-pulp contact with the fingers. This movement combines flexion, adduction and rotation of the first metacarpal at its carpometacarpal joint.

The thenar muscles are supplied by the recurrent branch of the median nerve (Figs. 3.37 & 3.38).

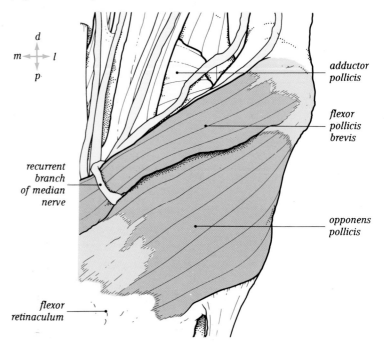

adductor
pollicis

flexor
pollicis
brevis

recurrent
branch
of median
nerve

opponens
pollicis

flexor
retinaculum

Fig. 3.38 *Opponens pollicis and flexor pollicis brevis exposed by removal of abductor pollicis brevis.*

HYPOTHENAR MUSCLES

Abductor, flexor and opponens digiti minimi (Fig. 3.39) form the hypothenar eminence and attach proximally to the pisiform, the hook of the hamate and the adjacent part of the flexor retinaculum. Abductor digiti minimi passes from the pisiform to the base of the proximal phalanx of the little finger and abducts the digit, moving it medially in the plane of the palm. Flexor digiti minimi attaches between the hamate and base of the proximal phalanx of the little finger and flexes the metacarpal and proximal phalanx of the little finger. Opponens digiti minimi passes from the hamate to the shaft of the fifth metacarpal and on contraction deepens the hollow of the palm.

The hypothenar muscles are supplied by the deep branch of the ulnar nerve (Fig. 3.39).

digital branches of ulnar nerve

tendons of flexor digitorum superficialis

abductor digiti minimi

opponens digiti minimi

flexor retinaculum

flexor digiti minimi

deep branch of ulnar nerve

Fig. 3.39 *Hypothenar muscles exposed by removal of the palmar fascia and aponeurosis.*

DEEP MUSCLES

The deep muscles of the hand consist of adductor pollicis, the palmar and dorsal interossei, and the lumbricals.

Adductor pollicis (Fig. 3.40) has transverse and oblique heads. The transverse head attaches to the shaft of the third metacarpal bone, and the oblique head to the trapezoid, capitate and bases of the second and third metacarpals. Both heads pass laterally to attach to the base of the proximal phalanx of the thumb by a common tendon which usually contains a sesamoid bone. The muscle adducts and flexes the thumb at its carpometacarpal and metacarpophalangeal joints and is supplied by the deep branch of the ulnar nerve (see Fig. 3.48).

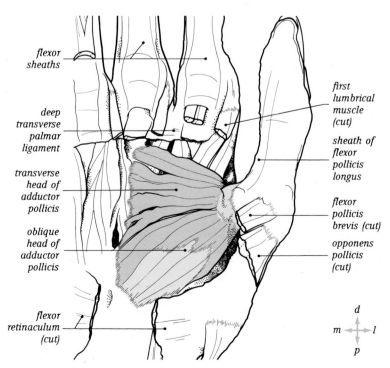

flexor sheaths

deep transverse palmar ligament

transverse head of adductor pollicis

oblique head of adductor pollicis

flexor retinaculum (cut)

first lumbrical muscle (cut)

sheath of flexor pollicis longus

flexor pollicis brevis (cut)

opponens pollicis (cut)

Fig. 3.40 *Adductor pollicis. The muscles of the thenar eminence, long flexor tendons, and palmar and digital vessels and nerves have been removed.*

PALM AND DIGITS

The interossei consist of three palmar and four dorsal muscles (Fig. 3.41). Each palmar interosseous muscle (Fig. 3.42) arises by a single head from the anterior border of the shaft of the second, fourth or fifth metacarpal. Each dorsal interosseous muscle (Fig. 3.43) arises by two heads from the contiguous sides of the shafts of the adjacent metacarpals. Distally the tendon of each interosseous muscle attaches to the base of the proximal phalanx and to the extensor expansion of the appropriate digit (see Fig. 3.45).

The interossei move the fingers in the plane of the palm (coronal plane); movement of a finger away from the long axis of the middle finger is called abduction while movement towards the middle finger is adduction. The palmar interossei adduct and the dorsal interossei abduct the fingers. In addition, the interossei flex the metacarpophalangeal joints and extend the

Fig. 3.41 *Palmar and dorsal interossei exposed by removal of the long flexor tendons and adductor pollicis. The dorsal interossei have much more bulk than the palmar interossei.*

Fig. 3.42 *Palmar interossei. The dorsal interossei and deep transverse palmar ligaments have been excised.*

interphalangeal joints. All the interossei are supplied by the deep branch of the ulnar nerve (see Fig. 3.48).

The lumbricals are four small muscles attaching proximally to the tendons of flexor digitorum profundus (Fig. 3.44). Distally each lumbrical attaches to the radial side of the extensor expansion of the appropriate finger. The muscles extend the interphalangeal joints and flex the metacarpophalangeal joints. The first and second lumbricals usually have only one head each and are supplied by the median nerve whereas the third and fourth (medial) usually have two heads and are supplied by the ulnar nerve.

Fig. 3.43 *Dorsal interossei exposed by removal of deep fascia and tendons of extensor digitorum.*

Fig. 3.44 *Removal of the tendons of flexor digitorum superficialis has revealed the attachments of the lumbrical muscles to the tendons of flexor digitorum profundus.*

DIGITAL EXTENSOR EXPANSIONS

Each finger possesses an extensor expansion or hood (Fig. 3.45) which receives the tendons of the appropriate long extensor muscle(s), interossei and lumbricals. The broad proximal part of the expansion overlies the metacarpophalangeal joint. Distally the expansion tapers and attaches by a central slip to the base of the middle phalanx and by two marginal slips to the base of the distal phalanx.

BLOOD VESSELS

The arterial supply to the hand is derived from branches of the ulnar and radial arteries, which form superficial and deep palmar arches linking the two main arteries and ensuring a rich blood supply to the palm and fingers.

The ulnar artery enters the hand superficial to the flexor retinaculum and gives a deep branch accompanying the deep branch of the ulnar nerve. The main artery continues as the superficial palmar arch (Fig. 3.46) which passes distally to the level of the thumb web, lying deep to the palmar aponeurosis but anterior to the digital nerves and flexor tendons. Laterally the superficial palmar arch is completed by a branch of the radial artery and gives four palmar digital branches which supply the adjacent sides of the fingers (Fig. 3.47) and medial side of the little finger.

The radial artery enters the palm from the dorsum of the hand between the two heads of the first dorsal interosseous muscle (see Fig. 3.43). The artery gives branches to the thumb and index finger and continues as the deep palmar arch (Fig. 3.48), which lies over the bases of the metacarpal bones, deep to the flexor tendons about 1cm proximal to the superficial arch. The deep arch, completed medially by the deep branch of the ulnar artery, provides perforating branches, which anastomose with dorsal metacarpal arteries, and three palmar metacarpal arteries, which anastomose with the palmar digital arteries of the superficial arch. Other vessels such as dorsal metacarpal arteries from the dorsal carpal arch may provide an important supply of blood to the hand.

Most venous blood from the fingers and palm drains into superficial veins on the dorsum of the hand to enter the cephalic or basilic veins.

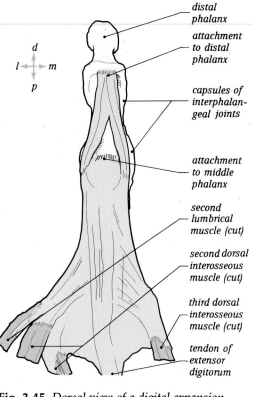

Fig. 3.45 *Dorsal view of a digital expansion which has been flattened proximally to show the attachments of lumbrical and interosseous muscles.*

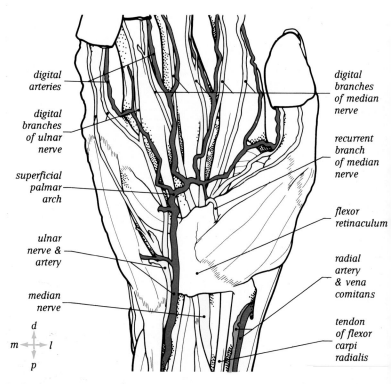

Fig. 3.46 *Superficial vessels and nerves of the palm. Skin, superficial fascia and the palmar aponeurosis have been removed.*

NERVES

Innervation of the anterior aspect of the hand is shared by the ulnar and median nerves. The ulnar nerve supplies more intrinsic muscles than the median nerve, which supplies a larger area of skin.

The ulnar nerve (Fig. 3.46) enters the palm superficial to the flexor retinaculum and terminates as digital and deep branches. The digital branches supply the skin of the medial one-and-one-half digits. A corresponding area of the palm is supplied by palmar branches which arise from the ulnar nerve in the forearm. The deep branch of the ulnar nerve (Fig. 3.48) accompanies the deep palmar arch and supplies the three hypothenar muscles, the medial two lumbricals, all the interossei and adductor pollicis. The ulnar nerve also supplies palmaris brevis.

The median nerve traverses the carpal tunnel and terminates as digital and recurrent branches. The digital branches (Fig. 3.46) supply skin overlying the lateral three-and-one-half digits and usually the lateral two lumbricals. A corresponding area of the palm is supplied by palmar branches arising from the median nerve in the forearm. The recurrent branch of the median nerve (see Fig. 3.37) supplies the three thenar muscles.

In the palm the digital branches of the ulnar and median nerves lie deep to the superficial palmar arch (Fig. 3.46), but in the fingers they lie anterior to the digital arteries arising from the superficial arch (Fig. 3.47). Although there may be overlapping and variability of innervation of the ring and middle fingers, the skin on the anterior surface of the thumb is always supplied by the median nerve and that of the little finger by the ulnar nerve. The palmar digital branches of the median and ulnar nerves also supply the nail beds of their respective digits.

Fig. 3.47 *Palmar digital vessels and nerves of the fingers.*

Labels: connective tissue of pulp space; digital arteries; digital branches of median nerve; fibrous flexor sheath; lumbrical muscle; tendon of flexor digitorum superficialis; superficial palmar arch

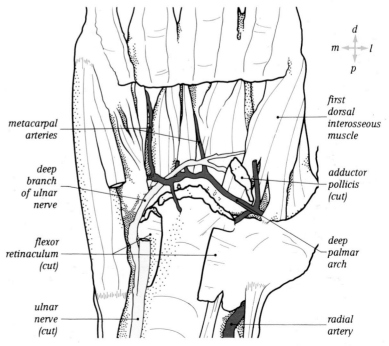

Labels: metacarpal arteries; deep branch of ulnar nerve; flexor retinaculum (cut); ulnar nerve (cut); first dorsal interosseous muscle; adductor pollicis (cut); deep palmar arch; radial artery

Fig. 3.48 *Deep palmar arch and deep branch of ulnar nerve. The long flexor tendons and muscles of the thenar eminence have been removed, and adductor pollicis and the hypothenar muscles divided.*

3.25

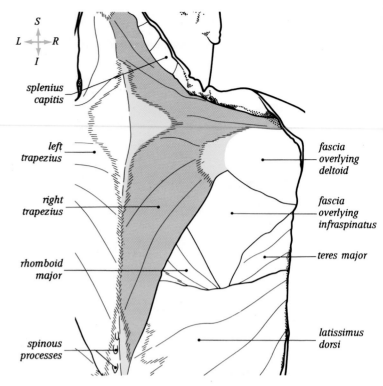

Fig. 3.49 *The trapezius muscles have fascial attachments to the cervical and upper thoracic spinous processes and, in this dissection, are asymmetric inferiorly.*

Three muscles connect the root of the upper limb to the anterior chest wall and are usually dissected with the thorax. For this reason, pectoralis major and minor and serratus anterior are described with the thoracic wall (see page 2.5. Only the posterior group of muscles attaching the limb and its girdle to the vertebral column are described here, namely trapezius, latissimus dorsi, levator scapulae and the rhomboids.

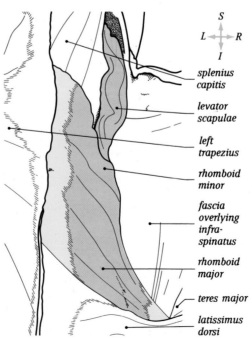

Fig. 3.50 *Levator scapulae and rhomboids exposed by removal of trapezius. Latissimus dorsi partly obscures the inferior angle of the scapula.*

TRAPEZIUS

Trapezius (Fig. 3.49) is a large superficial muscle overlying the dorsum of the neck and thorax. Its upper fibres attach to the ligamentum nuchae, the external occipital protuberance and the superior nuchal line and pass downwards and laterally to the acromion of the scapula and the lateral part of the clavicle. These fibres produce elevation of the scapula as in shrugging the shoulder. When the scapula is fixed they produce lateral flexion of the neck. The middle fibres of trapezius run horizontally from the ligamentum nuchae and upper thoracic spinous processes to the acromion and spine of the scapula and retract the scapula. Fibres of the lower part of the muscle attach to the lower thoracic spinous processes superficial to latissimus dorsi (Figs. 3.49 & 3.52) and pass upwards and laterally to the spine of the scapula. These fibres depress the scapula. Acting together the upper and lower parts of trapezius produce rotation of the scapula, turning the glenoid fossa superiorly to permit full abduction of the limb (see page 3.40). In the neck the anterior edge of the muscle forms one of the boundaries of the posterior triangle. The accessory nerve crosses the triangle (see Fig. 7.6) and enters the deep surface of trapezius, providing motor fibres. Proprioceptive fibres are derived from the cervical plexus.

Fig. 3.51 *Latissimus dorsi. The anterior border lies parallel to the cut skin edge and the thoracic attachment has been exposed by removal of trapezius.*

LEVATOR SCAPULAE AND RHOMBOIDS

These three muscles are covered by trapezius. Levator scapulae (Fig. 3.50) ascends from the medial border of the scapula above the root of the spine to the transverse processes of the upper four cervical vertebrae. The fibres of the rhomboids incline upwards and medially (Fig. 3.50). Rhomboid minor attaches to the medial border of the scapula at the root of its spine and to the spinous processes of the seventh cervical and first thoracic vertebrae. Rhomboid major passes between the remainder of the medial border of the scapula and the spines of the second to fifth thoracic vertebrae.

All three muscles elevate the scapula and assist in scapular rotation during adduction of the upper limb. The dorsal scapular nerve (C5) (see brachial plexus, page 3.8) supplies the rhomboids and may innervate levator scapulae which is also supplied by branches from the cervical plexus (C3 & C4).

LATISSIMUS DORSI

Latissimus dorsi (Fig. 3.51) is a large triangular muscle overlying much of the dorsal aspect of the trunk. The muscle attaches to the spinous processes of the lower six thoracic vertebrae and through the lumbar fascia to the spines of the lumbar vertebrae and the sacrum. The most inferior fibres attach to the posterior part of the iliac crest. Fibres also attach to the lower four ribs and to the inferior angle of the scapula. All the fibres converge on a narrow tendon in the posterior fold of the axilla. The tendon winds round the lower border of teres major to attach to the intertubercular sulcus of the humerus.

The muscle is a powerful adductor and extensor of the humerus at the shoulder joint, particularly when the upper limb is abducted and flexed. Latissimus dorsi is also a medial rotator at the shoulder joint and assists with rotation and retraction of the scapula. In movements such as rising from an armchair, if the humerus is fixed, both muscles contract to raise the trunk. This action is particularly important in patients with paralysed lower limbs. The latissimus dorsi is supplied by a single neurovascular bundle which contains the thoracodorsal nerve (a branch of the posterior cord of the brachial plexus; see Fig. 3.15) and the thoracodorsal vessels, which are branches of the subscapular vessels. In reconstructive surgery, the muscle and its overlying skin may be mobilized on this neurovascular pedicle to provide a large myocutaneous flap.

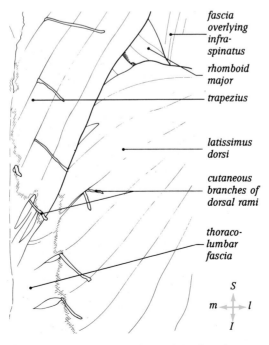

Fig. 3.52 *Cutaneous branches of the dorsal rami of the spinal nerves penetrate both trapezius and latissimus dorsi. These branches supply skin on the dorsum of the trunk.*

SHORT SCAPULAR MUSCLES

These five short muscles span the shoulder (glenohumeral) joint, attaching to the scapula and to the proximal part of the humerus.

ROTATOR CUFF MUSCLES

This important group of four muscles, namely subscapularis, supraspinatus, infraspinatus and teres minor, is intimately related to the shoulder joint. By attaching not only to the tubercles of the humerus but also to the capsule of the joint, they hold the humeral head firmly in the glenoid fossa and help stabilize the joint.

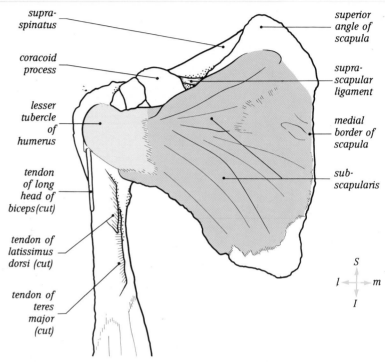

Fig. 3.53 *Anterior view of subscapularis. The attachment of serratus anterior to the medial border of the scapula has been excised.*

Subscapularis

Subscapularis (Fig. 3.53) attaches proximally to the medial part of the costal surface of the scapula. Its tendon, separated from the neck of the scapula by the subscapular bursa, is attached to the lesser tubercle of the humerus. The muscle is supplied by the subscapular nerves from the posterior cord of the brachial plexus. Subscapularis produces medial rotation of the arm at the shoulder joint.

Supraspinatus

Supraspinatus (Fig. 3.54) attaches to the supraspinous fossa of the scapula and to the superior facet of the greater tubercle of the humerus. The subacromial bursa lies above the tendon of supraspinatus, separating the tendon and the capsule of the shoulder joint from the coracoacromial arch. The muscle initiates abduction of the shoulder joint, and damage to its tendon produces pain during the early stages of this movement.

Fig. 3.54 *Superior view of supraspinatus after removal of the acromion of the scapula.*

Infraspinatus

Infraspinatus (Fig. 3.55) arises from the infraspinous fossa and its tendon inserts into the middle facet of the greater tubercle of the humerus. The muscle is covered by a strong fascial membrane. A bursa sometimes separates the tendon from the neck of the scapula.

Supraspinatus and infraspinatus are supplied by the suprascapular nerve which arises from the upper trunk of the brachial plexus and passes beneath the suprascapular ligament (Fig. 3.53).

Teres minor

Teres minor (Figs. 3.55 & 3.56) attaches to the posterior surface of the scapula along the upper part of the lateral edge and to the inferior facet of the greater tubercle of the humerus. It is supplied by the axillary nerve.

Both infraspinatus and teres minor laterally rotate the humerus at the shoulder joint.

TERES MAJOR

Teres major (Fig. 3.56) is a short bulky muscle which attaches to the lower part of the posterior surface of the scapula. Distally the muscle attaches below the lesser tubercle of the humerus to the medial lip of the intertubercular sulcus (Fig. 3.53). Teres major is supplied by the lower subscapular nerve and adducts and medially rotates the humerus at the shoulder joint.

The interval between teres minor and teres major (Fig. 3.56) is divided by the long head of triceps into a laterally located quadrilateral space and a medial triangular space. The axillary nerve and posterior circumflex humeral vessels pass through the quadrilateral space (see Fig. 3.59). The triangular space transmits the circumflex scapular vessels.

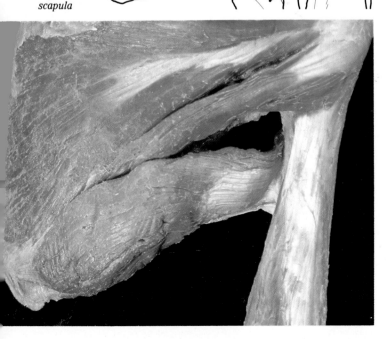

Fig. 3.55 *Posterior view of infraspinatus and teres minor. Teres major has been removed.*

Labels: supra-spinatus; tendons fused with capsule of shoulder joint; teres minor; surgical neck of humerus; lateral head of triceps; long head of triceps; spine of scapula (cut); infra-spinatus; medial border of scapula; sub-scapularis; attachment of teres major; inferior angle of scapula

Fig. 3.56 *Posterior view of teres major and teres minor. The long head of triceps has been excised.*

Labels: infra-spinatus; teres major; teres minor; inter-muscular space; lateral head of triceps

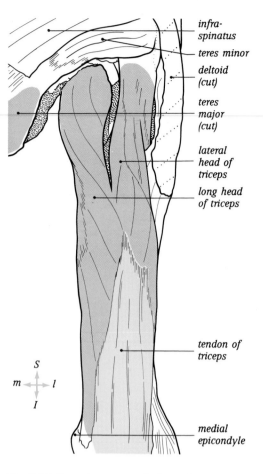

The posterior compartment of the arm contains triceps brachii, the radial nerve accompanied by the profunda brachii artery with its venae comitantes, and the ulnar nerve.

TRICEPS BRACHII

Proximally this muscle attaches to the scapula and the humerus by three heads. The tendon of the long head (Fig. 3.57) attaches to the infraglenoid tubercle of the scapula, and the lateral head attaches to the posterior aspect of the shaft of the humerus above the spiral groove. Both the long and lateral heads lie superficial to the medial head (Fig. 3.58) which has an extensive origin from the lateral and medial intermuscular septa and from the shaft of the humerus below the spiral groove. Distally the three heads fuse and triceps attaches by a single tendon to the olecranon process of the ulna. Frequently, a bursa lies deep to the tendon, separating it from the capsule of the elbow joint. The three heads are supplied separately by branches of the radial nerve. Triceps is a powerful extensor of the elbow joint. The long head alone spans the shoulder joint and may assist in stabilizing that joint, particularly in full abduction.

Fig. 3.57 *Posterior aspect of triceps. Teres major and the posterior fibres of deltoid have been excised.*

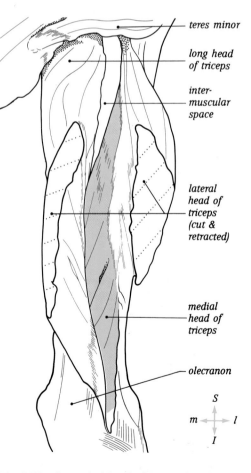

VESSELS AND NERVES
Radial nerve

The radial nerve, a terminal branch of the posterior cord, leaves the axilla by passing through the triangular space below teres major and between the humerus and the long head of triceps (Fig. 3.59). In the posterior compartment the nerve passes between the medial and lateral heads of triceps and in the spiral groove is intimately related to the shaft of the humerus (Fig. 3.60). It then leaves the posterior compartment by piercing the lateral intermuscular septum to reach the lateral part of the cubital fossa in front of the elbow joint (see Fig. 3.24). In the arm the radial nerve gives muscular branches to the medial and lateral heads of triceps and to brachioradialis and extensor carpi radialis longus, and cutaneous branches to the lateral aspect of the arm and the posterior aspect of the forearm. The branch to the long head of triceps usually arises in the axilla.

Profunda brachii artery

The profunda brachii artery, a proximal branch of the brachial artery (see Fig. 3.13), supplies the posterior compartment and accompanies the radial nerve in the spiral groove of the humerus (Fig. 3.60). It gives muscular branches and contributes to the anastomosis around the elbow joint. The venae comitantes of the profunda brachii artery drain into the axillary vein.

Ulnar nerve

The ulnar nerve passes from the anterior to the posterior compartment by piercing the medial intermuscular septum at about midarm level (see Fig. 3.19), and descends between the septum and the medial head of triceps. At the elbow it passes posterior to the medial epicondyle of the humerus, medial to the joint, and enters the forearm between the humeral and ulnar heads of flexor carpi ulnaris. The nerve gives no branches in the arm.

Fig. 3.58 *The medial head of triceps has been exposed by removal of deltoid, and division and retraction of the lateral head.*

Fig. 3.59 *The interval between the long head of triceps and the humerus, divided by teres major into quadrilateral and triangular spaces.*

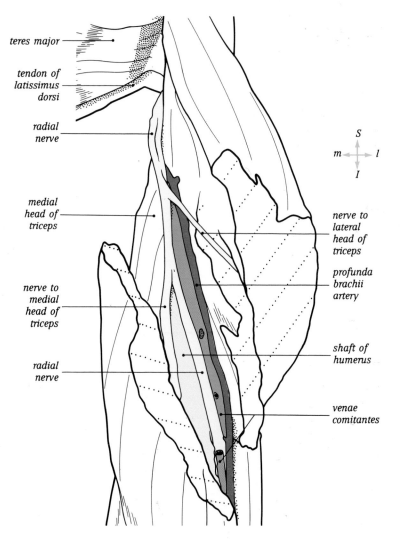

Fig. 3.60 *The radial nerve and profunda brachii artery in the spiral groove, seen after retraction of the cut lateral head. The long head has been excised.*

POSTERIOR COMPARTMENT OF FOREARM

The posterior compartment of the forearm lies behind the radius and ulna and the intervening interosseous membrane. It contains the extensor muscles of the wrist and fingers, the extensors and long abductor of the thumb, and also brachio-radialis, supinator and anconeus. The muscles are supplied by the posterior interosseous artery and nerve (deep branch of the radial nerve), assisted by the radial nerve itself. The compartment is enclosed by a layer of deep fascia which attaches to the subcutaneous border of the ulna. In the region of the wrist the fascia is thickened to form the extensor retinaculum (Fig. 3.61). The extensor tendons, invested by synovial sheaths, pass deep to the retinaculum in compartments formed by fibrous septa (see Fig. 3.92) and enter the hand.

extensor
digitorum

extensor
carpi
ulnaris

abductor
pollicis
longus

extensor
retinaculum

extensor
pollicis
longus

extensor
digitorum

extensor
indicis

Fig. 3.61 *Extensor retinaculum exposed by removal of superficial and investing layers of fascia. The fibres of the retinaculum run obliquely, passing medially and inferiorly from the radius towards the hamate and pisiform bones.*

3.32

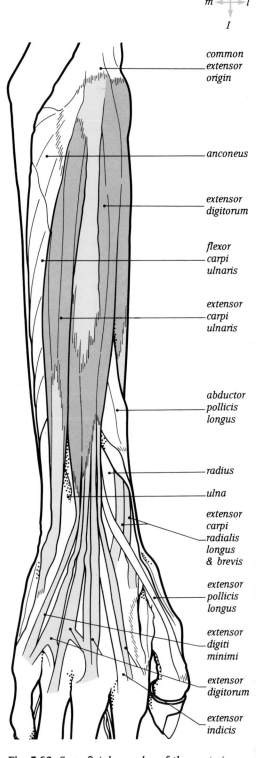

common
extensor
origin

anconeus

extensor
digitorum

flexor
carpi
ulnaris

extensor
carpi
ulnaris

abductor
pollicis
longus

radius

ulna

extensor
carpi
radialis
longus
& brevis

extensor
pollicis
longus

extensor
digiti
minimi

extensor
digitorum

extensor
indicis

Fig. 3.62 *Superficial muscles of the posterior compartment exposed by removal of investing fascia and the extensor retinaculum. Flexor and extensor carpi ulnaris lie edge-to-edge along the subcutaneous border of the ulna.*

SUPERFICIAL MUSCLES

Four superficial extensors attach proximally to the anterior surface of the lateral humeral epicondyle at the common extensor origin. Extensor carpi radialis brevis (Fig. 3.63) passes distally to the base of the third metacarpal and is an extensor and abductor of the wrist. Extensor digitorum (Figs. 3.61 & 3.62) has four tendons which pass to the fingers and form the dorsal expansions or extensor hoods (see Fig. 3.45). On the dorsum of the hand these tendons are interconnected by fibrous bands. The muscle is an extensor of the fingers and the wrist joint. Extensor digiti minimi (Fig. 3.62) attaches via two tendons to the dorsal expansion of the little finger and assists in extension of this finger. Extensor carpi ulnaris

(Fig. 3.62) attaches proximally to both the common extensor origin and the posterior surface of the ulna. Distally it attaches to the base of the fifth metacarpal bone. The muscle is an extensor and adductor of the wrist. These four superficial extensors span the elbow but, since their attachments are close to the axis of movement, do not act effectively on that joint. They are innervated by the posterior interosseous (deep branch of the radial) nerve.

Two other superficial muscles, brachioradialis and extensor carpi radialis longus, arise from the lateral supracondylar ridge of the humerus and are innervated directly from the main trunk of the

radial nerve. Brachioradialis (Figs. 3.63 & 3.64) arises from the upper two-thirds of the ridge and attaches distally to the radial styloid process. The muscle is a flexor of the elbow joint and rotates the forearm from full pronation or supination into an intermediate position. Extensor carpi radialis longus (Figs. 3.62 & 3.63) arises from the lower third of the supracondylar ridge and attaches distally to the base of the second metacarpal bone. The muscle is an extensor and abductor of the wrist joint. In addition to their primary roles, the three carpal extensors provide an essential contribution to the power grip by fixing the wrist in an optimum position while the long flexors act on the fingers.

brachialis

triceps

brachio-
radialis

extensor
carpi
radialis
longus

extensor
carpi
radialis
brevis

shaft
of ulna

tendon of
abductor
pollicis
longus
(cut)

radial
artery

brachialis

radial
nerve

biceps
tendon
(cut)

brachio-
radialis

flexor
carpi
radialis

extensor
carpi
radialis
longus
tendon

radial
artery

abductor
pollicis
longus
tendon (cut)

thenar
muscles

hypo-
thenar
muscles

Fig. 3.63 *Extensors carpi radialis longus and brevis, and brachioradialis after removal of abductor pollicis longus and extensors pollicis longus and brevis.*

Fig. 3.64 *Brachioradialis (anterior aspect). The muscle forms the lateral boundary of the cubital fossa and covers the radial artery and the superficial branch of the radial nerve in the forearm.*

DEEP MUSCLES

The proximal attachments of four of the deep muscles are illustrated in Fig. 3.65. The tendon of extensor indicis (Fig. 3.66) passes distally medial to that of extensor digitorum and attaches to the extensor expansion of the index finger. The extensor pollicis longus tendon passes distally around the ulnar (medial) side of the dorsal tubercle of the radius (Fig. 3.66), then across the radial extensors of the carpus to attach to the base of the distal phalanx of the thumb (Fig. 3.67). The muscle extends the thumb and its

carpometacarpal joint. The tendons of extensor pollicis brevis and abductor pollicis longus (Fig. 3.67) lie together as they cross the radial carpal extensors and brachioradialis. Extensor pollicis brevis attaches to the base of the proximal phalanx of the thumb, which it extends. Abductor pollicis longus attaches to the base of the first metacarpal bone, which it extends and abducts.

Although these four deep muscles act primarily on the joints of the hand, they also span the wrist joint;

but their actions here are weak. They are all innervated by the posterior interosseous (deep branch of the radial) nerve.

Extension of the thumb creates a hollow on the posterolateral aspect of the wrist called the 'anatomical snuff box' (Fig. 3.68). It is limited anteriorly by the tendons of abductor pollicis longus and extensor pollicis brevis and posteriorly by extensor pollicis longus. Superficial to the snuff box lie the origin of the cephalic vein and branches of the radial nerve supplying the dorsum of the hand. The tendons of the two radial carpal extensors and the radial artery pass through the snuff box. The bony floor comprises the radial styloid process, scaphoid, trapezium and base of the first metacarpal bone. Fracture of the scaphoid bone often produces pain, swelling and tenderness in the snuff box.

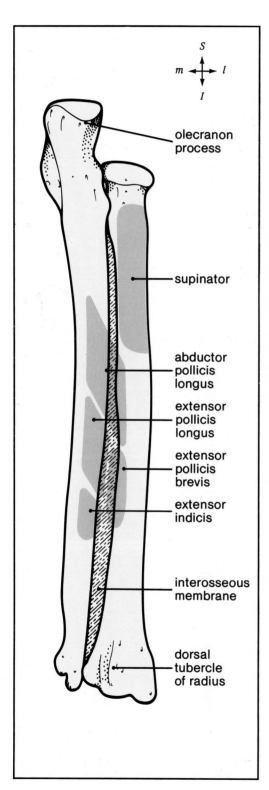

Fig. 3.65 *Attachments of the deep layer of posterior compartment muscles to the radius, ulna and interosseous membrane.*

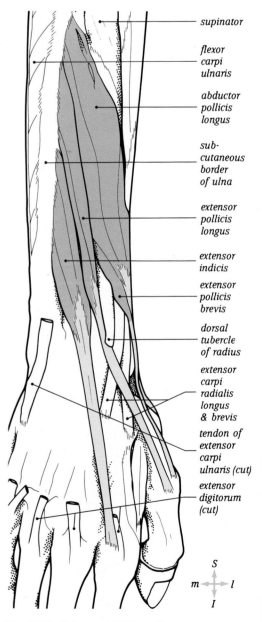

Fig. 3.66 *Extensor indicis and extensors pollicis longus and brevis, after division of extensor digitorum. The tendon of extensor indicis lies on the ulnar (medial) side of the index tendon of extensor digitorum.*

supinator

brachio-
radialis

extensor
carpi
radialis
brevis

sub-
cutaneous
border
of ulna

abductor
pollicis
longus
& tendon

extensor
pollicis
brevis
& tendon

extensor
indicis

extensor
carpi
radialis
longus

radial
artery

extensor
pollicis
longus

S
P ← → A
I

Fig. 3.67 *Abductor pollicis longus and
extensors pollicis longus and brevis. At the wrist
the radial carpal extensors are crossed by the
tendons of these three muscles passing to the
thumb.*

extensor
digitorum

abductor
pollicis
longus

brachio-
radialis

extensor
pollicis
brevis

extensor
carpi
radialis
brevis

extensor
carpi
radialis
longus

radial
artery

extensor
pollicis
longus

S
P ← → A
I

Fig. 3.68 *Boundaries and contents of the
'anatomical snuff box' (coloured magenta) exposed
by removal of its fascial roof.*

3.35

Supinator, also a deep muscle, consists of oblique and transverse heads (Fig. 3.69). The oblique head attaches to the lateral epicondyle and collateral ligament, while the transverse head is attached to the supinator crest of the ulna. Both heads wind laterally around the proximal part of the radius and attach to its anterior surface. The muscle supinates the forearm and is supplied by the posterior interosseous nerve, which passes between the two heads of the muscle (Fig. 3.70).

VESSELS

In the cubital fossa the common interosseous branch of the ulnar artery divides into larger anterior and smaller posterior interosseous arteries, which pass distally into their respective compartments of the forearm. The posterior interosseous artery (Fig. 3.70) lies between and supplies the superficial and deep groups of muscles. Near the wrist a branch of the anterior interosseous artery penetrates the interosseous membrane to assist in the supply of the distal part of the posterior compartment. In addition, muscles on the lateral aspect of the compartment may receive blood from branches of the radial artery. The arteries of the compartment are accompanied by venae comitantes which drain into veins accompanying the brachial artery.

On the dorsum of the wrist the radial artery enters the anatomical snuff box from the anterior compartment of the forearm deep to the tendons of abductor pollicis longus and extensor pollicis brevis (see Fig. 3.68). The artery crosses the floor of the snuff box and leaves the dorsum of the hand by penetrating the first dorsal interosseous muscle to enter the palm.

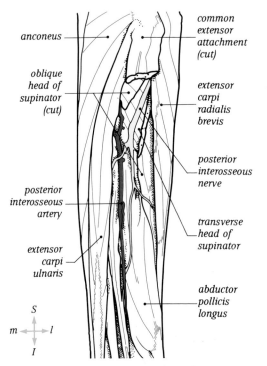

Fig. 3.69 *Supinator, revealed by removal of the other muscles of the posterior compartment. The posterior interosseous nerve passes between the transverse and oblique heads of the muscle.*

Fig. 3.70 *Posterior interosseous artery and nerve, exposed by division of extensor digitorum. The specimen is partly pronated so the radial border of the forearm faces anteriorly.*

NERVES

The posterior compartment of the forearm is supplied by the radial nerve, which leaves the arm by penetrating the lateral intermuscular septum. Anterior to the elbow the nerve lies between brachialis and brachioradialis and divides into superficial and deep branches (Fig. 3.69). The superficial branch continues distally through the forearm covered by brachioradialis, leaving the posterior border near the wrist and crossing the snuff box to terminate as cutaneous branches on the dorsum of the hand (Fig. 3.71). The deep branch, the posterior interosseous nerve, arises from the radial nerve at the level of the neck of the radius and enters the posterior compartment by passing between the two heads of supinator (Fig. 3.70). Initially it accompanies the posterior interosseous artery but distally lies more deeply on the interosseous membrane. The posterior interosseous nerve gives branches to the elbow, radioulnar and wrist joints, and supplies all the posterior compartment muscles except brachioradialis and extensor carpi radialis longus, which are supplied directly by the radial nerve from branches arising in the arm, and anconeus, which is supplied by the branch of the radial nerve to the medial head of triceps.

DORSUM OF HAND

The dorsum of the hand is innervated by branches of the radial and ulnar nerves (Fig. 3.71). The superficial branch of the radial nerve usually supplies the skin of the lateral three and one-half digits (excluding the nail beds) and a corresponding part of the dorsum of the hand. The skin over the remainder of the posterior aspect of the hand and the medial one and one-half fingers (excluding the nail beds) is supplied by dorsal branches of the ulnar nerve which arise in the anterior compartment and pass around the medial aspect of the wrist.

Much of the venous blood from the digits and the palm drains into a network of vessels which often form a superficial venous arch on the dorsum of the hand.

At the wrist the tendons of extensor digitorum lie deep to the extensor retinaculum (Fig. 3.72) invested by a single synovial sheath. On the dorsum of the hand the tendons diverge to reach the fingers.

Skin on the dorsum of the hand is elastic and freely mobile on the underlying loose connective tissue. Infection or injury of the hand frequently results in swelling of these lax dorsal tissues.

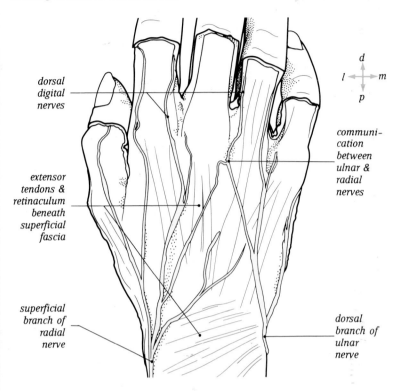

Fig. 3.71 *Cutaneous branches of the radial and ulnar nerves on the dorsum of the hand after removal of the superficial veins.*

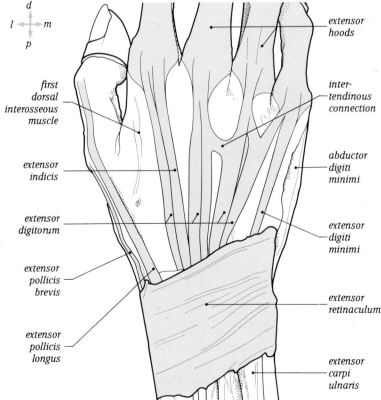

Fig. 3.72 *Extensor retinaculum and extensor tendons exposed by removal of superficial fascia. The tendons pass through fibro-osseous tunnels deep to the retinaculum and are enveloped by synovial sheaths (here removed) which continue beyond the edges of the retinaculum.*

3.37

CLAVICULAR AND SHOULDER JOINTS

Three joints contribute to the considerable mobility of the arm; movement occurs between the humerus and the scapula at the shoulder (glenohumeral) joint, and the scapula moves on the chest wall through the joints at each end of the clavicle. Although few muscles attach to the clavicle, the numerous muscles attached to the scapula and upper humerus all contribute to movement at the clavicular joints. Indeed, movement at the shoulder joint is almost always associated with movement at the sternoclavicular and acromioclavicular joints.

CLAVICULAR JOINTS

The sternoclavicular and acromioclavicular joints are subcutaneous and easily palpable in the living subject. Each has a tubular capsule lined by synovial membrane.

At the sternoclavicular joint (Fig. 3.73), the medial end of the clavicle articulates with the notch on the upper border of the manubrium and with the first costal cartilage. The joint is partitioned by an intracapsular disc of fibrocartilage which attaches superiorly to the clavicle, inferiorly to the first costal cartilage and around its periphery to the capsule. There are two accessory ligaments. Above the capsule is the interclavicular ligament which joins the medial ends of the clavicles. Just lateral to the joint is the costoclavicular (rhomboid) ligament which attaches the clavicle firmly to the first costal cartilage. Stability depends on the disc and accessory ligaments which limit both medial displacement and elevation of the medial end of the clavicle. The sternoclavicular joints are separated from the origins of the brachiocephalic veins and other structures in the root of the neck by the sternohyoid and sternothyroid muscles.

At the acromioclavicular joint (Fig. 3.74) the lateral end of the clavicle articulates with the medial aspect of the acromion of the scapula. The joint capsule attaches to the edges of the articular surfaces which lie obliquely, the clavicular facet facing laterally and inferiorly. Stability of the joint is provided mostly by the strong coracoclavicular ligament linking the coracoid process and the undersurface of the clavicle near its lateral end. This ligament consists of conoid and trapezoid parts.

Fig. 3.73 *Sternoclavicular joints. On the left side, the joint capsule and subclavius have been excised to reveal the cartilaginous disc and costoclavicular ligament.*

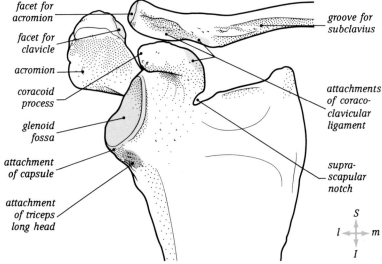

Fig. 3.74 *Oblique anterior view of scapula and lateral part of clavicle. The bones have been separated to show the articular surfaces of the acromioclavicular joint and the sites of attachment of the coracoclavicular ligament.*

Both the sternoclavicular and acromioclavicular joints are supplied by branches of the supraclavicular nerves (C3 & C4).

The lateral end of the clavicle may be elevated or depressed and drawn forwards or backwards. The axes of these movements occur at the costoclavicular and coracoclavicular ligaments rather than through the clavicular joints. Thus, the medial end of the clavicle is elevated during depression of the scapula and moves posteriorly when the scapula is protracted. Full abduction of the upper limb requires rotation of the scapula so that the glenoid fossa tilts upwards. Rotation of the clavicle through forty degrees at the sternoclavicular joint supplements the twenty

degrees of movement available at the acromioclavicular joint, permitting the scapula to rotate through about sixty degrees. The principal muscles of scapular rotation are trapezius and serratus anterior. Protraction is produced by pectoralis minor and serratus anterior and retraction by trapezius and the rhomboids.

The clavicle forms a strut which supports the scapula against the medial pull of muscles such as pectoralis major and latissimus dorsi. The clavicular joints are stabilized by their accessory ligaments which are so strong that trauma, such as falling onto the outstretched limb, is more likely to fracture the clavicle than rupture the ligaments.

SHOULDER JOINT

The shoulder (glenohumeral) joint is synovial, of the ball-and-socket type, and is capable of a wide range of movement. The hemispherical head of the humerus is directed medially and backwards and articulates with the much smaller glenoid fossa of the scapula (Fig. 3.75). The fossa faces anterolaterally and is slightly deepened by the glenoid labrum, a cartilaginous lip round its edge.

The joint capsule (Fig. 3.76) forms a loose sleeve attaching medially to the glenoid labrum. Its humeral attachment is around the anatomical neck except inferiorly on the medial side where it descends to the level of the surgical neck.

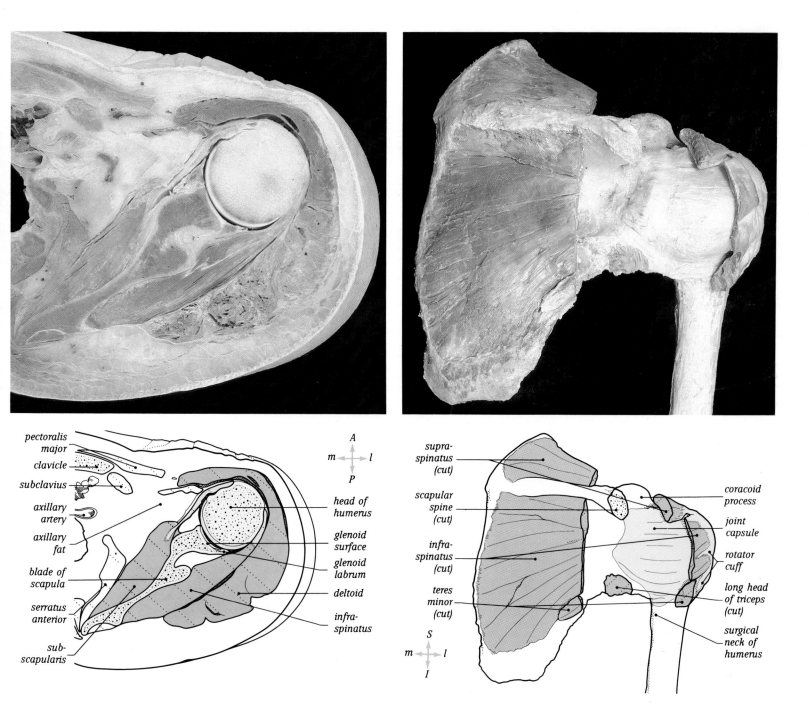

Fig. 3.75 *Transverse section at the level of the humeral head showing the relations of the shoulder joint.*

Fig. 3.76 *Posterior aspect of the shoulder joint. The acromion and parts of the rotator cuff muscles have been excised to reveal the joint capsule.*

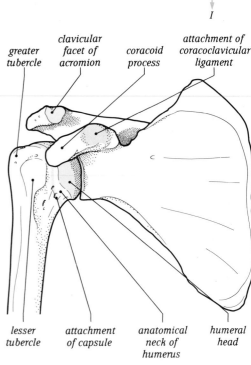

greater tubercle | *clavicular facet of acromion* | *coracoid process* | *attachment of coracoclavicular ligament*

lesser tubercle | *attachment of capsule* | *anatomical neck of humerus* | *humeral head*

Fig. 3.77 *Anterior view of scapula and upper end of humerus. The head of the humerus is partly obscured by the overlying coracoid process of the scapula.*

greater tubercle | *anatomical neck* | *attachment of capsule* | *clavicular facet of acromion* | *attachment of coracoclavicular ligament*

inter-tubercular sulcus | *lesser tubercle* | *coracoid process* | *attachment of coracoacromial ligament* | *humeral head*

Fig. 3.78 *Superior view of scapula and upper end of humerus. The acromion and coracoacromial ligament prevent upward displacement of the humeral head.*

Synovial membrane lines the fibrous capsule and covers the intracapsular part of the humeral shaft (Fig. 3.77). The cavity of the joint usually communicates with the subscapular bursa through a deficiency in the anterior part of the capsule. Indistinct thickenings in the capsule form the glenohumeral ligaments. Between the greater and lesser tubercles (Fig. 3.78) the capsule forms the transverse humeral ligament beneath which the tendon of the long head of biceps enters the joint from the intertubercular groove. The tendon is surrounded by a tubular sheath of synovial membrane as it passes over the humeral head to attach to the supraglenoid tubercle (Fig. 3.79).

The joint is intimately related to subscapularis, supraspinatus, infraspinatus and teres minor (Figs. 3.79 & 3.80) whose tendons fuse with the capsule to form the rotator cuff (see Fig. 3.76). Above the joint is the coracoacromial arch formed by the coracoid process, the acromion and the intervening coracoacromial ligament. The arch is separated from supraspinatus by the subacromial bursa.

Articular nerves are derived from the suprascapular and subscapular nerves and also from the axillary nerve which passes very close to the joint. As this nerve leaves the axilla through the quadrilateral space (see Fig. 3.59), it lies immediately inferior to the capsule. The vascular supply is provided by branches of the circumflex humeral and suprascapular arteries.

Flexion of the shoulder joint (up to one hundred and eighty degrees) is produced mainly by the clavicular fibres of pectoralis major and the anterior fibres of deltoid. Extension (limited to about forty-five degrees) is produced by latissimus dorsi and the posterior fibres of deltoid. At the shoulder joint itself, about one hundred and twenty degrees of abduction is possible, produced by supraspinatus and deltoid; simultaneous rotation of the scapula through sixty degrees permits full elevation of the arm above the head. Adduction, produced by teres major, latissimus dorsi and pectoralis major, is limited by the area of the articular surface of the humerus. Medial rotation is produced by pectoralis major, subscapularis, teres major and the anterior fibres of deltoid, and lateral rotation by infraspinatus, teres minor and the posterior fibres of deltoid.

Fig. 3.79 *Lateral aspect of scapula showing the pear-shaped glenoid fossa. The positions of the supraspinous, infraspinous and subscapular fossae can be appreciated.*

Fig. 3.80 *The scapular component of a disarticulated shoulder joint showing the relations and internal features of the joint.*

Although the coracoacromial arch prevents upward displacement of the humerus, stability of the shoulder joint relies principally on the rotator cuff muscles which hold the humeral head firmly in the glenoid fossa. Despite the labrum, the glenoid fossa is a shallow socket. The capsular ligaments are lax in most positions and tighten only near the extremes of movement. Dislocation of the joint, either traumatic or associated with weakness of the short muscles, is therefore relatively common and may result in damage to the axillary nerve.

ELBOW JOINT

The elbow is a synovial hinge joint between the distal end of the humerus and the proximal ends of the radius and ulna (Fig. 3.81). Laterally the capitulum of the humerus articulates with the slightly concave upper surface of the head of the radius. Medially the trochlea of the humerus articulates with the deep trochlear notch of the ulna.

The joint capsule (Figs. 3.82 & 3.83) attaches to the shaft of the humerus above the radial and coronoid fossae anteriorly, to the margins of the olecranon fossa posteriorly and distally to the annular ligament of the proximal radioulnar joint and to the margins of the trochlear notch of the ulna. Synovial membrane lines the capsule and also clothes the underlying pads of fat which project into the radial, coronoid and olecranon fossae of the humerus. The cavity of the elbow joint is continuous with that of the proximal radioulnar joint.

There are two collateral ligaments (Figs. 3.82 & 3.83). The lateral (radial) collateral ligament passes between the lateral epicondyle and the annular ligament. The medial (ulnar) collateral ligament attaches proximally to the medial epicondyle whilst distally its fibres diverge and attach to the medial aspects of the coronoid and olecranon processes of the ulna. Stability of the joint depends on the integrity of these collateral ligaments which hold the trochlea of the humerus firmly in the trochlear notch.

Rotation of the ulna is prevented by the shape of the articular surfaces of the trochlea. Dislocation of the joint is usually associated with ligamentous or bony injury.

Only flexion and extension occur at the elbow joint. Flexion (about one hundred and fifty degrees) is produced mainly by biceps and brachialis with a contribution from brachioradialis when the elbow is partially flexed. Extension is produced by triceps assisted by anconeus. The flexors and extensors of the wrist and hand arising from the humerus close to the joint do not contribute significantly to elbow movements.

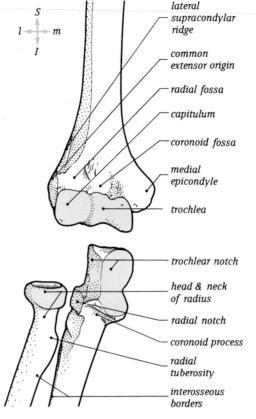

Fig. 3.81 *The bones which form the elbow and proximal radioulnar joints.*

Behind the elbow joint lies the tendon of triceps (Fig. 3.84). Immediately anterior to the capsule are brachialis and the tendon of biceps in the cubital fossa (see Fig. 3.24). The brachial artery and median nerve are separated from the capsule by brachialis. The ulnar nerve lies behind the medial epicondyle in contact with the medial collateral ligament.

The elbow receives blood from the anastomosis around the joint formed by branches of the brachial, radial and ulnar arteries. The vessels supplying the joint are accompanied by articular nerves derived from branches of the musculocutaneous, radial, ulnar (and sometimes the median) nerves.

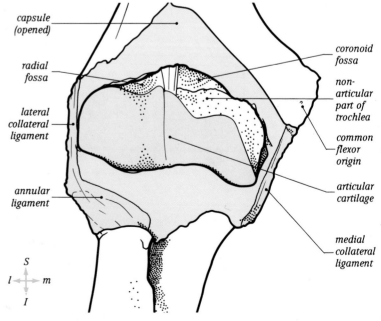

Fig. 3.82 *Anterior aspect of elbow joint. The capsule has been opened to expose the interior of the joint.*

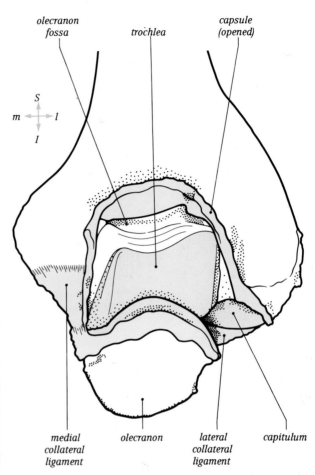

olecranon
fossa

trochlea

capsule
(opened)

S

m ← → l

I

medial
collateral
ligament

olecranon

lateral
collateral
ligament

capitulum

Fig. 3.83 *Posterior aspect of flexed elbow joint. The capsule has been opened to reveal the olecranon fossa.*

S

P ← → A

I

triceps
brachii

fat pad in
olecranon
fossa

capsule
of elbow
joint

brachialis

biceps
brachii

brachio-
radialis

olecranon
& bursa

humerus

head of
radius

supinator

annular
ligament

radial
nerve

Fig. 3.84 *Oblique longitudinal section of elbow (extended) and proximal radioulnar joints showing the articular surfaces and relations of the joints.*

RADIOULNAR JOINTS

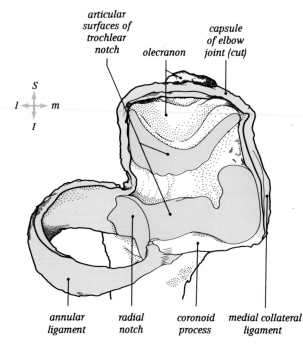

Fig. 3.85 Anterior view of proximal end of ulna with attached annular ligament showing articular surfaces of trochlear and radial notches.

Fig. 3.86 Anterior view of distal ends of radius and ulna. The bones have been separated to reveal the ulnar notch.

The radius and ulna articulate at the proximal and distal radioulnar joints which are synovial. At the proximal joint the head of the radius articulates with the radial notch of the ulna (see Fig. 3.81). The head and neck are encircled by the annular ligament which attaches to the anterior and posterior margins of the notch on the ulna (Fig. 3.85) and blends with the capsule and radial collateral ligament of the elbow. Thus, the cavity of the proximal joint is continuous with that of the elbow.

The distal radioulnar joint occurs between the head of the ulna and the ulnar notch of the radius (Fig. 3.86). A triangular cartilage attaches the ulnar styloid process to the distal end of the radius and separates the cavity of the distal joint from that of the wrist.

The annular ligament of the proximal joint and the triangular cartilage of the distal joint prevent separation of the radius and ulna, yet allow the radius to rotate freely. In addition, the shafts of the bones are joined by the interosseous membrane whose fibres incline downwards and medially from the interosseous border of the radius to that of the ulna. The membrane may be regarded as a fibrous radioulnar joint.

The movements of supination and pronation occur through approximately one hundred and eighty degrees at the radioulnar joints. During pronation the radius rotates across the ulna and twists the forearm and hand so that the palm faces posteriorly. Supination returns the limb to the anatomical position. The axis of the movement passes through the head of the radius and the styloid process of the ulna. Supination is the more powerful movement and is produced by biceps and supinator, although biceps is ineffective when the elbow is fully extended. Pronation is produced by pronator teres and pronator quadratus. Also, when the elbow is flexed, brachioradialis rotates the forearm and returns the limb to the midposition from the extremes of supination or pronation.

In a fall onto the hand, the interosseous membrane may transmit force from the radius to the ulna, protecting the radial head from compression against the capitulum of the humerus. However, the membrane does not oppose distraction and a sudden tug on the hand may dislocate the radial head downwards from within the annular ligament of the proximal radioulnar joint.

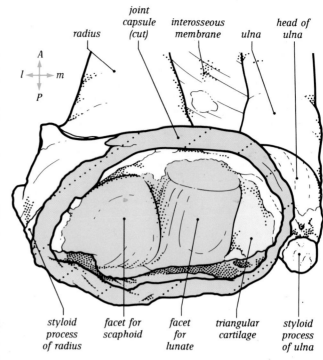

Fig. 3.87 *Articular surface of the distal end of the radius and adjacent triangular cartilage, exposed by removal of the carpal bones.*

Fig. 3.88 *Coronal section of the wrist joint showing articular surfaces and triangular cartilage.*

Mobility of the hand on the forearm is provided by a series of synovial joints. Most of the movement occurs at the radiocarpal (wrist) joint which is supplemented by movement between the carpal bones themselves.

RADIOCARPAL JOINT

At the radiocarpal joint the distal end of the radius and the attached triangular cartilage articulate with the proximal row of carpal bones including, from lateral to medial, the scaphoid, lunate and triquetral

(Fig. 3.87). The triangular cartilage attaches to the radius and the root of the ulnar styloid process and separates the cavity of the radiocarpal joint from that of the inferior radioulnar joint (Fig. 3.88). The capsule, lined by synovial membrane, attaches to the edges of the articular surfaces and is strengthened on each side by collateral ligaments which pass from the styloid processes of the ulna and radius to the adjacent carpal bones. The movements of this joint are considered on page 3.47.

CARPUS

The carpal bones are arranged in two rows: a proximal row, consisting of, from lateral to medial, scaphoid, lunate, triquetral and pisiform; and a distal row of trapezium, trapezoid, capitate and hamate bones (Fig. 3.89).

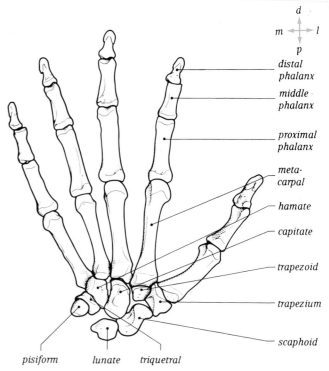

distal phalanx
middle phalanx
proximal phalanx
meta-carpal
hamate
capitate
trapezoid
trapezium
scaphoid
pisiform   lunate   triquetral

Fig. 3.89 *Bones of the hand. Adjacent bones, particularly in the carpus, have been slightly separated to reveal their articular surfaces.*

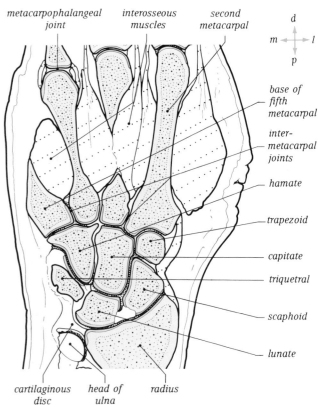

metacarpophalangeal joint   interosseous muscles   second metacarpal

base of fifth metacarpal
inter-metacarpal joints
hamate
trapezoid
capitate
triquetral
scaphoid
lunate
cartilaginous disc   head of ulna   radius

Fig. 3.90 *Coronal section of the hand showing the joints of the carpal region. The thumb and little finger lay anterior to the plane of section.*

INTERCARPAL JOINTS

The joints between the carpal bones are supported by anterior, posterior and interosseous ligaments. The cavities of these joints usually communicate (Fig. 3.90) and function as a single unit called the 'midcarpal joint'.

The pisiform, a sesamoid bone in the tendon of flexor carpi ulnaris, has a separate joint with the triquetral (Fig. 3.91), and is firmly anchored distally to the hook of the hamate and base of the fifth metacarpal bone by pisohamate and pisometacarpal ligaments (see Fig. 3.41). The relations of the intercarpal joints are illustrated in Fig. 3.91.

MOVEMENTS

Movements at the radiocarpal and intercarpal joints are complementary, allowing flexion, extension, adduction and abduction of the hand on the forearm. Although the long flexors and extensors of the digits act on the radiocarpal and intercarpal joints, flexion is due principally to the two carpal flexors, and extension to the three carpal extensors. Adduction is produced mainly by the simultaneous contraction of the flexors and extensors on the ulnar side of the forearm and abduction by contraction of the muscles on the radial side.

Fig. 3.91 *Transverse section through the carpus showing the carpal tunnel and its contents.*

The radiocarpal and intercarpal joints are stabilized by the extensors and flexors of the wrist during action of the long flexors and/or extensors of the digits. In many activities, movement between the hand and forearm combines extension and abduction, achieved by the two radial carpal extensors.

CARPAL TUNNEL

The carpal tunnel is a fibro-osseous passage linking the anterior compartment of the forearm with the palm of the hand. The walls of the tunnel consist anteriorly of the flexor retinaculum and posteriorly of the two rows of carpal bones which form a deep groove on their flexor surface. The retinaculum (Fig. 3.92) lies transversely across the anterior aspect of the wrist, attaching to the trapezium and scaphoid laterally, and to the pisiform and hook of the hamate medially. The tendon of palmaris longus gains partial attachment to the retinaculum and enters the hand in front of the carpal tunnel (see Fig. 3.33). The tendon is accompanied on its medial side by the ulnar artery and nerve which pass lateral to the pisiform but medial to the hook of the hamate. However, the median nerve and the other tendons entering the palm pass deep to the flexor retinaculum and traverse the carpal tunnel.

Within the tunnel (see Fig. 3.91) the tendons of flexor digitorum superficialis lie anterior to those of flexor digitorum profundus. These tendons all possess a common synovial sheath which is usually in continuity with the digital synovial sheath of the little finger but not with those of the other fingers. The tendon of flexor pollicis longus also traverses the tunnel invested by a separate synovial sheath which continues into the thumb. The tendon of flexor carpi radialis lies laterally in a groove on the trapezium, isolated from the main part of the carpal tunnel.

The median nerve traverses the tunnel immediately deep to the flexor retinaculum, lying approximately at the midpoint of the wrist close to the tendon of palmaris longus, anterior to the tendon of flexor pollicis longus and medial to the flexor carpi radialis tendon. Compression of the median nerve may occur within the carpal tunnel, giving rise to a condition called 'carpal tunnel syndrome'. The syndrome may be treated operatively by dividing the flexor retinaculum to decompress the tunnel.

thenar muscles

flexor retinaculum

ulnar artery

flexor carpi ulnaris (cut)

flexor carpi radialis (cut)

flexor digitorum superficialis

ulnar nerve

median nerve

flexor digitorum profundus

flexor pollicis longus

radial artery & nerve

Fig. 3.92 *Flexor retinaculum and the superficial relations and structures entering the carpal tunnel.*

The carpometacarpal, metacarpophalangeal and interphalangeal joints are synovial and allow the hand to perform its various functions, including the intricate movements involved in gripping objects.

CARPOMETACARPAL JOINTS

There are three separate carpometacarpal joints, one for the thumb and two for the fingers. The joint between the first metacarpal and trapezium (Fig. 3.93) possesses saddle-shaped articular surfaces and a lax capsule. This joint permits flexion and extension in a plane parallel to that of the palm, and adduction and abduction in a plane at right angles to that of the palm (and in the plane of the thumbnail). During opposition (the combined movements of medial rotation, adduction and flexion), the thumb rotates so that it may touch any of the fingers 'pulp-to-pulp'.

The remaining two carpometacarpal joints, those for the fingers, are plane joints and less mobile than the first. Laterally a joint cavity lies between the second and third metacarpals and the trapezoid and capitate whilst medially the fourth and fifth metacarpals articulate with the hamate (see Fig. 3.90). These carpometacarpal joints communicate with the three plane (intermetacarpal) joints which lie between the bases of the medial four metacarpals.

METACARPOPHALANGEAL JOINTS

These joints occur between the rounded heads of the metacarpals and concave bases of the proximal phalanges (see Fig. 3.89). Each joint capsule is reinforced at the sides by collateral ligaments and is thickened anteriorly to form a fibrocartilaginous plate. The plates of the medial four digits are interconnected by the deep transverse ligament of the palm. The joints permit flexion, extension, adduction and abduction. Because the collateral ligaments tighten during flexion, adduction and abduction are possible only in the extended position.

INTERPHALANGEAL JOINTS

Each of these joints possesses a capsule reinforced by collateral ligaments (Fig. 3.94). However, posteriorly the capsule is deficient and is replaced by the extensor expansion (Fig. 3.95). These are hinge joints in that they allow only flexion and extension.

The carpometacarpal, metacarpophalangeal and interphalangeal joints are supplied by branches of adjacent vessels and nerves traversing the palm and fingers.

d
m ← → l
p

head of
first
metacarpal

shaft

base

trapezium

nutrient
foramina

groove for
flexor
carpi
radialis

Fig. 3.93 *Trapezium and metacarpal of thumb separated to show the saddle-shaped articular surfaces of the carpometacarpal joint.*

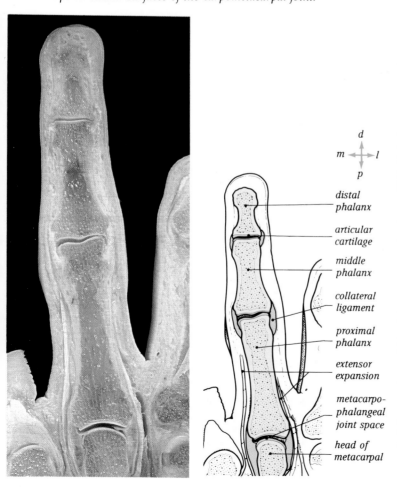

d
m ← → l
p

distal
phalanx

articular
cartilage

middle
phalanx

collateral
ligament

proximal
phalanx

extensor
expansion

metacarpo-
phalangeal
joint space

head of
metacarpal

Fig. 3.94 *Coronal section of a finger. The interphalangeal and metacarpophalangeal joint spaces are exaggerated by slight extension of the specimen.*

nail   distal   middle
plate   phalanx   phalanx

d
P ← → A
p

articular
cartilage

tendon of
flexor
digitorum
profundus

extensor
expansion

proximal
phalanx

tendon of
flexor
digitorum
super-
ficialis

head of
metacarpal

Fig. 3.95 *Sagittal section of a finger to show the capsules and relations of the joints.*

CUTANEOUS NERVES

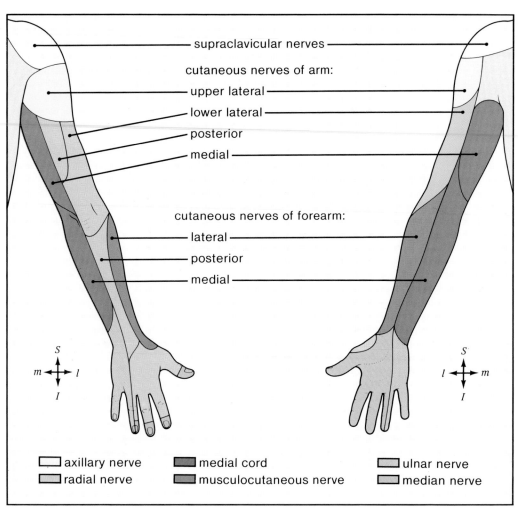

The cutaneous innervation of the upper limb, except for the supraclavicular nerves, derives from the brachial plexus (Fig. 3.96). Each cutaneous nerve supplies an area of skin which is variable from one person to another. There is considerable overlapping of innervation by adjacent nerves; therefore damage to a single nerve usually produces anaesthesia of only the central part of the area of skin it supplies.

Fig. **3.96** *Typical distribution of cutaneous nerves in the upper limb.*

4
ABDOMEN

ANTERIOR ABDOMINAL WALL

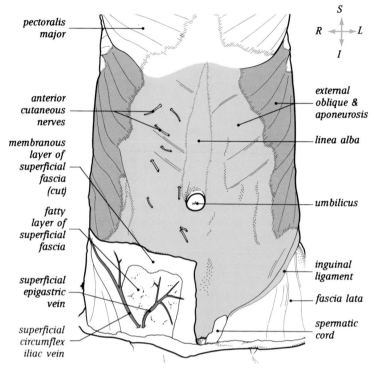

Fig. 4.1 *External oblique muscles and aponeuroses. Some superficial fascia, veins and cutaneous nerves have been preserved on one side.*

The skin and superficial fascia of the anterior abdominal wall overlie four muscles which move the trunk, control intra-abdominal pressure and support the abdominal contents. Deep to the muscles are the transversalis fascia, extraperitoneal fat and the parietal peritoneum.

SKIN AND SUPERFICIAL FASCIA
The midline umbilicus marks the site of former attachment of the umbilical cord. In a lean person it usually lies midway between the xiphisternum and the symphysis pubis, at the level of the fourth lumbar vertebra, but its position is variable.

The superficial fascia has an outer fatty layer which is particularly thick in obese individuals, and a deeper membranous layer which lies on the external oblique muscle (Fig. 4.1). Although thin over most of the abdominal wall, the membranous layer becomes substantial inferiorly. Laterally it descends into the thigh and attaches to the fascia lata while medially it continues around the external genitalia into the perineum (see page 5.24).

The superficial fascia receives its blood from small branches of the arteries that supply the abdominal muscles. The superficial veins drain either upwards towards the axillae or downwards to the groins. The nerve supply to the skin is segmental and is provided by cutaneous branches of the lower thoracic spinal nerves and the first lumbar nerve (Fig. 4.2).

MUSCLES
On each side of the midline there are four principal muscles. Three of these are flat muscles, arranged in layers in the lateral part of the abdominal wall. External oblique is the most superficial, internal oblique lies deep to it and the deepest layer is transversus abdominis. As each of these muscles is traced anteriorly and medially its fleshy part gives way to an aponeurosis (Fig. 4.1). The aponeuroses of the flat muscles form a sheath around the fourth muscle, rectus abdominis. In the midline the aponeuroses from both sides interdigitate to form the linea alba whilst inferiorly they attach to the pubic crest. These muscles are innervated by the lower six thoracic nerves and the first lumbar nerve (see page 4.7).

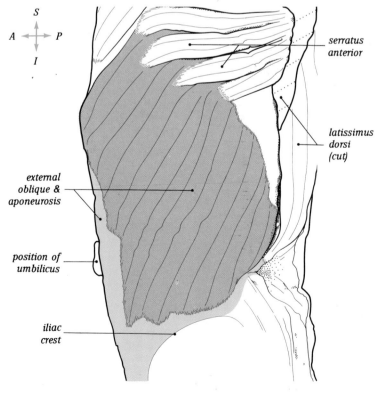

Fig. 4.2 *Schematic representation of the cutaneous innervation of the abdominal wall. To reveal the extent of each dermatome, those with even numbers are depicted on one side and those with odd numbers on the other. T10 is shown on both sides to exemplify the concept of overlapping.*

Immediately above the groin, the inguinal canal traverses the lowest part of the abdominal wall and transmits the spermatic cord in the male and the round ligament of the uterus in the female (see page 4.10).

External oblique

The muscle fibres of external oblique slope downwards and forwards (Fig. 4.3). Superiorly a series of fleshy slips attaches to the outer surfaces of the lower eight ribs, the upper slips interdigitating with serratus anterior, the lower ones with latissimus dorsi. The most posterior fibres attach inferiorly to the iliac crest; elsewhere the fibres give way to the aponeurosis which passes medially in front of rectus abdominis to reach the linea alba. The aponeurosis possesses a free lower border which extends from the anterior superior iliac spine to the pubic tubercle and forms the inguinal ligament (Fig. 4.1) which marks the boundary between the abdominal wall and the anterior aspect of the thigh.

Immediately above the medial end of the inguinal ligament, the external oblique aponeurosis presents an aperture, the superficial inguinal ring, which is the medial opening of the inguinal canal (see page 4.8).

Fig. 4.3 *The left external oblique showing its attachments to the lower ribs and the iliac crest.*

Fig. 4.4 *Most of the left external oblique has been excised to reveal the underlying internal oblique muscle.*

Fig. 4.5 *Left internal oblique and attachments revealed by removal of the external oblique. In this specimen the costal attachments of serratus anterior include the ninth rib.*

Internal oblique

Internal oblique attaches to the lateral two-thirds of the inguinal ligament, to the anterior part of the iliac crest and to the lumbar (thoracolumbar) fascia (Fig. 4.5), through which it is anchored to the lumbar vertebrae. Most of its fibres slope forwards and upwards. The uppermost fibres attach to the costal margin between the ninth and twelfth ribs while the remainder give way to the aponeurosis of the muscle (Fig. 4.4).

Some aponeurotic fibres reach the linea alba by passing anterior to rectus abdominis whilst others pass behind rectus (see below). The lowest fibres arch medially and downwards, contributing to the roof of the inguinal canal. They unite with the underlying fibres of transversus to form the conjoint tendon which descends to the pectineal line on the pubic bone.

Transversus abdominis

The upper part of this muscle arises from the inner aspects of the lower six costal cartilages (see Fig. 4.7) by fleshy slips which interdigitate with the costal attachments of the diaphragm. The middle part of the muscle fuses with the lumbar fascia while the lowest fibres attach to the iliac crest and the lateral half of the inguinal ligament. Most of the fibres run horizontally forwards and are replaced, near the lateral border of rectus, by an aponeurosis (Figs. 4.6 & 4.8). The upper part of the aponeurosis reaches the linea alba by passing posterior to rectus abdominis while the inferior part passes anterior to it (see below).

The lowest fibres of transversus abdominis attach to the lateral part of the inguinal ligament and arch over the inguinal canal and, fusing with those of the overlying internal oblique, contribute to the conjoint tendon.

Rectus abdominis

Rectus abdominis runs vertically on each side of the linea alba from the pubis to the front of the chest wall (Fig. 4.6). The inferior attachment is to the anterior aspect of the pubic symphysis and to the pubic crest. The muscle widens superiorly and attaches to the anterior surfaces of the fifth, sixth and seventh costal cartilages. Its gently convex lateral border forms a surface feature called the linea semilunaris. Rectus abdominis is characterized by transverse tendinous intersections, usually at the levels of the xiphisternum, the umbilicus and midway between the two.

Rectus sheath

Rectus abdominis is enclosed in a sheath formed by the aponeuroses of the flat abdominal muscles. The anterior wall of the sheath, which is anchored to the tendinous intersections, covers the entire length of the muscle (Fig. 4.4). By contrast, the posterior wall is not attached to the muscle and falls short of its superior and inferior extremities. Superiorly the posterior wall of the sheath terminates at the costal margin, above which rectus is in direct contact with the costal cartilages. Inferiorly the posterior wall continues only a short distance below the umbilicus where it thins out or ends abruptly. In the latter case the posterior wall has a recognizable inferior margin, the arcuate line (see Fig. 4.8), below which the posterior surface of rectus is in direct contact with the transversalis fascia.

The composition of the rectus sheath varies at different levels. The anterior wall above the costal margin consists solely of the external oblique aponeurosis, but from that level down to the level of the arcuate line it is supplemented by the anterior layer of the internal oblique aponeurosis. Above the arcuate line the posterior wall of the sheath consists of transversus abdominis and the posterior layer of the internal oblique aponeurosis. Below the level of the arcuate line all three aponeuroses pass anterior to rectus and form the anterior wall.

In addition to rectus abdominis, the rectus sheath contains the small triangular pyramidalis muscle, the superior and inferior epigastric vessels (Figs. 4.6 & 4.8) and the terminal parts of the lower six intercostal nerves which supply rectus and the overlying skin.

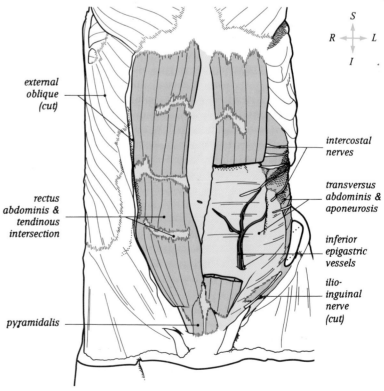

Fig. 4.6 *Rectus abdominis muscles and neurovascular plane. The anterior walls of both rectus sheaths, the left oblique muscles and part of the left rectus abdominis have been removed.*

4.5

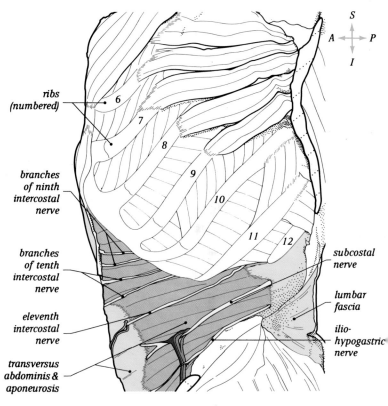

Fig. 4.7 *Removal of the external and internal oblique muscles have revealed the transversus abdominis muscle and aponeurosis. Running across its surface are the lower intercostal, subcostal and iliohypogastric nerves.*

ACTIONS OF ABDOMINAL MUSCLES

The abdominal muscles flex the lumbar spine, rectus abdominis being particularly powerful in this action. Lateral flexion and rotation of the trunk are produced by coordinated contraction of the oblique muscles on both sides of the midline. Acting collectively, the abdominal muscles increase intra-abdominal pressure and, if the respiratory passages are open, the diaphragm is pushed upwards as in forced expiration, sneezing and coughing. Increased abdominal pressure with the airway closed (straining) occurs when lifting heavy objects and during defecation, parturition and vomiting.

STRUCTURES DEEP TO MUSCLES

The deep surfaces of transversus and rectus abdominis are covered by the transversalis fascia, which forms part of a complete fascial sheet lying deep to the muscles surrounding the peritoneal cavity. Several names are given to this continuous fascial sheet and are derived from the muscles to which the fascia relates. For example, the diaphragmatic and iliac fasciae cover the diaphragm and iliacus respectively. Above the midpoint of the inguinal ligament an aperture in the transversalis fascia (the deep inguinal ring) forms the lateral opening of the inguinal canal.

Deep to the transversalis fascia is the extraperitoneal fat, which contains four vestigial structures converging on the umbilicus. Descending from the liver is the round ligament (ligamentum teres; see page 4.13), the remnant of the left umbilical vein. Ascending in the midline from the urinary bladder is the urachus, the remnant of the embryonic allantois (Fig. 4.8). Inclining upwards from each side of the pelvis is the obliterated umbilical artery.

The deepest layer of the abdominal wall is the parietal peritoneum (Fig. 4.8). Although the peritoneum and the abdominal musculature are adherent in most areas, they are only loosely attached between the pubis and umbilicus. Therefore, an enlarging bladder intervenes between them and the organ can be approached surgically through the abdominal wall without traversing the peritoneal cavity.

NERVES AND VESSELS

The skin, muscles and parietal peritoneum of the anterior abdominal wall are innervated by the lower six thoracic nerves and the first lumbar nerve.

Lower thoracic nerves

At the costal margin, thoracic nerves seven to eleven leave their intercostal spaces and enter the neurovascular plane of the abdominal wall between transversus abdominis and internal oblique (Fig. 4.7). The seventh and eighth nerves slope upwards, the ninth runs horizontally and the tenth and eleventh incline downwards. The nerves pierce rectus abdominis and the anterior layer of the rectus sheath to emerge as anterior cutaneous branches which supply the overlying skin (see Fig. 4.1).

The subcostal nerve (T12) takes the line of the twelfth rib across the posterior abdominal wall. It continues around the flank in the neurovascular plane and terminates in a similar manner to the lower intercostal nerves.

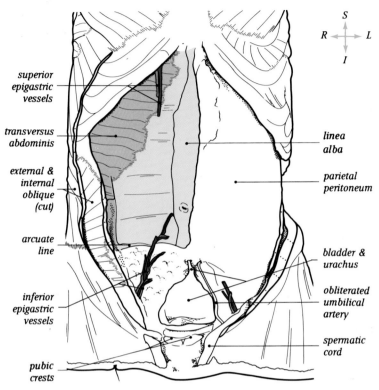

Fig. 4.8 *On the right, most of the oblique muscles and all of rectus abdominis have been excised to reveal the posterior wall of the rectus sheath. On the left, all the muscles have been removed to show the parietal peritoneum. The bladder is enlarged.*

The seventh to twelfth thoracic nerves give off lateral cutaneous nerves which further divide into anterior and posterior branches. The anterior branches supply skin as far forwards as the lateral edge of rectus abdominis while the posterior branches supply skin overlying latissimus dorsi. The lateral cutaneous branch of the subcostal nerve is distributed to the skin on the side of the buttock.

First lumbar nerve
The first lumbar nerve divides into upper and lower branches, the iliohypogastric and ilioinguinal nerves. The iliohypogastric nerve reaches the neurovascular plane in the loin and divides just above the iliac crest into two terminal branches. The lateral cutaneous branch supplies the side of the buttock and the anterior cutaneous branch supplies the suprapubic region.

The ilioinguinal nerve leaves the neurovascular plane by piercing internal oblique above the iliac crest (see Fig. 4.4). It continues between the two oblique muscles and accompanies the spermatic cord (or round ligament of the uterus) in the inguinal canal. Emerging from the superficial inguinal ring, it gives cutaneous branches to skin on the medial side of the root of the thigh, the proximal part of the penis and front of the scrotum (or the mons pubis and the anterior part of the labium majus).

Blood vessels
The blood supply to the abdominal wall is provided by the superior and inferior epigastric arteries, supplemented by the musculophrenic artery and the lower posterior intercostal arteries. The superior epigastric artery descends behind rectus abdominis and may anastomose with the inferior epigastric artery (Fig. 4.8). The latter vessel arises from the external iliac artery immediately above the inguinal ligament and inclines upwards and medially, passing just medial to the deep inguinal ring (Figs. 4.6 & 4.8). The inferior epigastric artery enters the rectus sheath by passing in front of its posterior wall at the arcuate line. From the anterior ends of the lower two or three intercostal spaces, posterior intercostal arteries continue forwards in the neurovascular plane.

Venous drainage of the deeper layers of the abdominal wall is via venae comitantes of the respective arteries. Blood from the superficial tissues drains into veins, lying in the superficial fascia, which run towards the axilla and groin. Dilatation of the subcutaneous veins is an important clinical sign in patients with obstruction of venous flow within the abdomen, for example, within the inferior vena cava or the liver.

Lymphatics
Lymph from the abdominal wall above the level of the umbilicus drains upwards. Lymphatics from the skin and superficial fascia accompany the subcutaneous veins and drain into the axillary nodes, while those from the deeper tissues follow the course of the superior epigastric artery to the internal thoracic nodes. The superficial lymphatics of the lower half of the abdominal wall pass to the superficial inguinal nodes while the deeper lymph vessels follow the course of the inferior epigastric artery to reach the external iliac nodes.

INGUINAL CANAL

Fig. 4.9 *Position of the inguinal canal and its superficial and deep rings in relation to the inguinal ligament, the pubis and the iliac crest.*

- anterior superior iliac spine & inguinal ligament
- deep inguinal ring
- superficial inguinal ring
- pubic tubercle
- pubic symphysis & crest
- spermatic cord
- root of penis

The inguinal canal is about 4cm long and passes obliquely through the flat muscles of the abdominal wall just above the medial half of the inguinal ligament (Fig. 4.9). In the male the canal conveys the spermatic cord (comprising the vas deferens and the vessels and nerves of the testis). In the female the canal is narrower and contains the round ligament of the uterus.

Laterally the canal communicates with the abdominal cavity via the deep inguinal ring. This aperture in the transversalis fascia lies at the midinguinal point, halfway between the anterior superior iliac spine and the pubic symphysis. Medially the canal opens into the subcutaneous tissues at the superficial inguinal ring, an aperture in the external oblique aponeurosis immediately above the pubic tubercle (Fig. 4.10). Continuous with the margins of the superficial ring is a thin sleeve surrounding the spermatic cord, the external spermatic fascia (Fig. 4.11).

BOUNDARIES
The canal possesses a floor, a roof, an anterior and a posterior wall. The gutter-shaped floor is formed by the inguinal ligament (Fig. 4.12), the inturned lower edge of the external oblique aponeurosis. The ligament attaches laterally to the anterior superior iliac spine and medially to the pubic tubercle and the pectineal line of the pubis. The expanded medial end of the inguinal ligament, the lacunar ligament, lies in the floor of the medial end of the canal and its concave lateral edge forms the medial boundary of the femoral ring (see Fig. 4.13).

- external oblique aponeurosis
- superficial inguinal rings
- ilio-inguinal nerve (cut)
- cremasteric fascia
- external spermatic fascia
- inguinal ligament
- fascia lata
- long saphenous vein

S / R ↔ L / I

Fig. 4.10 *Removal of the skin and superficial fascia reveals both superficial inguinal rings (male specimen). On one side the external spermatic fascia has been removed to show the margins of the superficial ring.*

4.8

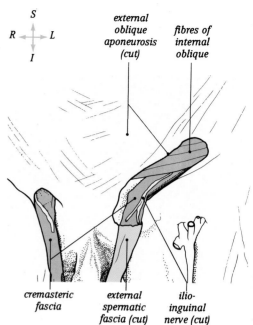

external oblique aponeurosis (cut)   fibres of internal oblique

cremasteric fascia   external spermatic fascia (cut)   ilio-inguinal nerve (cut)

Fig. 4.11 *External spermatic fascia and a strip of the external oblique aponeurosis have been removed to show the spermatic cord and ilioinguinal nerve within the canal.*

The roof is formed by the lowest fibres of internal oblique and transversus abdominis (Fig. 4.12). These fibres arch over the canal and pass medially and downwards to form the conjoint tendon which attaches to the crest and pectineal line of the pubis. The anterior wall of the canal is formed by the external oblique aponeurosis, supplemented laterally by fibres of internal oblique that attach to the lateral part of the inguinal ligament (Fig. 4.11). The posterior wall is formed by the transversalis fascia, reinforced medially by the conjoint tendon. Deep to the transversalis fascia are the inferior epigastric vessels which lie just medial to the deep ring (see Fig. 4.13).

The inguinal canal is a site of potential weakness in the abdominal wall through which intra-abdominal structures may pass, producing an inguinal hernia (see below). However, several features of the canal's anatomy minimize this weakness. The obliquity of the canal ensures that the superficial and deep inguinal rings do not overlie one another (Fig. 4.9). Furthermore, the strongest part of the anterior wall lies in front of the deep ring and the strongest part of the posterior wall lies behind the superficial ring. Hence, when pressure within the abdomen rises, the anterior and posterior walls of the canal are firmly opposed. In addition, when the abdominal muscles contract, the canal is compressed by the descent of fibres of internal oblique and transversus abdominis in its roof.

external oblique aponeurosis (cut)

internal oblique (cut)

conjoint tendon

lacunar ligament

pampiniform plexus

testicular artery

transversus abdominis

transversalis fascia

internal spermatic fascia

testicular artery & veins

vas deferens

pubic tubercle

Fig. 4.12 *Lower fibres of internal oblique and part of the spermatic cord have been excised to reveal the posterior wall and floor of the canal.*

CONTENTS

In the male, the canal contains the spermatic cord (see Fig. 4.11). In the female, it transmits the round ligament of the uterus (Fig. 4.14), a fibromuscular cord running from the body of the uterus to the subcutaneous tissues of the labium majus. Lymphatics from part of the body of the uterus accompany the round ligament and terminate in the superficial inguinal nodes (see Fig. 6.2).

In both sexes the ilioinguinal nerve (see Fig. 4.4) lies deep to the external oblique aponeurosis close to the inguinal ligament. The nerve runs medially in the anterior wall of the canal and emerges through the superficial ring (Figs. 4.10 & 4.14).

INGUINAL HERNIAS

The inguinal canal is the commonest site for an abdominal hernia. Two types of inguinal hernia are recognized. The direct type passes through the conjoint tendon into the medial part of the canal. By contrast, the indirect (oblique) type traverses the deep ring and turns medially along the canal. Hernias of both types may emerge through the superficial ring and descend into the scrotum or labium majus. Direct and indirect hernias are distinguished by their relationships to the inferior epigastric vessels. A direct hernia lies on the medial side of these vessels while the indirect type enters the inguinal canal lateral to them.

In the male, an indirect hernia may pass along the canal within a patent processus vaginalis, giving rise to an 'infantile inguinal hernia'.

inferior epigastric vessels (cut)

trans. versalis fascia

deep inguinal ring

femoral & genito-femoral nerves

external iliac artery & vein

lacunar ligament

pectineal line

bladder

vas deferens

femoral ring

ureters

testicular vessels

Fig. 4.13 *Superior view of the male pelvis to show the deep inguinal ring, the femoral ring and the lacunar ligament.*

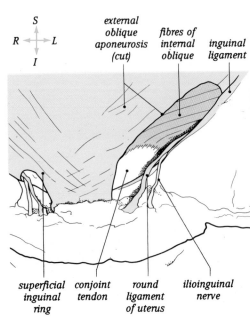

external oblique aponeurosis (cut)

fibres of internal oblique

inguinal ligament

superficial inguinal ring

conjoint tendon

round ligament of uterus

ilioinguinal nerve

Fig. 4.14 *Superficial ring and inguinal canal in the female showing the round ligaments of the uterus.*

SCROTUM

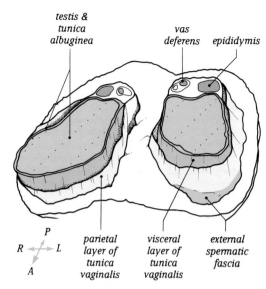

Fig. 4.15 *Transverse section through scrotum. The spermatic fasciae are trimmed flush with the superficial fascia.*

The scrotum is a pouch of skin and fascia derived from the anterior abdominal wall and contains the testes, epididymides and the lower parts of the spermatic cords (Fig. 4.15).

SKIN AND SUPERFICIAL FASCIA

The skin of the scrotum is supplied anteriorly by the external pudendal vessels and innervated by the ilioinguinal nerve. The remainder of the scrotal skin is supplied by branches of the internal pudendal vessels and branches of the pudendal nerve and posterior cutaneous nerve of thigh. Lymph drains to the superficial inguinal nodes.

Deep to the skin lies the superficial fascia, continuous superiorly with the superficial fascia of the abdominal wall. The scrotal superficial fascia, which contains smooth muscle called the dartos, forms a median septum, dividing the pouch into right and left sides.

SPERMATIC FASCIAE

Deep to the superficial fascia of each side of the scrotum lie three layers of spermatic fascia (Fig. 4.16). Each layer takes the form of a sleeve derived from one of the layers of the abdominal wall.

The outermost sleeve, the external spermatic fascia, begins at the superficial inguinal ring and is continuous with the external oblique aponeurosis (see Fig. 4.10). The intermediate sleeve is the cremasteric fascia and muscle, continuous within the inguinal canal with the internal oblique muscle (see Fig. 4.11). The transversalis fascia of the abdominal wall (see Fig. 4.12) provides the deepest sleeve, the internal spermatic fascia, which commences at the deep inguinal ring. These three fascial layers surround the components of the spermatic cord and continue downwards to enclose the testis and epididymis.

SPERMATIC CORD

The spermatic cord runs from the deep inguinal ring into the scrotum, terminating posterior to the testis. The cord comprises the vas deferens and the vessels and nerves of the testis and epididymis (see Fig. 4.17) surrounded by the layers of spermatic fascia (Fig. 4.16).

The principal artery of the spermatic cord is the testicular artery, a branch of the abdominal aorta (see Fig. 4.77). Also present is the artery to the vas (see Fig. 4.18), often arising from the superior vesical artery within the pelvic cavity. The veins draining the testis and epididymis form a network, the pampiniform plexus. Occasionally these veins become dilated, a condition known as a varicocele. From this plexus, one or two veins continue through the deep inguinal ring and ascend the posterior abdominal wall with the testicular artery (see Fig. 4.13). The testicular vessels are accompanied by a plexus of autonomic nerves and by lymph vessels which terminate in the aortic lymph nodes.

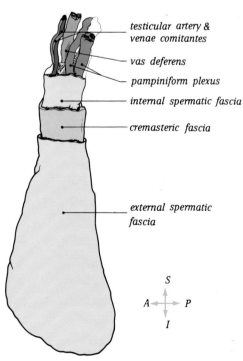

testicular artery & venae comitantes

vas deferens

pampiniform plexus

internal spermatic fascia

cremasteric fascia

external spermatic fascia

Fig. 4.16 *Left testis and spermatic cord within their fascial sleeves.*

TUNICA VAGINALIS

The tunica vaginalis is a closed serous sac which covers the medial, anterior and lateral surfaces of the testis and the lateral aspect of the epididymis (Figs. 4.15 & 4.17). Like the peritoneum from which it is derived, the tunica vaginalis has parietal and visceral layers separated by a small quantity of serous fluid. An excessive accumulation of fluid in the sac produces a swelling (hydrocele) anterior to the testis.

In the fetus the processus vaginalis links the tunica vaginalis with the peritoneal cavity. Usually the processus closes before birth, but occasionally it remains patent.

TESTIS

The testis is an ovoid organ approximately 5cm long in the adult, suspended by the spermatic cord in the lower part of the scrotum with its superior pole tilted slightly forwards (Fig. 4.18). The testis has a thick fibrous capsule, the tunica albuginea, which is covered laterally, anteriorly and medially by the visceral layer of the tunica vaginalis (see Fig. 4.15). The posterior surface of the organ, devoid of a covering of tunica vaginalis, is pierced by the efferent ducts, branches of the testicular artery and numerous small veins that form the pampiniform plexus (Figs. 4.18 & 4.19).

EPIDIDYMIS

The epididymis consists of a narrow, highly convoluted duct applied to the posterior surface of the testis (Fig. 4.19). Its broad superior part, the head, overhangs the upper pole of the testis from which it receives several efferent ducts (Fig. 4.18). The body of the epididymis tapers into the tail which is continuous with the vas deferens. The epididymis is supplied by branches of the testicular artery and drained by the pampiniform plexus.

VAS DEFERENS

The vas (ductus) deferens is approximately 25cm long and connects the tail of the epididymis with the ejaculatory duct in the prostate gland. The vas ascends behind the testis on the medial side of the epididymis and continues upwards in the cord. When the upper part of the scrotum is palpated, the vas can be distinguished from the accompanying testicular vessels by its firm consistency.

After traversing the inguinal canal, the vas runs backwards across the pelvic brim and along the lateral wall of the pelvis (see Fig. 4.13) before terminating in the ejaculatory duct (see page 5.14).

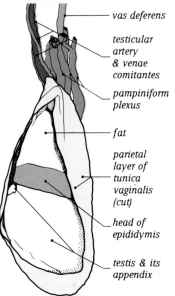

vas deferens

testicular artery & venae comitantes

pampiniform plexus

fat

parietal layer of tunica vaginalis (cut)

head of epididymis

testis & its appendix

Fig. 4.17 *Anterolateral part of the parietal layer of the tunica vaginalis has been removed to reveal the testis and head of the epididymis. This testis bears a vestigial tag, the appendix of the testis.*

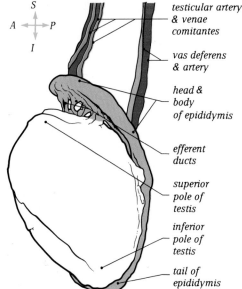

testicular artery & venae comitantes

vas deferens & artery

head & body of epididymis

efferent ducts

superior pole of testis

inferior pole of testis

tail of epididymis

Fig. 4.18 *Lateral aspect of testis and epididymis after removal of the tunica vaginalis and pampiniform plexus. The head of the epididymis has been lifted to display the efferent ducts.*

testicular artery

head of epididymis

vas deferens

pampiniform plexus (cut)

body of epididymis

tail of epididymis

Fig. 4.19 *Posterior view of testis, epididymis and vas deferens.*

PERITONEUM

The peritoneum is a serous membrane with parietal and visceral layers which encloses a space, the peritoneal cavity. The parietal peritoneum lines the walls of the abdomen and pelvis while the visceral layer covers many of the abdominal and pelvic organs. In the male the peritoneal cavity is a closed sac, but in the female it communicates with the interior of the uterus and vagina via a microscopic channel through each uterine tube. Normally, the peritoneal cavity contains only a few millilitres of serous fluid, but in certain diseases several litres of fluid (ascites) can accumulate.

The peritoneal cavity comprises the greater and lesser sacs. The greater sac is very extensive and can be traced from the diaphragm above into the pelvic cavity below. The lesser sac (omental bursa) is located in the upper part of the abdomen behind the stomach and communicates with the greater sac through a narrow opening, the epiploic foramen.

PARIETAL PERITONEUM

The parietal peritoneum is applied to the inner aspect of the abdominal and pelvic walls (Fig. 4.20) and continues superiorly across most of the undersurface of the diaphragm. The peritoneum lining the anterior abdominal wall is raised into several folds or ridges. Below the umbilicus the remnant of the urachus often raises a midline ridge, on each side of which the obliterated umbilical artery may produce a further peritoneal fold (Fig. 4.21). Above the umbilicus the round ligament of the liver (Fig. 4.20) is contained in a large fold of peritoneum, the falciform ligament, which attaches the liver to the anterior abdominal wall and the diaphragm (see Fig. 4.45).

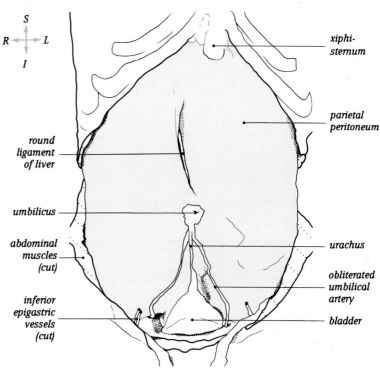

Fig. 4.20 *Removal of muscles and fascia of the anterior abdominal wall reveals the parietal peritoneum and extraperitoneal structures.*

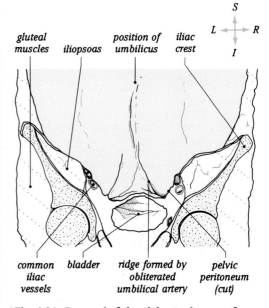

Fig. 4.21 *Removal of the abdominal organs from a coronal section shows the parietal peritoneum from within.*

Posteriorly the peritoneum covers several organs which lie on the muscles of the posterior abdominal wall (Fig. 4.22). These retroperitoneal organs include the ascending and descending parts of the colon, the kidneys, ureters and suprarenal glands, and most of the pancreas and duodenum. Also lying behind the peritoneum are the aorta and its branches, and the inferior vena cava and its tributaries.

Nerve supply
The parietal peritoneum of the abdominal wall is innervated by the lower thoracic and first lumbar nerves. The lower thoracic nerves also innervate the peritoneum covering the periphery of the diaphragm. Inflammation of this peritoneum consequently gives rise to pain in the lower thoracic wall and abdominal wall. By contrast, the peritoneum on the central part of the diaphragm receives sensory branches from the phrenic nerves (C3, C4 & C5) and irritation here may produce pain referred to the region of the shoulder (the fourth cervical dermatome; see page 1.17).

Fig. 4.22 *Transverse section through the abdomen at the level of the second lumbar vertebra shows the relationship of the peritoneum to the retroperitoneal structures.*

VISCERAL PERITONEUM AND MESENTERIES
Most of the abdominal organs have a covering of visceral peritoneum and are suspended within the abdominopelvic cavity by mesenteries. Although organs possessing mesenteries are often termed 'intraperitoneal', they do not lie within the peritoneal cavity but merely project into it.

Mesenteries consist of double layers of peritoneum containing the vessels and nerves of the 'intraperitoneal' organs. Most mesenteries attach to the posterior abdominal wall where their peritoneal layers are continuous with the parietal peritoneum. Typical examples include the mesenteries of the small intestine (see Fig. 4.25) and the transverse mesocolon.

The omenta or mesenteries of the stomach, however, do not attach to the abdominal wall but to other organs. The lesser curvature of the stomach is connected to the liver by the lesser omentum while the upper part of the greater curvature is attached to the spleen by the gastrosplenic ligament (see Figs. 4.27 & 4.28). The major portion of the greater curvature gives attachment to the greater omentum.

Fig. 4.23 *Greater sac after removal of most of the parietal peritoneum. In this specimen the greater omentum is adherent to the right side of the diaphragm, concealing the right lobe of the liver and the gall bladder.*

The greater omentum is an apron-like fold of peritoneum with a free lower border (Fig. 4.23). Hanging behind the anterior abdominal wall and in front of most of the small intestine, this omentum is usually a conspicuous feature when the peritoneal cavity is opened. Superiorly it attaches to both the transverse colon (Fig. 4.24) and the greater curvature of the stomach, enclosing the inferior part of the lesser sac (see below). The free inferior border of the omentum ascends on the right as far as the first part of the duodenum while on the left it merges with the gastrosplenic ligament. The position of the greater omentum is influenced by previous episodes of intra-abdominal disease since it tends to adhere to sites of inflammation.

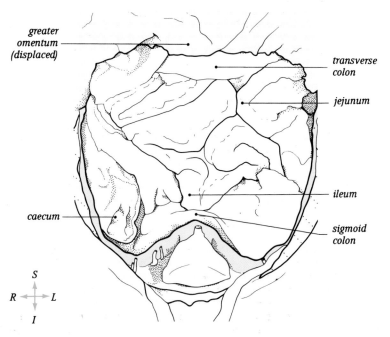

Fig. 4.24 *Greater omentum has been turned upwards to display the contents of the infracolic compartment of the greater sac.*

4.15

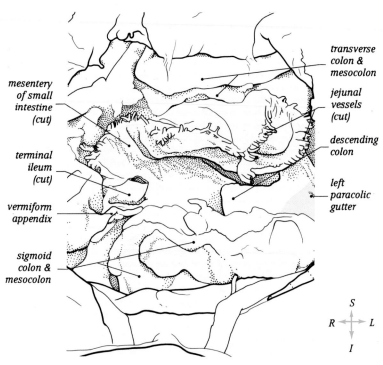

mesentery
of small
intestine
(cut)

terminal
ileum
(cut)

vermiform
appendix

sigmoid
colon &
mesocolon

transverse
colon &
mesocolon

jejunal
vessels
(cut)

descending
colon

left
paracolic
gutter

Fig. 4.25 *Infracolic compartment of the greater sac. Removal of the jejunum and ileum has revealed their mesenteries. The descending colon is more medially placed than usual.*

The transverse mesocolon (Fig. 4.25) has a long horizontal root, attached across the posterior aspect of the abdomen and principally to the pancreas. This mesocolon slopes downwards and forwards into the greater sac, dividing it into supracolic and infracolic compartments. Along its lower margin, close to the anterior abdominal wall, runs the transverse colon.

INFRACOLIC COMPARTMENT OF GREATER SAC

This compartment lies below and behind the transverse mesocolon and is usually covered anteriorly by the greater omentum. The infracolic compartment consists of right and left spaces separated by the mesentery of the small intestine (Fig. 4.25). The root of this mesentery begins to the left of the midline near the transverse mesocolon and slopes downwards into the right iliac fossa. The mesentery is extensively folded and is attached to the jejunum and ileum. The left infracolic space communicates directly with the cavity of the pelvis. By contrast, the right infracolic space is confined inferiorly by the attachment of the lower part of the mesentery.

Behind the peritoneum on either side of the infracolic compartment lie the ascending and descending parts of the colon. Lateral to these are grooves covered by peritoneum, the right and left paracolic gutters.

Another mesentery, the sigmoid mesocolon, lies in the left lower part of the infracolic compartment. Its root is shaped like an inverted V with its apex overlying the bifurcation of the left common iliac vessels and the left ureter. Behind the sigmoid mesocolon lies the intersigmoid fossa which ends blindly at the apex of the V but is continuous inferiorly with the pelvic cavity.

Small folds of peritoneum produce additional peritoneal fossae (or recesses) near the fourth part of the duodenum (paraduodenal fossae) and the caecum (retrocaecal and ileocaecal fossae).

Nerve supply

The autonomic nerves that supply the abdominal organs also innervate the visceral peritoneum surrounding the organs. Pain conveyed by these nerves tends to be deeply felt and poorly localized.

SUPRACOLIC COMPARTMENT OF GREATER SAC

The supracolic compartment lies above and in front of the transverse mesocolon (Fig. 4.26). Its superior part intervenes between the diaphragm and the liver and is divided by the falciform ligament into two subphrenic spaces. The compartment includes the deep recess between the right lobe of the liver and the right kidney (the hepatorenal space) and extends across the midline below the left lobe of the liver and in front of the stomach.

LESSER SAC

The lesser sac (omental bursa) is the small part of the peritoneal cavity behind the stomach (Fig. 4.26; see also Fig. 4.28). It communicates with the greater sac through a narrow opening, the aditus or epiploic foramen, which lies between the first part of the duodenum and the undersurface of the liver (Fig. 4.27).

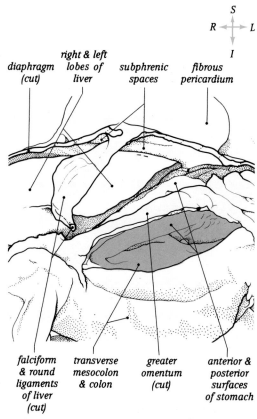

S
R ⟷ *L*
I

diaphragm
(cut)

right & left
lobes of
liver

subphrenic
spaces

fibrous
pericardium

falciform
& round
ligaments
of liver
(cut)

transverse
mesocolon
& colon

greater
omentum
(cut)

anterior &
posterior
surfaces
of stomach

Fig. 4.26 *Supracolic compartment of the greater sac. After removal of most of the greater omentum, the greater curve of the stomach has been displaced upwards to show the position of the lesser sac (coloured magenta).*

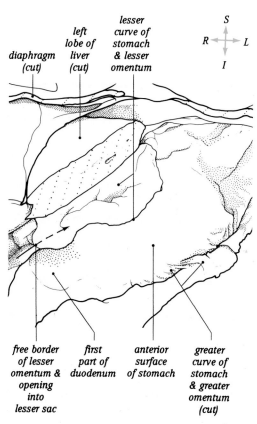

S
R ⟷ *L*
I

diaphragm
(cut)

left
lobe of
liver
(cut)

lesser
curve of
stomach
& lesser
omentum

free border
of lesser
omentum &
opening
into
lesser sac

first
part of
duodenum

anterior
surface
of stomach

greater
curve of
stomach
& greater
omentum
(cut)

Fig. 4.27 *Lesser omentum and opening into the lesser sac after removal of part of the left lobe of the liver.*

superior pole of right kidney

right suprarenal gland

liver

inferior vena cava

opening into lesser sac

portal vein, bile duct & hepatic artery

spleen

left suprarenal gland

lienorenal ligament

aorta & coeliac artery

gastrosplenic ligament

greater curve of stomach

lesser curve of stomach & lesser omentum

P

R — L

A

Fig. 4.28 *Transverse section at the level of the disc between the twelfth thoracic and first lumbar vertebrae showing the lesser sac and its opening. In this specimen the left kidney lies lower than usual.*

The lesser sac is isolated from the greater sac by the stomach and several peritoneal folds. One of these folds, the lesser omentum, connects the lesser curvature of the stomach to the posterior surface of the liver (see Fig. 4.27). Two further folds, the gastrosplenic and lienorenal ligaments, attach the spleen to the greater curvature of the stomach and the left kidney respectively (Fig. 4.28).

The lesser sac extends upwards behind the stomach and the caudate lobe of the liver as far as the diaphragm. On the left it continues to the hilum of the spleen, terminating between the gastrosplenic and lienorenal ligaments. Inferiorly the lesser sac usually extends a short distance below the greater curvature of the stomach between the gastric and colic attachments of the greater omentum.

STOMACH

The stomach is the dilated portion of the gut in which the early stages of digestion take place. It lies in the upper part of the abdomen beneath the left dome of the diaphragm (Fig. 4.29). Proximally the stomach joins the oesophagus at the cardiac orifice and distally it is continuous with the duodenum at the pylorus. Between these two relatively fixed points, the organ varies considerably in size, shape and location in response to its muscle tone, the quantity and nature of its contents and the position of the individual. Usually the loaded stomach is J-shaped and lies in the left hypochondrium, the epigastrium and umbilical region of the abdomen.

STRUCTURE

The oesophagus pierces the diaphragm and has a short intra-abdominal course before joining the stomach at the cardiac orifice. This junction lies a little to the left of the midline at about the level of the eleventh thoracic vertebra.

The stomach has two surfaces, anterior and posterior, which meet at two curved borders, the curves or curvatures (Fig. 4.30). The lesser curve extends from the cardiac orifice downwards and to the right to reach the upper border of the pylorus. A notch, the incisura angularis, is usually present on the lesser curve towards its pyloric end. The greater curve is longer and begins at the cardiac notch on the left side of the cardiac orifice. It arches upwards and to the left before descending along the left and inferior aspects of the organ to reach the inferior border of the pylorus.

inferior vena cava (cut)
oesophagus
liver (cut)
lesser omentum
anterior surface of stomach

aorta
left dome of diaphragm (cut)
gastrosplenic ligament
spleen
transverse colon

Fig. 4.29 *Stomach and some of its relations seen after removal of the anterior half of the diaphragm and left lobe of the liver, and dissection of the greater omentum.*

The pylorus is normally situated just to the right of the midline at the level of the first lumbar vertebra, on the transpyloric plane.

By convention the stomach is described as having three parts, the fundus, the body and the antrum (Fig. 4.30). The fundus lies above an imaginary horizontal plane passing through the cardiac orifice while the antrum lies to the right of the incisura angularis. The body lies between the fundus and the antrum and is the largest part of the stomach. The cavity of the antrum tapers to the right into a narrow passage, the pyloric canal.

The mucosal lining presents numerous longitudinal folds or rugae which are most prominent when the stomach is empty (Fig. 4.30). There is a well developed smooth muscle coat which is thickened around the pyloric canal and pylorus to form the pyloric sphincter.

cardiac notch

fundus
cardiac orifice
body
greater curve
lesser curve
rugae
incisura angularis
muscle coat

pyloric orifice & sphincter
pyloric canal
antrum

Fig. 4.30 *Longitudinal section through the stomach.*

RELATIONS

The anterior surface of the stomach lies in contact with the diaphragm, the anterior abdominal wall and the left and quadrate lobes of the liver. Posterolateral to the fundus lies the gastric surface of the spleen (see Fig. 4.29). The remainder of the stomach's relations are situated posteriorly and collectively form the stomach bed. This includes the diaphragm, left suprarenal gland, upper part of the left kidney, the splenic artery, pancreas, transverse mesocolon and sometimes the transverse colon (Fig. 4.31). However, these structures are separated from the stomach by the lesser sac (see below).

Omenta and lesser sac

Peritoneum covers both surfaces of the stomach. Attached to the curves are double layers of peritoneum which form the lesser and greater omenta.

The lesser omentum extends from the liver (see Fig. 4.27) to the lesser curve of the stomach and also attaches to the abdominal oesophagus and the commencement of the duodenum (see Fig. 4.29). Near the lesser curve it contains the left and right gastric vessels (Fig. 4.32), accompanied by lymphatics and autonomic nerves, while its free border encloses the portal vein, the bile duct and the hepatic artery.

liver (cut)
anterior surface of stomach
posterior surface of stomach
pancreas (deep to peritoneum)
right gastroepiploic vessels
transverse mesocolon & colon

a short gastric artery
gastrosplenic ligament
left gastroepiploic artery
spleen
lesser sac

Fig. 4.31 *Lesser sac and stomach bed seen after removal of the greater omentum and lifting the greater curve upwards.*

caudate lobe of liver
right crus of diaphragm
anterior vagal trunk
oesophageal artery & vein

bile duct, hepatic artery & portal vein
right gastric artery
pancreas
left gastric artery & vein

Fig. 4.32 *Dissection of the lesser omentum shows structures along the lesser curve of the stomach.*

The greater omentum hangs from the distal part of the greater curve and from the first part of the duodenum. Near the greater curve it contains the left and right gastroepiploic vessels (Fig. 4.31). To the left the greater omentum is continuous with the gastrosplenic ligament which connects the proximal part of the greater curve to the hilum of the spleen.

The lesser sac (the omental bursa) lies behind the stomach and the lesser omentum (Fig. 4.31). Its opening (the epiploic foramen) lies above the first part of the duodenum, immediately posterior to the free border of the lesser omentum. From here the lesser sac extends to the left as far as the hilum of the spleen where it is limited by the gastrosplenic and lienorenal ligaments. Superiorly it reaches the undersurface of the diaphragm behind the caudate lobe of the liver. Inferiorly the sac extends a short distance below the greater curve between the two peritoneal folds that constitute the greater omentum.

BLOOD SUPPLY
Coeliac and gastric arteries

The stomach is supplied by several arteries which are all derived from branches of the coeliac artery and which anastomose extensively with each other. The coeliac artery (Fig. 4.33) is a short, wide vessel arising from the anterior aspect of the aorta just below the diaphragm. It divides into three branches, namely the left gastric, the hepatic and the splenic arteries.

The left gastric artery is the smallest branch, passing upwards and to the left behind the lesser sac to reach the oesophagus, then descending along the lesser curve within the lesser omentum (Fig. 4.32). Its branches include two or three to the lower oesophagus which ascend through the oesophageal opening of the diaphragm. Other branches supply the cardiac region and lesser curve of the stomach.

The hepatic artery gives rise to the right gastric and gastroduodenal arteries. The right gastric artery (Fig. 4.32) arises above the first part of the duodenum and runs to the left within the lesser omentum, supplying the lesser curve and anastomosing with the left gastric artery. One of the branches of the gastroduodenal artery is the right gastroepiploic artery (Fig. 4.31). This vessel runs to the left within the greater omentum, parallel to the greater curve, giving numerous branches to the antrum and body of the stomach.

Fig. 4.33 *Stomach and most of the pancreas removed to reveal the coeliac artery and its branches.*

The splenic artery is the largest branch of the coeliac artery (Fig. 4.33). It runs a tortuous course to the left along the superior border of the pancreas, initially behind the lesser sac and then within the lienorenal ligament, and terminates near the hilum of the spleen. It provides collateral branches to the pancreas and terminal branches to the spleen and stomach. There are several gastric branches which pass to the greater curve by way of the gastrosplenic ligament. Most of these vessels supply the fundus of the stomach and are called short gastric arteries (Fig. 4.31). However, one branch, the left gastroepiploic artery, continues downwards and to the right within the greater omentum. It follows the greater curve, supplies the body of the stomach and may anastomose with the right gastroepiploic artery.

VENOUS DRAINAGE

The veins of the stomach accompany the gastric arteries and drain into the portal venous system, the portal vein itself receiving the right and left gastric veins. The splenic vein receives the short gastric and left gastroepiploic veins while the right gastroepiploic vein usually enters the superior mesenteric vein. The oesophageal tributaries of the left gastric vein (Fig. 4.32) take part in an important portacaval anastomosis (see page 4.38) with tributaries of the azygos venous system within the thorax.

NERVE SUPPLY

In the thorax the vagus nerves form a plexus on the surface of the oesophagus. From this plexus emerge two principal nerves, the anterior and posterior vagal trunks, which enter the abdomen on the respective surfaces of the oesophagus. The anterior vagal trunk (Fig. 4.32), derived mostly from the left vagus nerve, gives branches to the anterior surface of the stomach including the pyloric region. Branches from the posterior trunk, whose origin is mainly from the right vagus nerve, pass to the posterior surface of the stomach and also to the coeliac plexus (see pages 4.50 & 4.51). The parasympathetic innervation of the stomach by the vagus nerves is important in relation to both secretion and motility of the organ.

SPLEEN

The spleen is a lymphoid organ lying in the left hypochondrium posterior to the stomach. The fresh spleen is purple in colour, of soft and delicate consistency and rather variable in size and shape. Since it lies entirely behind the midaxillary line and under cover of the left lower ribs, the normal spleen cannot be palpated in the living subject, even during full inspiration.

SURFACE FEATURES

The spleen is oval in shape when viewed from its anterior aspect (Fig. 4.34) and its long axis lies parallel to the left tenth rib. The two extremities of the organ are connected by superior and inferior borders. The superior border often possesses one or more notches near its anterior end while the inferior

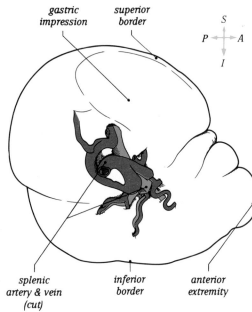

Fig. 4.34 *Visceral surface of the spleen.*

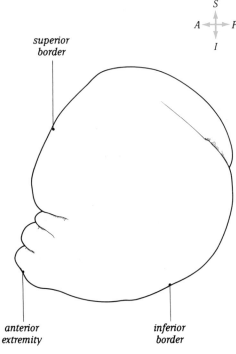

Fig. 4.35 *Diaphragmatic surface of the spleen. This specimen has several well-defined notches on its superior border and, in addition, a single notch on the inferior border.*

border is usually smooth. The organ has two easily distinguishable surfaces. The diaphragmatic surface faces backwards and laterally and is smoothly convex (Fig. 4.35). The visceral surface faces anteromedially and is characterized by ridges and depressions. The most prominent feature, the hilum, is perforated by numerous blood vessels together with lymphatics and nerves. The depressions on either side of the hilum accommodate adjacent organs.

RELATIONS

The spleen is an intraperitoneal organ and most of its capsule is covered by peritoneum of the greater sac. However, there is a small bare area near the hilum which gives attachment to two peritoneal folds or ligaments. The lienorenal ligament runs medially to reach the left kidney while the gastrosplenic ligament connects the spleen to the greater curve of the stomach. Part of the lesser sac lies between these two ligaments and extends to the left as far as the splenic hilum (see Fig. 4.28).

Arching above the spleen and descending posterior and lateral to it, the left dome of the diaphragm is responsible for movements of the organ during ventilation (Fig. 4.36). The diaphragm separates the spleen from the left lung and pleura and from the ninth, tenth and eleventh ribs.

The depression on the visceral surface of the spleen above the hilum is termed the gastric impression since it accommodates part of the posterior surface of the stomach. Below the medial half of the hilum is the renal impression which abuts the superior pole of the left kidney.

Near the lateral extremity of its visceral surface the spleen may possess a small colic impression which lies against the colic flexure. The tail of the pancreas extends laterally into the lienorenal ligament and its tip may reach the splenic hilum (Fig. 4.36).

BLOOD SUPPLY

The splenic artery is a direct branch of the coeliac artery. It follows a tortuous course along the upper border of the pancreas, giving off several pancreatic branches. The artery traverses the lienorenal ligament and divides into its terminal branches near the hilum of the spleen. Several splenic branches enter the hilum, while the short gastric arteries and the left gastroepiploic artery enter the gastrosplenic ligament to supply the fundus and greater curve of the stomach respectively.

Veins accompany the terminal branches of the splenic artery and unite adjacent to the hilum of the spleen to form the splenic vein. Running to the right, this vein lies posterior to the tail of the pancreas within the lienorenal ligament and continues retroperitoneally posterior to the body of the gland and inferior to the splenic artery. It then crosses the anterior aspects of the left kidney and renal vessels and receives several small tributaries from the pancreas. Posterior to the neck of the pancreas the splenic vein unites with the superior mesenteric vein to form the portal vein and, close to its termination, is usually joined from below by the inferior mesenteric vein.

Fig. 4.36 *Spleen and its vessels and relationship to the diaphragm, pancreas and left kidney. The stomach, part of the colon and all peritoneum have been removed.*

spleen

oesophagus (cut)

splenic artery & vein

tail of pancreas

left kidney

left renal vein

inferior mesenteric vein

duodenum (cut)

colon (cut)

DUODENUM

The duodenum, the proximal portion of the small intestine, begins at the pylorus and terminates at the duodenojejunal flexure. Deeply placed in the epigastric and umbilical regions of the abdomen, it curves round the head of the pancreas and is shaped like the letter C (Fig. 4.37). Unlike the remainder of the small intestine, the duodenum is mostly retroperitoneal and therefore relatively immobile. The duodenal lumen receives bile and pancreatic secretions via the bile duct and the pancreatic ducts.

PARTS AND STRUCTURE

The duodenum is conventionally described as consisting of four parts (Fig. 4.37). The first (superior) part begins slightly to the right of the midline at the level of the first lumbar vertebra (on the transpyloric plane) and passes upwards, backwards and to the right. In clinical practice its initial segment is often termed the duodenal bulb or duodenal cap. The second (descending) part runs vertically to the level of the third lumbar vertebra. The third (horizontal) part runs transversely to the left across the midline, arching forwards across the inferior vena cava and aorta. The fourth (ascending) part slopes upwards and to the left and terminates at the level of the second lumbar vertebra by turning sharply forwards at the duodenojejunal flexure.

Close to the pylorus the duodenal mucosa is smooth but in the second and subsequent parts of the organ it is raised to form numerous circular folds, the plicae circulares (Fig. 4.38).

lesser omentum

liver

first part of duodenum

pylorus

gall bladder

second part of duodenum

pancreas

transverse mesocolon & colon (cut)

inferior vena cava

inferior mesenteric vein

duodenojejunal flexure

fourth part of duodenum

jejunal arteries (cut)

superior mesenteric vein & artery (cut)

third part of duodenum

Fig. 4.37 *Duodenum and some related structures. The liver and gall bladder have been slightly displaced.*

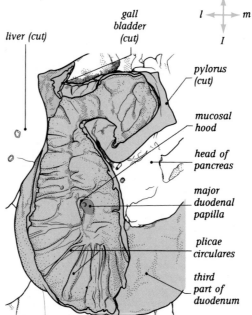

liver (cut)

gall bladder (cut)

pylorus (cut)

mucosal hood

head of pancreas

major duodenal papilla

plicae circulares

third part of duodenum

Fig. 4.38 *First and second parts of the duodenum opened to show the plicae circulares and the major duodenal papilla.*

The bile duct and main pancreatic duct approach the second part of the duodenum near its midpoint from the posteromedial aspect (Fig. 4.39). They usually pierce the duodenal wall in proximity and commonly open into a single chamber, the hepatopancreatic ampulla (ampulla of Vater). The ampulla raises a projection, the major duodenal papilla, on the internal aspect of the duodenum. Bile and pancreatic secretions enter the duodenal lumen through the tip of this papilla via a minute opening controlled by a ring of smooth muscle, the sphincter of Oddi. Immediately above the major duodenal papilla there is often a prominent mucosal fold forming a hood (Fig. 4.38) which may serve as a guide to the location of the papilla, particularly during endoscopic examinations. The pancreas usually possesses a second and smaller duct, the accessory pancreatic duct, which enters the second part of the duodenum at the minor duodenal papilla, about 2cm proximal to the major papilla.

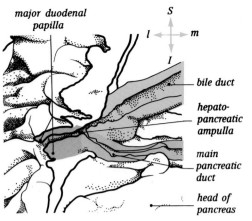

major duodenal papilla

S
l ⟷ *m*
I

bile duct

hepato-pancreatic ampulla

main pancreatic duct

head of pancreas

Fig. 4.39 *Terminal portions of the bile and main pancreatic ducts and the hepatopancreatic ampulla have been opened.*

RELATIONS

Most of the duodenum is retroperitoneal. However, the initial 2cm have peritoneal relationships similar to the stomach in that the lesser and greater omenta attach respectively to the superior and inferior borders. This short segment is relatively mobile and lies immediately inferior to the opening into the lesser sac (Fig. 4.37).

Anterior relations of the proximal portion of the duodenum include the liver and gall bladder. Crossing in front of the second part are the transverse colon and mesocolon (Fig. 4.37), below which lie coils of jejunum and ileum. Running obliquely across the third part of the duodenum are the superior mesenteric vessels (Fig. 4.37) contained in the root of the mesentery of the small intestine. Adjacent to the fourth part there are often folds of peritoneum which may form small recesses, the paraduodenal fossae.

Posteriorly the first part of the duodenum is related to the portal vein, the bile duct and the gastroduodenal artery (Fig. 4.40). The second part lies in front of the hilum of the right kidney and the right renal vessels while the third part crosses the right ureter and gonadal vessels, the inferior vena cava, aorta and origin of the inferior mesenteric artery (Fig. 4.40). The fourth part ascends in front of the left psoas muscle, the left gonadal and renal vessels and the inferior mesenteric vein.

Within the concavity of its C-shaped curve, all parts of the duodenum are related to the pancreas (Figs. 4.37 & 4.40).

BLOOD SUPPLY

The gastroduodenal branch of the hepatic artery descends behind the first part of the duodenum and divides into right gastroepiploic and superior pancreaticoduodenal branches (Fig. 4.40). The latter vessel, which is often duplicated, runs in the interval between the duodenum and head of the pancreas and supplies the portion of the duodenum proximal to the major papilla.

The remainder of the duodenum is supplied by the inferior pancreaticoduodenal branch of the superior mesenteric artery (Fig. 4.40), given off as the superior mesenteric artery emerges from between the neck and uncinate process of the pancreas. The inferior pancreaticoduodenal artery runs to the right between the duodenum and pancreas, supplying both structures and anastomosing with the superior pancreaticoduodenal artery. The veins draining the duodenum follow the arterial supply and terminate in the portal venous system.

hepatic artery

portal vein

branch to pylorus

pyloric canal (cut & displaced)

gastroduodenal artery

superior pancreatico-duodenal arteries

right kidney

right gastroepiploic artery (cut)

inferior vena cava

S
R ⟷ *L*
I

superior mesenteric vein & artery (cut)

inferior pancreatico-duodenal arteries

inferior mesenteric vein & artery

aorta

Fig. 4.40 *Arterial supply and some relations of the duodenum. The first part of the duodenum has been displaced laterally to reveal the gastroduodenal artery, bile duct and portal vein.*

PANCREAS

The pancreas is both an exocrine and an endocrine gland. Most of its substance is involved in producing pancreatic juice which is conveyed by a duct system into the second part of the duodenum. In addition, microscopic clumps of endocrine tissue, the islets of Langerhans, are dispersed throughout the gland.

MORPHOLOGY AND LOCATION

The pancreas is a long narrow lobulated organ, deeply located on the posterior abdominal wall. It lies approximately on the transpyloric plane (L1 vertebral level) and slopes slightly upwards from right to left. Its extremities lie in the right and left paravertebral gutters while the intermediate portion is thrust forwards in the midline by the prominence of the vertebral column and aorta.

The gland is divided into four parts, from right to left, the head, neck, body and tail (Fig. 4.41). The head is the broadest part and is surrounded by the loop of the duodenum. Projecting to the left from its lower portion is the uncinate process. The neck is indented posteriorly by the portal and superior mesenteric veins. The body, of fairly uniform width, extends to the left and is continuous with the tail which tapers as it approaches the hilum of the spleen. The tail is contained within the lienorenal ligament but all other parts are retroperitoneal.

In cross-section the pancreas is triangular. It has well-defined superior and inferior borders and a blunt anterior border to which is attached the transverse mesocolon. The inferior half of the gland is related to the infracolic compartment of the peritoneal cavity while the upper half lies in the floor of the lesser sac and contributes to the stomach bed.

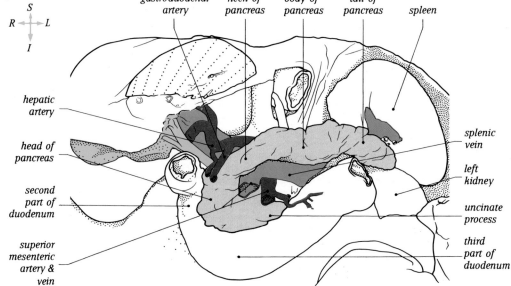

Fig. 4.41 *Principal relations and parts of the pancreas.*

RELATIONS

Surrounded by the loop of the duodenum, the head of the pancreas lies anterior to the inferior vena cava, the right renal vessels and the terminal portion of the bile duct, which is sometimes embedded within the substance of this part of the gland (Fig. 4.42). The anterior surface of the head is related to the first part of the duodenum, the transverse colon and the gastroduodenal artery (Fig. 4.41). The uncinate process lies immediately superior to the third part of the duodenum. The superior mesenteric vessels cross the anterior surface of the uncinate process and separate it from the neck of the gland which lies in front of the superior mesenteric vein and the commencement of the portal vein. The anterior surface of the neck is separated from the pylorus by the lesser sac (omental bursa).

The body of the pancreas crosses the aorta and usually covers the origins of its ventral branches, the coeliac artery whose hepatic and splenic branches are related to the superior border of the gland (Fig. 4.43) and the superior mesenteric artery which emerges at the lower border (Fig. 4.41). Further to the left the gland covers the left renal vessels and suprarenal gland, and the hilum of the left kidney. Immediately posterior to the body the splenic vein receives a major tributary, the inferior mesenteric vein (Figs. 4.42 & 4.43). The inferior border of the body is related to the duodenojejunal flexure, coils of jejunum and the left colic flexure. Overlying the anterior surface of the body are the transverse mesocolon, the stomach and lesser sac, and part of the lesser omentum.

The tail of the gland lies within the lienorenal ligament and is accompanied posteriorly by the splenic vessels (Fig. 4.43). It lies anterior to the visceral surface and hilum of the spleen and posterior to the stomach and lesser sac.

PANCREATIC DUCTS

The main pancreatic duct arises in the tail of the gland and traverses the body and neck to reach the head where it curves downwards and to the right to reach the medial wall of the second part of the duodenum (Fig. 4.42). The duct receives numerous tributaries and gradually increases in calibre from left to right. It pierces the intestinal wall at the greater duodenal papilla (see Fig. 4.39).

S
R ← → *L*
I

portal vein

hepatic artery

bile duct

second part of duodenum

main pancreatic duct

duodenojejunal flexure

inferior mesenteric vein

Fig. 4.42 *Dissection of the pancreas to expose the terminal portions of the bile and main pancreatic ducts.*

The main pancreatic duct and the bile duct usually enter the duodenal wall together and unite to form a common chamber, the ampulla of Vater, in which pancreatic juice and bile may mix before entering the duodenal lumen. There is usually a second and smaller duct, the accessory pancreatic duct, which opens into the duodenum about 2cm above the main duct, at the minor duodenal papilla.

BLOOD SUPPLY

This is derived from branches of the coeliac and superior mesenteric arteries. The head and uncinate process receive superior pancreaticoduodenal branches from the gastroduodenal artery (a branch of the hepatic artery; Fig. 4.41) and inferior pancreaticoduodenal branches from the superior mesenteric artery (see Fig. 4.40). The remainder of the gland is supplied by branches from the splenic artery (Fig. 4.42). The venous drainage of the pancreas passes into the portal system. Superior and inferior pancreaticoduodenal veins from the head of the gland pass respectively into the portal vein and the superior mesenteric vein. Veins from the remainder of the gland terminate in the splenic vein.

splenic artery & branches to pancreas

hepatic artery

S
R ← → *L*
I

portal vein

duodenojejunal flexure

splenic vein

left kidney

inferior mesenteric vein

Fig. 4.43 *Principal vascular relations of the body and tail of the pancreas.*

LIVER

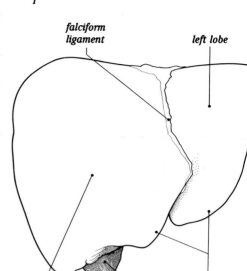

Fig. 4.44 Anterior view of the liver.

The liver is the largest organ in the body and lies in the upper part of the abdominal cavity just beneath the diaphragm and mostly under cover of the ribs. It fills the right hypochondrium and extends across the epigastrium into the left hypochondrium. The living organ is reddish-brown and very soft and delicate.

In the living subject the surface marking of the inferior margin of the liver coincides with the right costal margin as far anteriorly as the ninth costal cartilage and inclines across the abdomen to the eighth left costal cartilage. In life, a healthy liver is usually impalpable.

The liver has the shape of a wedge tapering towards the left (Fig. 4.44). Of its five surfaces the superior, the anterior and the right lateral merge with no distinct borders intervening. However, a sharp inferior margin separates the anterior from the inferior or visceral surface, which is directed obliquely downwards, backwards and to the left. The posterior surface blends with the visceral and superior surfaces at indistinct borders. Most of the surface area of the liver is clothed in peritoneum.

SURFACE FEATURES AND RELATIONS
Anterior and lateral surfaces
The anterior and lateral surfaces of the liver are smoothly convex to conform with the diaphragm and the anterior abdominal wall (Fig. 4.45). A two-layered fold of peritoneum, the falciform ligament, connects the anterior surface to the abdominal wall and demarcates the right and left lobes of the organ. In the free lower border of this ligament runs the fibrous remnant of the umbilical vein, the round ligament (ligamentum teres) of the liver, passing from the umbilicus to the visceral surface of the liver.

Fig. 4.45 Liver and some of its relations. In this specimen the greater omentum is adherent to the liver and stomach.

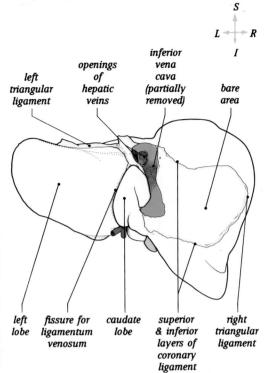

S
L ← → R
I

left
triangular
ligament

openings
of
hepatic
veins

inferior
vena
cava
(partially
removed)

bare
area

left
lobe

fissure for
ligamentum
venosum

caudate
lobe

superior
& inferior
layers of
coronary
ligament

right
triangular
ligament

Fig. 4.46 *Posterior view of the liver.*

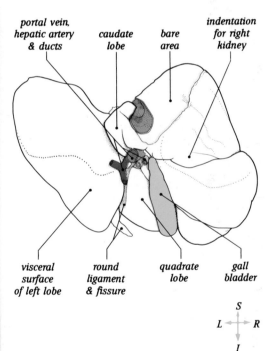

portal vein,
hepatic artery
& ducts

caudate
lobe

bare
area

indentation
for right
kidney

visceral
surface
of left lobe

round
ligament
& fissure

quadrate
lobe

gall
bladder

S
L ← → R
I

Fig. 4.47 *Inferior view of liver and gall bladder showing porta hepatis and visceral surface.*

Superior surface

This surface is gently convex on each side of a shallow depression related to the central tendon of the diaphragm. Above the liver the two layers of the falciform ligament diverge. One layer passes to the right and continues as the superior layer of the coronary ligament (Fig. 4.46); the other extends to the tip of the left lobe where it forms the left triangular ligament. The posterior layer of this ligament, when traced to the right, is continuous with the lesser omentum.

Visceral surface

This surface (Fig. 4.47) is divided into three areas by two vertical features, the gall bladder and the fissure for the round ligament, the upper ends of which are linked by a horizontal cleft. This cleft is the porta hepatis through which pass the branches of the hepatic artery and portal vein and the hepatic ducts. The round ligament ascends along its fissure to reach the portal vein. To the left of the fissure, the left lobe of the liver overlies the body of the stomach and lesser omentum. To the

right of the fissure is the small rectangular quadrate lobe which is related to the anterior aspects of the pyloric region of the stomach and the first part of the duodenum. To the right of the quadrate lobe is the gall bladder, embedded in its fossa. An indentation to the right of the gall bladder accommodates the upper pole of the right kidney. This surface of the right lobe is also related to the right colic flexure and the second part of the duodenum.

Posterior surface

This surface is also divided into three areas (see Fig. 4.46). Extending upwards from the left end of the porta hepatis is the fissure in which lies the ligamentum venosum, the fibrous remnant of the fetal ductus venosus. The lesser omentum attaches to the liver in the depths of this fissure and around the margins of the porta hepatis (Fig. 4.48). The portion of the liver to the left of the fissure covers the front of the abdominal oesophagus and the fundus of the stomach.

To the right of the fissure lies the caudate lobe, facing into the superior recess of the lesser sac. To the right of this lobe lies the inferior vena cava which usually grooves the liver deeply. Further to the right is the bare area (see Fig. 4.46) where the right lobe of the liver is in direct contact with the diaphragm and the right suprarenal gland with no intervening peritoneum. The bare area is bounded above and below by the two layers of the coronary ligament which converge laterally to form the right triangular ligament.

Labels on figure: posterior surface of stomach · coeliac artery (cut) · lesser omentum · caudate lobe · inferior vena cava (cut) · right lobe of liver · splenic artery (cut) · body of pancreas (cut) · inferior & splenic mesenteric veins · aorta (cut) · portal vein & hepatic artery · bile duct · superior mesenteric vein & artery (cut) · right kidney · S L R I

Fig. 4.48 *Posterior view of liver, stomach and lesser omentum. The spleen, left kidney, parts of the pancreas, aorta and inferior vena cava have been removed.*

SUBPHRENIC AND SUBHEPATIC SPACES

The arrangement of the various peritoneal ligaments around the liver produces several clinically important spaces in which fluids may accumulate. Between the liver and the diaphragm are the subphrenic spaces (see Fig. 4.45), separated from each other by the falciform ligament and the superior layer of the coronary ligament. The subhepatic spaces lie below and behind the liver, adjacent to either the stomach or the right kidney.

BILIARY APPARATUS
Ducts

Bile produced by the liver is collected by a system of canaliculi which drain into the right and left hepatic ducts. The two hepatic ducts emerge through the porta hepatis and soon unite to form the common hepatic duct. As this duct descends in the free border of the lesser omentum it is joined from the right by the cystic duct to form the (common) bile duct (Fig. 4.49).

Initially the bile duct lies in the free edge of the lesser omentum, to the right of the hepatic artery and in front of the portal vein. It then passes behind the first part of the duodenum with the gastroduodenal artery and curves to the right behind the head of the pancreas, sometimes grooving the gland (see Fig. 4.42). The bile duct pierces the wall of the second part of the duodenum in company with the main pancreatic duct (see Fig. 4.39).

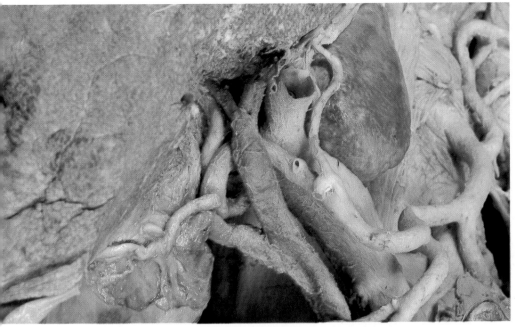

S
R ← → L
I

right &
left hepatic ducts

liver (cut)

common
hepatic duct

cystic artery

cystic duct

gall bladder

left branch of
portal vein

right & left branches
of hepatic artery

coeliac artery

portal vein

gastroduodenal
artery

bile duct

Fig. 4.49 *Porta hepatis including the right, left and common hepatic ducts and the cystic branch of the hepatic artery.*

Gall bladder

This is a hollow, pear-shaped organ in which bile from the liver is concentrated and stored (see Fig. 4.47). It lies against the visceral surface of the liver, often partially buried in its substance, and usually projects beyond the inferior margin to end blindly in a rounded fundus. The fundus normally makes contact with the anterior abdominal wall where the lateral edge (linea semilunaris) of the right rectus abdominis muscle crosses the costal margin. The body of the gall bladder is its widest part and tapers superiorly into the neck which continues as the cystic duct. This duct, through which bile enters and leaves, runs upwards towards the porta hepatis and then turns downwards to join the common hepatic duct. The undersurface of the gall bladder is covered by peritoneum continuous with that surrounding the liver. The body is usually related to the proximal part of the duodenum and the fundus often makes contact with the transverse colon.

The arterial supply to the gall bladder is provided by the cystic artery which usually springs from the right branch of the hepatic artery (Fig. 4.49) though its origin is variable. The cystic vein normally drains into the portal vein or its right branch.

HEPATIC BLOOD VESSELS

Blood is conveyed to the liver by the hepatic artery and the portal vein, both of which enter via the porta hepatis. Blood is drained by the hepatic veins embedded in the organ which enter the anterior aspect of the inferior vena cava immediately below the diaphragm (see Fig. 4.46). The hepatic artery, a branch of the coeliac artery (Fig. 4.50), runs retroperitoneally downwards and to the right to the superior border of the first part of the duodenum (Fig. 4.49). It then ascends in the free border of the lesser omentum on the left of the bile duct and anterior to the portal vein. Near the porta hepatis it divides into right and left branches to enter the liver with corresponding branches of the portal vein. The left branches of the artery and vein are distributed to the left, quadrate and most of the caudate lobes. The right branches supply the remainder of the liver.

Before dividing, the hepatic artery usually has two branches, the right gastric and the gastroduodenal arteries. The right gastric artery arises above the first part of the duodenum and runs to the left within the lesser omentum, supplying the lesser curve of the stomach. The larger gastroduodenal artery descends behind the first part of the duodenum alongside the bile duct. Its terminal branches are the superior pancreaticoduodenal artery (see Fig. 4.41) and the right gastroepiploic artery (see Fig. 4.31).

The hepatic artery also supplies the gall bladder via its cystic branch (Fig. 4.49).

S
R ← → L
I

right
& left
branches of
hepatic artery

bile duct

cystic duct

round ligament

right gastric
artery

first part of
duodenum

caudate
lobe of liver

left gastric
artery & vein

portal vein

gastroduodenal
artery

pancreas

stomach

Fig. 4.50 *Course and branches of the hepatic artery. The lesser omentum has been removed.*

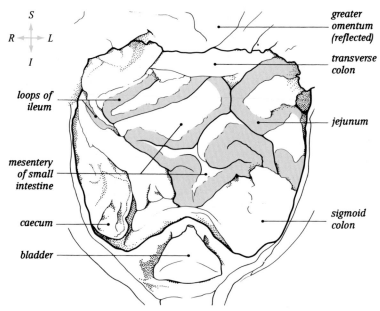

Fig. 4.51 *Jejunum and ileum. The greater omentum has been reflected upwards.*

Fig. 4.52 *Segments of jejunum (upper) and ileum (lower) opened to show their mucosae. Their mesenteries have been dissected to reveal the blood vessels.*

The jejunum and ileum constitute the major part of the small intestine. The jejunum commences at the duodenojejunal flexure and the ileum terminates at the ileocaecal valve. Between these two sites the small intestine is about 5 or 6 metres long and forms numerous loops that fill most of the infracolic compartment of the abdomen (Fig. 4.51). By convention the proximal two-fifths are called the jejunum and the remainder the ileum. However, no precise anatomical feature marks the junction between the two, there being a gradual morphological transition along the whole length of the small intestine.

STRUCTURE

As the small intestine is traced distally there is a gradual reduction in the size of the lumen. The terminal ileum is the narrowest region and it is here that foreign bodies may lodge. Mucosal folds (plicae circulares) are numerous in the proximal jejunum (Fig. 4.52) but diminish in both size and number so that in the distal ileum they are often absent. This difference in mucosal structure can be detected by palpation and may also be apparent on radiographs. The distribution of lymphoid tissue in the jejunum is diffuse whereas in the mucosa of the ileum it is arranged in discrete clumps (Peyer's patches).

ILEAL DIVERTICULUM

Within a metre of the ileocaecal valve the ileum occasionally possesses a diverticulum on its antimesenteric border. This diverticulum (Meckel's diverticulum) is the embryological remnant of the vitellointestinal duct and may be connected to the umbilicus. Inflammation of the diverticulum can give rise to clinical features similar to those of appendicitis.

MESENTERY

The jejunum and ileum are contained within the free border of the mesentery of the small intestine. This fan-shaped structure has a root about 15cm long attached to the posterior abdominal wall between the duodenojejunal flexure and the ileocaecal junction (Fig. 4.53). The mesentery divides the infracolic compartment of the peritoneal cavity into right and left infracolic spaces. Between its two peritoneal layers the mesentery contains a quantity of fat which is particularly abundant in the ileal portion. Embedded in this fat are numerous jejunal and ileal blood vessels (see below), lymphatic vessels and nodes, and autonomic nerves.

LOCATION AND RELATIONS

Because they are suspended from the mesentery, the jejunum and ileum possess considerable mobility and their coils can change position relative to adjacent organs. The jejunum usually occupies the central part of the abdomen, especially the umbilical region, while the ileum lies at a lower level, mostly in the hypogastrium and the pelvic cavity (Fig. 4.51). The terminal ileum usually ascends from the pelvis into the right iliac fossa to reach the medial aspect of the caecum (Fig. 4.53). The principal anterior relations of the jejunum and ileum are the greater omentum, the transverse colon and its mesocolon, and the anterior abdominal wall. Posteriorly the coils of small intestine overlie retroperitoneal structures on the posterior wall of the abdomen and pelvis and may also overlap the ascending, descending and sigmoid parts of the colon. Within the pelvis, loops of ileum may lie in contact with pelvic organs such as the rectum and urinary bladder and, in the female, with the uterus and its appendages.

Fig. 4.53 Mesentery of the small intestine. All of the jejunum and most of the ileum have been excised and the cut edge of mesentery trimmed to reveal the jejunal and ileal vessels.

SUPERIOR MESENTERIC VESSELS

The superior mesenteric artery supplies the intestine from the second part of the duodenum to the splenic flexure of the colon. The artery is an anterior branch of the abdominal aorta (see Fig. 4.76) at the level of the first lumbar vertebra, just below the coeliac artery. It descends in front of the left renal vein and behind the neck of the pancreas. Inclining to the right, the artery continues downwards in front of the uncinate process of the pancreas and across the third part of the duodenum to enter the root of the mesentery (Fig. 4.54).

Fig. 4.54 *Superior mesenteric artery and its branches. The jejunal and ileal veins have been removed.*

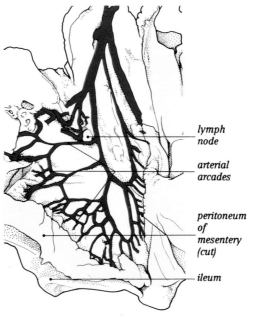

Fig. 4.55 *Ileal arteries and their arcades in the mesentery of the ileum.*

The superior mesenteric artery gives rise to middle colic and inferior pancreaticoduodenal branches before gaining the mesentery. As it descends in the root of the mesentery it furnishes the right colic artery which passes behind the peritoneum to supply the ascending colon. A further branch, also retroperitoneal, is the ileocolic artery which inclines downwards and to the right towards the caecum. The superior mesenteric artery also gives numerous branches to the jejunum and ileum. Within the mesentery these jejunal and ileal arteries anastomose, producing a series of arterial arcades which are more profuse in the ileal part of the mesentery (Fig. 4.55). The superior mesenteric artery terminates at the upper border of the terminal ileum where it anastomoses with the lower branch of the ileocolic artery and the distal ileal arteries.

The superior mesenteric vein begins above the terminal ileum and ascends in the root of the mesentery. It lies on the right of the superior mesenteric artery and its tributaries correspond to the branches of the artery. The vein terminates behind the neck of the pancreas by joining the splenic vein to form the portal vein. Close to its termination, it may be joined by the inferior mesenteric vein (see Fig. 4.65), but this more commonly enters the splenic vein.

CAECUM, APPENDIX AND COLON

The large intestine is approximately 1.5 metres long and comprises the caecum, appendix, colon, rectum and anal canal. The caecum and appendix lie in the right iliac fossa while the colon runs a circuitous course (Fig. 4.56) before descending into the pelvic cavity to become continuous with the rectum. Descriptions of the rectum and anal canal are given in the section on the pelvis.

The lumen of the intestine is relatively wide in the caecum and ascending colon but narrows gradually as the colon is traced towards the rectum. The outer longitudinal muscle coat of the caecum and colon is thickened to form three longitudinal bands, the taeniae coli (Fig. 4.57). Bulges (haustrations) of the gut wall between the taeniae correspond with sacculations on the mucosal surface. The peritoneal surface of the colon (but not of the appendix or caecum) is characterized by numerous fat-filled tags, the appendices epiploicae.

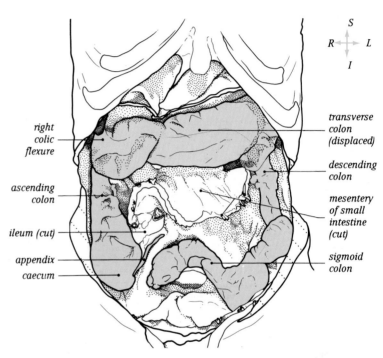

Fig. 4.56 Caecum, appendix and colon after removal of the greater omentum and most of the small intestine. The transverse colon has been raised.

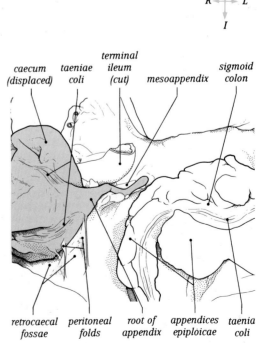

Fig. 4.57 Base of the appendix and retrocaecal folds and fossae after pulling the caecum forwards.

CAECUM

The ileum terminates by opening into the large intestine at a slit-like or oval aperture, the ileocaecal valve (Fig. 4.58). The caecum is the blind-ending portion of the large intestine below the level of the valve. The caecum and ascending colon are in direct continuity and the three taeniae coli descend along the outer surface of the caecum and converge on its posteromedial aspect at the root of the appendix.

The caecum usually lies in the right iliac fossa above the lateral half of the inguinal ligament (Fig. 4.59). Anteriorly it is related to the abdominal wall, the greater omentum and coils of ileum; posteriorly lie the iliacus and psoas muscles. The caecum may lie free in the iliac fossa, completely surrounded by peritoneum. Alternatively it may be attached to the iliac fossa by peritoneal folds forming a retrocaecal fossa (see Fig. 4.57). Rarely, the caecum is entirely retroperitoneal. On the medial side of the caecum, adjacent to the terminal ileum, small peritoneal folds may enclose one or more ileocaecal recesses.

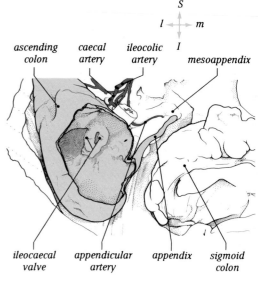

Fig. 4.58 *Ileocaecal valve revealed by removal of the anterior wall of the caecum. The mesoappendix has been dissected to show the appendicular artery.*

APPENDIX

The worm-like appendix is attached to the posteromedial wall of the caecum where the taeniae coli converge (see Fig. 4.57). It is a thick-walled tube with a narrow lumen and, although variable in length, usually measures approximately 10cm. The surface marking of the root of the appendix is relatively constant, lying one-third of the distance from the anterior superior iliac spine to the umbilicus.

The appendix usually possesses a mesentery, the mesoappendix (Fig. 4.58), which is attached to the mesentery of the ileum and confers upon the appendix a degree of mobility. Although it frequently lies behind the caecum (Fig. 4.60), in front of the iliacus or psoas muscle, it occasionally descends into the pelvis where its tip may lie adjacent to the bladder, the right ureter and, in the female, the ovary or uterine tube (Fig. 4.59). Rarely, the appendix lies anterior or posterior to the terminal ileum. It is a common site of infection (appendicitis) which may spread to adjacent structures.

COLON

The colon consists of ascending, transverse, descending and sigmoid parts (see Fig. 4.56). The ascending and descending parts are usually retroperitoneal while the transverse and sigmoid parts are suspended by mesenteries. The colon possesses two acute angulations, the right (hepatic) and left (splenic) flexures.

The ascending colon begins at the level of the ileocaecal valve and runs vertically upwards. At the right colic flexure under the right lobe of the liver, it becomes continuous with the transverse colon. Anterior to the ascending colon lie the abdominal wall, loops of ileum and often the greater omentum. Its posterior relations include the iliacus, transversus abdominis, quadratus lumborum and the right kidney.

The transverse colon extends from the right to the left colic flexure and is suspended by the transverse mesocolon. Typically its middle portion hangs downwards and crosses the umbilical region or hypogastrium. At the left colic flexure just below the splenic hilum, it turns inferiorly to become the descending colon. From right to left, the superior relations of the transverse colon include the liver and gall bladder and the greater curve of the stomach. Posteriorly lie the second part of the duodenum, the pancreas, loops of small intestine and the spleen. Anteriorly lie the greater omentum and the abdominal wall. The greater omentum attaches to both the transverse colon and the greater curve of the stomach (see page 4.15).

Fig. 4.59 *After removal of most of the small intestine, this appendix can be seen descending over the pelvic brim.*

The descending colon runs from the left flexure to the left iliac fossa and turns medially at the pelvic brim to continue as the sigmoid colon (see Figs. 4.56 & 4.62). The upper part of the descending colon is covered anteriorly by coils of jejunum while the lower part usually makes contact with the abdominal wall through which it is often palpable. Its posterior relations include the left kidney and the psoas, quadratus lumborum and iliacus muscles.

The sigmoid (pelvic) colon begins at the pelvic brim and terminates in front of the third sacral vertebra by joining the rectum. The sigmoid colon varies in length and is mobile on its mesentery, the sigmoid mesocolon. Its proximal portion usually runs to the right across the lower abdomen (see Fig. 4.56) and is related superiorly to loops of small intestine. The remainder of the sigmoid colon lies in the pelvic cavity in contact with the upper surfaces of the pelvic organs.

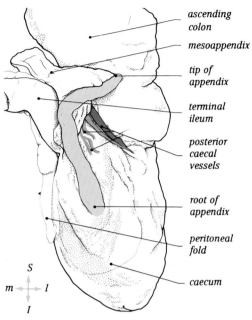

Fig. 4.60 *Posterior aspect of the caecum to show a retrocaecal appendix.*

BLOOD SUPPLY

The blood supply of the caecum, appendix, ascending colon and most of the transverse colon is provided by the superior mesenteric vessels. The remainder of the colon is supplied by the inferior mesenteric vessels.

Branches of superior mesenteric vessels

The origin and course of the superior mesenteric artery are described on page 4.34. Its branches to the large intestine vary considerably but usually include the middle colic, right colic, and ileocolic arteries (Fig. 4.61).

The middle colic artery enters the transverse mesocolon and divides into right and left branches which supply the proximal two-thirds of the transverse colon. The right colic artery reaches the ascending colon and divides into ascending and descending branches which supply the organ. The ileocolic artery has anterior and posterior caecal branches and also supplies the ascending colon and terminal ileum. The appendicular branch (Fig. 4.58) descends behind the terminal ileum, enters the mesoappendix and runs near its free border to the tip of the appendix. The arteries supplying the caecum and colon anastomose, often forming a continuous marginal artery (Fig. 4.61).

Veins corresponding to the branches of the superior mesenteric artery drain into the superior mesenteric vein (Fig. 4.61; see Fig. 4.64).

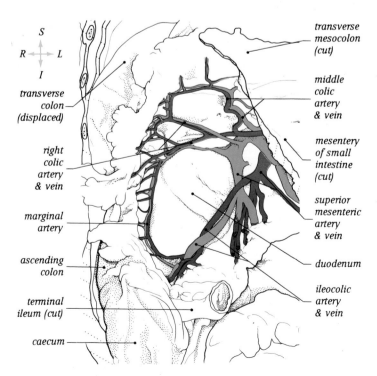

Fig. 4.61 *Blood supply to the caecum, ascending and transverse colon. The transverse mesocolon and the mesentery of the small intestine have been dissected to reveal the ileocolic, right colic and middle colic vessels.*

CAECUM, APPENDIX AND COLON

Inferior mesenteric vessels

The inferior mesenteric artery arises from the anterior aspect of the abdominal aorta 3 or 4cm above the bifurcation, often overlapped by the third part of the duodenum (Fig. 4.62). The artery runs retroperitoneally downwards and to the left to reach the pelvic brim. Here it crosses the common iliac vessels and continues into the pelvis as the superior rectal artery.

The first branch of the inferior mesenteric artery, the left colic artery, runs to the left and gives rise to ascending and descending branches. The former supplies the distal third of the transverse colon and the left colic flexure. The descending branch supplies the descending colon and the commencement of the sigmoid colon. The inferior mesenteric artery gives rise to several sigmoid arteries which reach the sigmoid colon via the mesocolon.

The branches of the inferior mesenteric artery are accompanied by tributaries of the inferior mesenteric vein (Fig. 4.62). The course and termination of this vessel are described with the portal venous system.

Fig. 4.62 *Blood supply to the left colic flexure, descending colon and sigmoid colon. Removal of peritoneum from the posterior abdominal wall to the left of the aorta displays the inferior mesenteric vessels.*

PORTAL VENOUS SYSTEM

The portal venous system drains blood from most of the alimentary tract including the abdominal oesophagus, stomach, small and large intestines, pancreas, and also from the spleen. Blood from these organs is drained by the superior mesenteric and splenic veins which unite to form the portal vein (Fig. 4.63). This large vein approaches the porta hepatis with the hepatic artery, and branches of both vessels enter the liver and further subdivide. After traversing the liver, blood from both sources is drained by the hepatic veins which enter the inferior vena cava.

TRIBUTARIES

The superior mesenteric vein (Fig. 4.64) receives blood from most of the small intestine and the proximal half of the large intestine. It drains the duodenum distal to the major papilla, the jejunum and ileum, the caecum and appendix, and the ascending and most of the transverse colon. The vein accompanies the superior mesenteric artery within the root of the mesentery and its tributaries generally correspond to the branches of the artery.

The splenic vein (Fig. 4.64) drains the spleen and parts of the pancreas and stomach. It arises at the hilum of the spleen and runs to the right in the lienorenal ligament behind the tail of the pancreas. The vein continues behind the body of the pancreas and usually receives the inferior mesenteric vein and other tributaries corresponding to the branches of the splenic artery.

The inferior mesenteric vein drains the upper part of the anal canal, the rectum, the sigmoid and descending parts of the colon and the distal part of the transverse colon. The vein initially accompanies the corresponding artery but in the latter part of its course it ascends the posterior abdominal wall independently, passing to the left of the duodenojejunal junction. The vessel usually terminates by joining the splenic vein behind the body of the pancreas (Fig. 4.63), but it may enter the superior mesenteric vein (Fig. 4.64).

PORTAL VEIN

The portal vein is formed behind the neck of the pancreas by the union of the superior mesenteric and splenic veins (Fig. 4.63). It runs upwards and to the right behind the gastroduodenal artery and the first part of the duodenum. The vein then enters the free border of the lesser omentum accompanied anteriorly by the bile duct and the hepatic artery (see Fig. 4.28). Near the porta hepatis the vein divides into left and right branches which enter the liver. Several small veins enter the portal vein directly, including the left and right gastric veins and the cystic vein.

PORTACAVAL ANASTOMOSES

There are numerous anastomoses between the tributaries of the portal venous system and those of the systemic venous system. In health, these portacaval anastomoses are microscopic; but if there is obstruction of blood flow through the portal vein or liver, they may dilate and give rise to characteristic clinical features. For example, in the wall of the lowest part of the oesophagus, veins draining into the left gastric vein communicate with tributaries of the azygos venous system. Portal vein obstruction can cause gross swelling of these oesophageal veins (oesophageal varices) which may bleed profusely.

Similarly, paraumbilical veins accompanying the round ligament of the liver communicate with the portal vein at the porta hepatis and with veins of the anterior abdominal wall around the umbilicus. Portal vein obstruction, therefore, may result in dilatation of the subcutaneous veins of the abdominal wall. Other sites of portacaval anastomoses include the anal canal and retroperitoneal parts of the intestine.

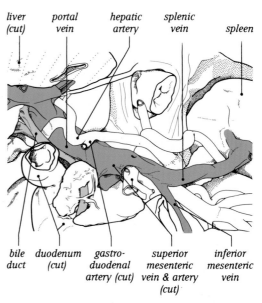

liver
(cut) portal
vein hepatic
artery splenic
vein spleen

bile
duct duodenum
(cut) gastro-
duodenal
artery (cut) superior
mesenteric
vein & artery
(cut) inferior
mesenteric
vein

Fig. 4.63 *Portal and splenic veins. Most of the pancreas has been removed and the first part of the duodenum turned aside.*

liver (cut) commencement
of portal vein splenic
vein &
artery short
gastric
veins (cut) spleen

first
part of
duodenum
(displaced) superior
mesenteric
vein jejunal
veins
(cut) superior
mesenteric
artery
(cut) inferior
mesenteric
vein

Fig. 4.64 *Tributaries of the portal vein. In this specimen the inferior mesenteric vein joins the superior mesenteric vein.*

KIDNEYS AND SUPRARENAL GLANDS

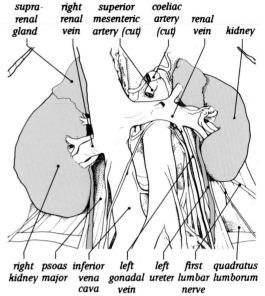

Fig. 4.65 *Kidneys, suprarenal glands and some of the vessels associated with them.*

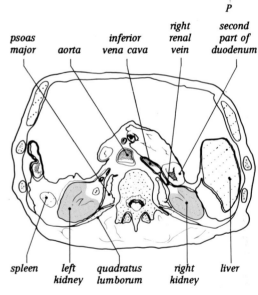

Fig. 4.66 *Transverse section at the level of the second lumbar vertebra showing the relationships of the kidneys to the lumbar vertebrae and some of the digestive organs.*

KIDNEYS

The two kidneys lie behind the peritoneum on either side of the upper lumbar vertebrae (Fig. 4.65). They are embedded in fat in the paravertebral gutters of the posterior abdominal wall and are placed obliquely with their anterior surfaces directed slightly laterally (Fig. 4.66). The left kidney usually lies at a higher level than the right.

Each kidney is bean-shaped, flattened anteroposteriorly and approximately 11 cm long. The anterior and posterior surfaces are gently convex and the superior and inferior poles are rounded. The lateral border is convex while the indented medial border bears an aperture, the hilum (Fig. 4.67), which is

Fig. 4.67 *Medial aspect of the right kidney showing the renal vessels passing through the hilum.*

Fig. 4.68 *Longitudinal section through the right kidney, seen from behind, showing the kidney substance and the contents of the renal sinus.*

Fig. 4.69 *Right kidney dissected from behind to show the renal pelvis and calices.*

traversed by the renal pelvis or ureter, the renal vessels, lymphatics and autonomic nerves. The hilum leads into a cavity within the kidney, the renal sinus (Fig. 4.68), which is occupied by the calices and renal pelvis, the renal blood vessels and a quantity of fat.

Covered by a thin capsule, the kidney comprises an outer cortex and an inner medulla. The medulla contains numerous pyramids whose apices project into the renal sinus as the renal papillae (Fig. 4.68). Urine discharged from the papillae is collected by about ten trumpet-shaped chambers, the minor calices (Fig. 4.69), which unite to form two or three major calices. These fuse into the single, funnel-shaped renal pelvis which lies posterior to most of the vessels and is continuous with the ureter.

Perirenal tissues

Each kidney is surrounded by a layer of perirenal fat enveloped in a thin sheet of connective tissue, the renal fascia (Fig. 4.70). This fascia also encloses the suprarenal gland and the proximal part of the ureter. From the inferior pole of the kidney, the renal fascia tapers downwards into the iliac fossa. Around the fascia is a further layer of fat (pararenal fat) lying against the posterior abdominal muscles and covered anteriorly by the peritoneum.

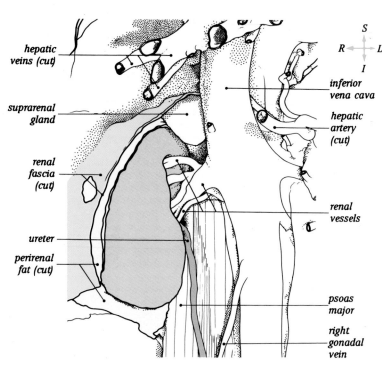

Fig. 4.70 *Right kidney and suprarenal gland seen within the renal fascia and perirenal fat, part of which has been removed.*

Relations of kidneys

The right and left kidneys have similar posterior relations (see Fig. 4.66). The superior poles lie against the diaphragm and the twelfth ribs, below which run the subcostal nerves and vessels. On the left the upper pole is also related, through the diaphragm, to the pleura and eleventh rib. The medial border of each kidney overlaps psoas major (see Fig. 4.65) while the inferolateral portion is related to quadratus lumborum and transversus abdominis, and to the first lumbar nerve.

The anterior relations of the kidneys are asymmetric. On the right, from above downwards, they include the bare area of the liver, the second part of the duodenum (see Fig. 4.66), the right flexure of the colon and coils of jejunum. The medial border of the right kidney is related to the inferior vena cava, the renal vessels and the upper part of the ureter (Fig. 4.70).

On the left, from above downwards, the anterior relations include the stomach and spleen, the splenic vessels, the tail of the pancreas, the left colic flexure and coils of jejunum. The medial border relates to the suprarenal gland, the renal and suprarenal vessels, the left gonadal vein and the proximal part of the ureter (see Fig. 4.73).

Renal vessels

At the level of the first lumbar vertebra, the aorta usually supplies one renal artery to each kidney (Fig. 4.71). Each artery lies behind the corresponding vein, and the artery on the right crosses behind the inferior vena cava. However, there are often supernumerary (anomalous, aberrant or accessory) renal arteries arising from the aorta above or below the typical vessel. Regardless of its origin, each renal artery divides as it approaches the kidney and all the branches usually traverse the hilum. However, a polar artery may occasionally be found entering the medial border of the organ above or below the hilum (see Figs. 4.67 & 4.73).

Several veins unite near the renal hilum, anterior to the arteries, forming the renal vein. On the right the vein runs a short course to terminate in the inferior vena cava. The left renal vein is longer and usually receives the suprarenal and gonadal veins before passing in front of the aorta to reach the inferior vena cava (see Fig. 4.65). Because of its termination, the left gonadal vein may become dilated if the renal vein is obstructed. In the male this can lead to swelling of the pampiniform plexus within the scrotum (varicocele).

Fig. 4.71 *Renal arteries exposed by removal of the renal veins and a portion of the inferior vena cava.*

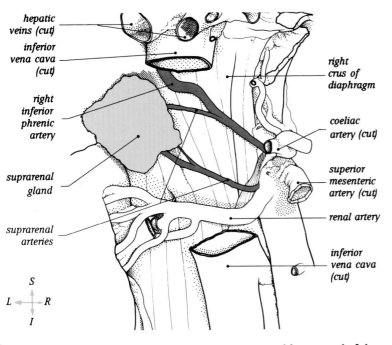

*hepatic
veins (cut)*

*inferior
vena cava
(cut)*

*right
inferior
phrenic
artery*

*suprarenal
gland*

*suprarenal
arteries*

*right
crus of
diaphragm*

*coeliac
artery (cut)*

*superior
mesenteric
artery (cut)*

renal artery

*inferior
vena cava
(cut)*

S

L ← → R

I

*inferior
phrenic
vein &
suprarenal
vein (cut)*

*suprarenal
arteries
(from aorta)*

*left
crus of
diaphragm*

*sympathetic
trunk*

*suprarenal
gland*

*polar
artery*

*renal
vein (cut)*

*psoas
major*

S

R ← → L

I

Fig. 4.72 *Right suprarenal gland and its arteries exposed by removal of the renal vein and a portion of the inferior vena cava.*

Fig. 4.73 *Left suprarenal gland and its vessels. The renal vein and inferior tip of the gland have been excised to reveal the suprarenal arteries.*

SUPRARENAL GLANDS

The suprarenal glands lie adjacent to the superior poles of the kidneys, embedded in the perirenal fat. On the right the gland is tetrahedral and occupies the angle between the superior pole of the kidney and the inferior vena cava (Fig. 4.72). The left gland is crescentic and is applied to the medial border of the kidney above the hilum (Fig. 4.73).

The blood supply to the suprarenal glands is provided by branches of the renal and inferior phrenic arteries and the aorta. The right suprarenal vein is very short and enters the inferior vena cava directly while that on the left descends to enter the left renal vein.

The medulla of each suprarenal gland is richly innervated by preganglionic sympathetic nerves from the adjacent part of the sympathetic trunk.

S
R — L
I

head of
pancreas

second
part of
duodenum

ileocolic
artery (cut)

ascending
colon

psoas
major
(covered
by psoas
fascia)

caecum
(cut)

testicular
vessels

ureter

common
iliac
artery

peritoneum
(cut)

Fig. 4.74 *Course of the right ureter within the abdomen showing some of its relations.*

ABDOMINAL AORTA

The aorta enters the abdomen behind the median arcuate ligament of the diaphragm at the level of the twelfth thoracic vertebra. It descends behind the peritoneum, inclining slightly to the left of the midline to its bifurcation in front of the fourth lumbar vertebra (Fig. 4.75). Throughout its course the abdominal aorta is accompanied by lymph vessels and nodes and is surrounded by a plexus of autonomic nerves (see pages 4.48–4.51).

Posterior to the aorta lie the left lumbar veins, the anterior longitudinal ligament and the lumbar vertebral bodies. Anterior relations, from above downwards, include the body of the pancreas, the splenic and left renal veins, the third part of the duodenum, the root of the mesentery and coils of small intestine.

To the right of the aorta lie the right crus of the diaphragm and the inferior vena cava (Fig. 4.75). On the left are the left diaphragmatic crus, suprarenal gland and kidney.

VISCERAL BRANCHES
Three arteries arise from the anterior aspect of the aorta to supply the alimentary organs while three pairs of lateral branches pass to the suprarenals, kidneys and gonads respectively.

The coeliac and superior mesenteric arteries arise at the levels of the twelfth thoracic and first lumbar vertebrae respectively whilst the smaller inferior mesenteric artery takes origin at the level of the third lumbar vertebra (Fig. 4.75). (For details of the course and distribution of each of these arteries, see pages 4.19–4.21; 4.32–4.38).

The suprarenal branches of the aorta (Fig. 4.75) are small and variable and are often supplemented by branches from the inferior phrenic and renal arteries (see Fig. 4.72; see also Fig. 4.79). The renal arteries usually arise at the level of the first lumbar vertebra but variations are common (see page 4.42).

The long and slender gonadal (testicular or ovarian) arteries usually arise from the aorta just below the renal arteries (Fig. 4.75). The gonadal artery on the right crosses in front of the inferior vena cava, and the arteries of both sides incline downwards and laterally through the retroperitoneal tissues on the psoas major muscles (Fig. 4.76). Each artery is accompanied by one or more gonadal veins and crosses anterior to the ureters but posterior to blood vessels supplying the intestines. Inferiorly the testicular artery follows the psoas major round the pelvic brim and enters the deep inguinal ring (see page 4.10). The ovarian artery crosses the external iliac vessels and pelvic brim to reach the ovary within the pelvis (see page 5.7).

ABDOMINAL PARTS OF URETERS
From the pelviureteric region each ureter descends through the retroperitoneal tissues of the posterior abdominal wall as far as the pelvic brim. Here it crosses in front of the external iliac vessels and continues down the lateral wall of the pelvis (see page 5.8). Within the abdomen the ureter lies on psoas major (see Fig. 4.70) behind which are the lumbar transverse processes, a relationship of radiological significance.

The right ureter commences behind the second part of the duodenum (Fig. 4.74) and is crossed by the root of the mesentery, the gonadal vessels and branches of the superior mesenteric artery and accompanying veins. This ureter is also related to coils of small intestine, and sometimes to the caecum and appendix. The left ureter is covered initially by the pancreas and is subsequently crossed by the gonadal vessels, branches of the inferior mesenteric artery and vein (see Fig. 4.62) and coils of small intestine and sigmoid colon. At the pelvic brim, it passes behind the root of the sigmoid mesocolon.

The blood supply to the abdominal part of the ureter is derived from branches of the renal artery, supplemented by minute peritoneal vessels.

PARIETAL BRANCHES
These vessels supply the diaphragm and the posterior walls of the abdomen and pelvis. The paired inferior phrenic arteries are the first branches of the aorta within the abdomen (Fig. 4.75; see Fig. 4.79) and often furnish small branches to the suprarenal glands before arching upwards and laterally on the abdominal surface of the diaphragm.

Four pairs of lumbar arteries usually arise from the posterolateral aspect of the aorta and supply the posterior abdominal wall (Fig. 4.76; see Fig. 4.77). The arteries on the right cross behind the inferior vena cava to curve round the side of the corresponding vertebral body deep to psoas major.

A single small vessel, the median sacral artery, arises from the back of the aortic bifurcation and descends behind the left common iliac vein to reach the anterior surface of the sacrum (see Fig. 4.77).

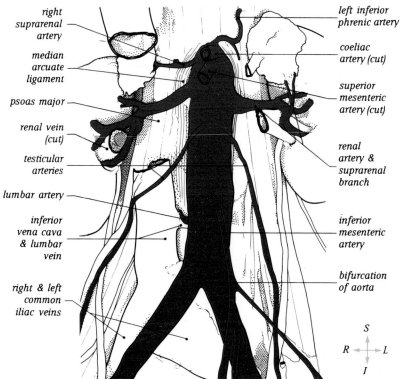

right
suprarenal
artery

left inferior
phrenic artery

median
arcuate
ligament

coeliac
artery (cut)

psoas major

superior
mesenteric
artery (cut)

renal vein
(cut)

renal
artery &
suprarenal
branch

testicular
arteries

lumbar artery

inferior
vena cava
& lumbar
vein

inferior
mesenteric
artery

right & left
common
iliac veins

bifurcation
of aorta

S

R —+— L

I

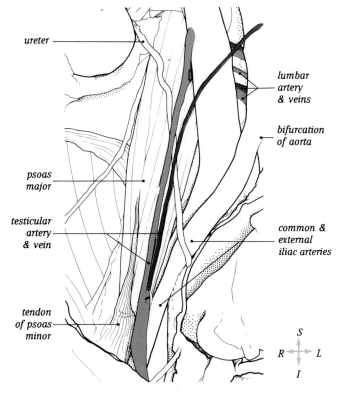

ureter

lumbar
artery
& veins

psoas
major

bifurcation
of aorta

testicular
artery
& vein

common &
external
iliac arteries

tendon
of psoas
minor

S

R —+— L

I

Fig. 4.75 *Abdominal aorta and its branches seen after removal of the renal veins and part of the inferior vena cava.*

Fig. 4.76 *Right testicular vessels within the abdomen. Several lumbar vessels are also seen.*

COMMON AND EXTERNAL ILIAC VESSELS

The aortic bifurcation gives rise to the two common iliac arteries which incline downwards and laterally on the medial aspects of psoas major (Fig. 4.77). The vessels terminate in front of the sacroiliac joints by dividing into internal and external iliac arteries. The right common iliac artery crosses in front of the left common iliac vein, while that on the left is crossed by the inferior mesenteric vessels. The ureter crosses either the lower end of the common iliac artery or the commencement of its external branch (Fig. 4.77). The internal iliac artery begins at the bifurcation of the common iliac artery and descends on the lateral wall of the pelvis (see page 5.21).

The external iliac artery curves round the pelvic brim (Fig. 4.77) and, passing behind the inguinal ligament, enters the thigh as the femoral artery (see page 6.6). The external iliac artery is accompanied on its medial side by the corresponding vein and posterolaterally by psoas major. The external iliac vessels are crossed by the ovarian vessels in the female and by the vas deferens in the male. Near the inguinal ligament the artery gives off the inferior epigastric artery which runs upwards and medially, medial to the deep inguinal ring (see Figs. 4.7 & 4.13).

Fig. 4.77 *Male pelvis and lower abdomen showing the common and external iliac vessels and some of their relations.*

Each external iliac vein begins behind the inguinal ligament as the continuation of the femoral vein (Fig. 4.77). It receives the inferior epigastric vein, ascends on the medial side of the corresponding artery and joins the internal iliac vein (see page 5.21) to form the common iliac vein. The two common iliac veins continue upwards and medially, passing behind the right common iliac artery, by which they may be compressed, before uniting to form the inferior vena cava.

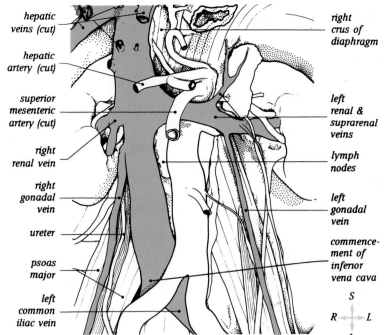

hepatic veins (cut)

hepatic artery (cut)

superior mesenteric artery (cut)

right renal vein

right gonadal vein

ureter

psoas major

left common iliac vein

right crus of diaphragm

left renal & suprarenal veins

lymph nodes

left gonadal vein

commence-ment of inferior vena cava

S
R ← → L
I

Fig. 4.78 *Course and principal tributaries of the inferior vena cava.*

The inferior vena cava is formed at the level of the fifth lumbar vertebra, a little to the right of the midline (Fig. 4.78). It ascends the posterior abdominal wall and pierces the central tendon of the diaphragm to enter the thorax at the level of the eighth thoracic vertebra (see page 2.34).

Behind the inferior vena cava lie the lumbar vertebral bodies, the anterior longitudinal ligament, the right sympathetic chain and right psoas major muscle. In addition, the right renal and right lumbar arteries cross behind the vena cava (see Figs. 4.75 & 4.76) and most of the right suprarenal gland lies posterior to the vessel (Fig. 4.79).

Near its commencement the inferior vena cava is covered anteriorly by peritoneum and coils of small intestine. Superiorly it is crossed by the root of the mesentery, the right gonadal artery (see Fig. 4.76) and the third part of the duodenum (see Fig. 4.40). It continues behind the opening into the lesser sac (see Fig. 4.28) and then grooves the posterior surface of the liver (see Fig. 4.48) before piercing the diaphragm.

To the right of the vena cava lie the gonadal vessels, the ureter, the kidney and renal vessels (Fig. 4.78) and the right lobe of the liver. To the left lie the aorta with its associated lymph nodes, the right crus of the diaphragm and the caudate lobe of the liver.

TRIBUTARIES

The venous drainage of the suprarenal glands, the kidneys and the gonads is asymmetric. On the right, each of these organs is drained by a vein that passes directly into the inferior vena cava (Figs. 4.78 & 4.79); but on the left, the renal vein receives the suprarenal and gonadal veins before crossing in front of the aorta to reach the vena cava. Immediately prior to its passage through the diaphragm the inferior vena cava receives several large hepatic veins (Fig. 4.79).

The parietal tributaries of the inferior vena cava drain the diaphragm and the posterior pelvic and abdominal walls. The lumbar and median sacral veins (see Figs. 4.76 & 4.77) accompany the corresponding arteries, the upper lumbar veins often communicating with the renal, suprarenal, azygos and hemiazygos veins. Two or more inferior phrenic veins drain the undersurface of the diaphragm (Fig. 4.79).

hepatic veins (cut)

inferior phrenic veins

inferior vena cava (cut)

right suprarenal vein

left inferior phrenic vein & artery

left gastric artery

right inferior phrenic artery

S
R ← → L
I

Fig. 4.79 *Upper part of inferior vena cava showing its tributaries. In this specimen the left inferior phrenic artery arises from the left gastric artery.*

Fig. 4.80 *The common and external iliac arteries are accompanied by a chain of lymphatic vessels and nodes.*

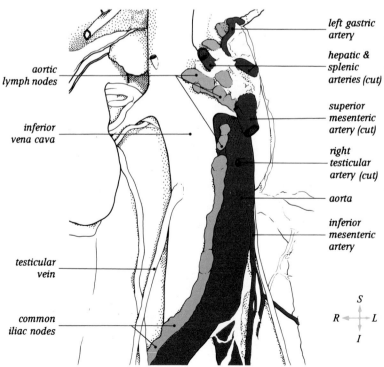

Fig. 4.81 *Removal of the autonomic nerves and retroperitoneal connective tissues reveals the lymphatic vessels and nodes lying on the right side of the aorta.*

Fig. 4.82 *Cisterna chyli revealed by removal of parts of the crura and a segment of aorta.*

The lymphatic vessels and nodes of the abdomen drain the abdominal and pelvic organs as well as the pelvic walls and the lower part of the abdominal wall. (The upper part of the abdominal wall is drained by the internal thoracic and axillary nodes; see page 4.7.) In addition, the abdominal lymphatics receive lymph from the lower limbs and the perineum.

Some lymph nodes are situated adjacent to the organs they drain and include those of the liver and spleen and in the hila of the kidneys. The lymphatic vessels draining most of the abdominal organs accompany blood vessels and pass to nodes grouped around the aorta. Often lymph passes through intermediate nodes situated along the courses of the arteries. Most lymph from the abdominal walls and viscera eventually drains into the thoracic duct.

Because of their deep position, most intra-abdominal lymph nodes are not palpable in the living subject, even when enlarged.

ILIAC LYMPH NODES
The external iliac nodes (Fig. 4.80) receive lymph from the lower limb and perineum via the deep inguinal nodes. In addition, the iliac nodes drain the deeper layers of the abdominal wall below the level of the umbilicus via lymphatic vessels accompanying the inferior epigastric vessels. Lymph from the superficial tissues of the lower abdominal wall reaches the external iliac nodes having passed first to superficial and then to deep inguinal nodes.

The internal iliac nodes drain the pelvic walls and floor and some of the pelvic organs, including the bladder, prostate and uterus. However, lymph from the rectum, sigmoid colon and ovaries drains to the aortic nodes.

From the external and internal iliac nodes, lymph passes to nodes alongside the common iliac artery (Fig. 4.80) and subsequently to the aortic nodes.

AORTIC NODES
The major abdominal lymphatic vessels and their associated nodes are arranged alongside the aorta (Fig. 4.81). The nodes on each side of the aorta receive lymph from the common iliac nodes, posterior abdominal wall, gonads, kidneys and suprarenal glands, while nodes lying immediately anterior to the aorta drain the digestive organs.

Nodes around the origin of the inferior mesenteric artery drain lymph from the upper half of the anal canal, the rectum, and the sigmoid and descending parts of the colon. Nodes lying adjacent to the origins of the superior mesenteric and coeliac arteries drain the spleen, pancreas, liver, stomach, small intestine and the large intestine as far as the splenic flexure.

CISTERNA CHYLI
Efferent lymphatics from the aortic nodes drain into the cisterna chyli (Fig. 4.82). This fusiform sac lies at the level of the upper two lumbar vertebrae, adjacent to the right crus of the diaphragm. It lies behind the right border of the aorta and opens superiorly into the thoracic duct. The duct ascends through the aortic opening of the diaphragm and continues through the thorax to drain into the great veins in the root of the neck (see page 2.35).

AUTONOMIC NERVES OF ABDOMEN

The autonomic innervation to the abdominal viscera is provided by perivascular plexuses of nerves accompanying the arterial supply to each organ. The plexuses comprise sympathetic and parasympathetic fibres of both motor and sensory type. The autonomic nerves control glandular secretion, smooth muscle activity and vasomotor tone; they are also sensory, mediating the distension of hollow organs and the tension on mesenteries.

PARASYMPATHETIC NERVES

Most of the parasympathetic supply is provided by the vagus (X cranial) nerves, but there are small contributions to the distal part of the colon from branches of the pelvic splanchnic nerves which arise from the sacral spinal nerves. The vagi and the pelvic splanchnic nerves carry preganglionic parasympathetic fibres which synapse with postganglionic fibres in the walls of the relevant organs.

From the oesophageal plexus (see page 2.34) two or more vagal trunks (gastric nerves) emerge and accompany the oesophagus through the diaphragm. The anterior trunk, derived mostly from the left vagus nerve (Fig. 4.83), enters the abdomen in front of the oesophagus and gives branches to the anterior surface of the stomach and to the liver. The posterior trunk, derived mostly from the right vagus, descends behind the oesophagus and supplies the posterior surface of the stomach and the coeliac plexus. From this plexus some vagal fibres pass inferiorly to the root of the superior mesenteric artery. The perivascular plexuses that accompany branches of the coeliac and superior mesenteric arteries convey these vagal fibres to all parts of the digestive system as far distally as the splenic flexure of the colon.

The remainder of the large intestine receives its parasympathetic supply from branches of the pelvic splanchnic nerves (nervi erigentes). These ascend through plexuses in the pelvis (see page 5.18) and cross the left common iliac vessels in the root of the sigmoid mesocolon to reach the root of the inferior mesenteric artery. By accompanying branches of this artery, parasympathetic fibres from the sacral segments of the spinal cord supply the descending and sigmoid parts of the colon and the rectum.

SYMPATHETIC NERVES

The sympathetic system in the abdomen comprises two ganglionated trunks and a network of nerves (the aortic or prevertebral plexuses) covering the surface of the aorta.

Each sympathetic trunk enters the abdomen behind the medial arcuate ligament of the diaphragm (Fig. 4.84) and descends along the medial border of psoas major, the trunk on the right lying posterior to the inferior vena cava. Each trunk passes behind the common iliac vessels and crosses the pelvic brim at the ala of the sacrum.

Within the abdomen each trunk bears five lumbar ganglia. Only the upper two ganglia receive fibres from the central nervous system. These preganglionic sympathetic fibres are conveyed in white rami communicantes arising from the first and second lumbar spinal nerves. Some preganglionic fibres synapse in the sympathetic trunk while others pass into branches of the trunk and synapse nearer the target organs.

Each ganglion of the trunk gives a branch, a grey ramus commmunicans, to the corresponding spinal nerve. The postganglionic sympathetic fibres in the grey rami are distributed to the body wall and the lower limb. In addition, the ganglia supply branches (containing both pre- and postganglionic fibres) to the abdominal and pelvic organs. Branches from the upper ganglia reinforce the aortic plexuses whilst the lumbar splanchnic nerves descend from the lower ganglia and cross anterior to the common iliac vessels (Fig. 4.85). The lumbar splanchnic nerves from the right and left trunks unite below the bifurcation of the aorta to form the hypogastric plexus from which branches descend to reach the pelvic autonomic plexuses (see page 5.18).

AORTIC PLEXUSES

The dense network of autonomic nerves (both parasympathetic and sympathetic) that invests the abdominal aorta (Fig. 4.85) has several component plexuses which are named according to the larger branches of the aorta. These are the coeliac, aorticorenal, renal, superior mesenteric, intermesenteric and inferior mesenteric plexuses. From these perivascular plexuses, nerves are distributed to the abdominal organs.

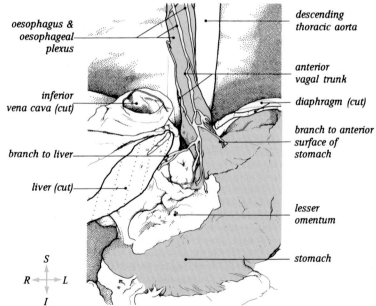

Fig. 4.83 *Anterior vagal trunk revealed by removal of part of the diaphragm and exposure of the lower oesophagus.*

Labels (Fig. 4.83): oesophagus & oesophageal plexus; inferior vena cava (cut); branch to liver; liver (cut); descending thoracic aorta; anterior vagal trunk; diaphragm (cut); branch to anterior surface of stomach; lesser omentum; stomach; S R—L I

The parasympathetic fibres in the aortic plexuses are derived mainly from the posterior vagal trunk which enters the abdomen on the wall of the oesophagus while the sympathetic fibres are provided principally by the

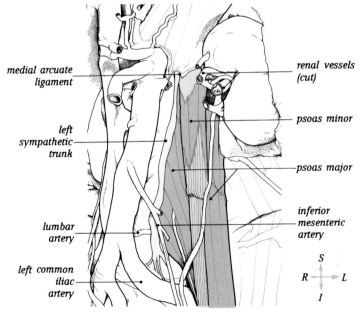

medial arcuate ligament

renal vessels (cut)

left sympathetic trunk

psoas minor

psoas major

lumbar artery

inferior mesenteric artery

left common iliac artery

S
R — L
I

Fig. 4.84 *Lumbar portion of the left sympathetic trunk after removal of the aortic plexuses of nerves.*

splenic & hepatic arteries (cut)

left kidney & suprarenal gland

coeliac plexus

superior mesenteric artery (cut) & plexus

renal plexus

intermesenteric plexus

inferior mesenteric artery & plexus

psoas fascia

lumbar splanchnic nerves

S
R — L
I

Fig. 4.85 *Aortic plexuses of autonomic nerves after removal of aortic nodes and lymph vessels.*

thoracic splanchnic nerves (see page 2.36). These branches of the thoracic portions of the sympathetic trunks pierce the crura of the diaphragm to reach the coeliac plexus. Additional sympathetic fibres are provided by the upper

ganglia of the lumbar sympathetic chain. Within the aortic plexuses are numerous small ganglia in which the pre- and postganglionic sympathetic fibres synapse.

Fig. 4.86 *Removal of the abdominal contents reveals the muscles and nerves of the posterior abdominal wall. On one side some iliac and psoas fasciae have been preserved.*

Fig. 4.87 *Iliacus and psoas major, seen after removal of the inguinal ligament and part of sartorius, attach to the lesser trochanter of the femur. The psoas minor tendon descends to the iliopubic eminence of the hip bone.*

Posterior to the abdominal cavity lie the lumbar spine, the psoas, iliacus and quadratus lumborum muscles, and associated fasciae and nerves (Fig. 4.86). The posterior abdominal wall extends inferiorly to the pelvic brim and superiorly to the attachment of the diaphragm (see page 4.56) while laterally it merges with the anterolateral abdominal wall. The lumbar spine and the postvertebral muscles (erector spinae) are considered on pages 4.59 & 4.60.

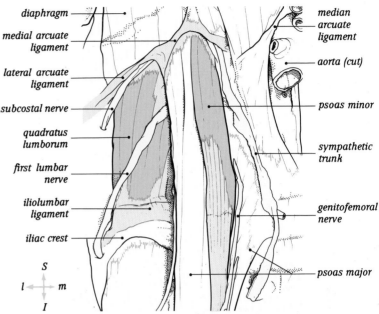

diaphragm —

medial arcuate ligament

lateral arcuate ligament

subcostal nerve —

quadratus lumborum

first lumbar nerve

iliolumbar ligament

iliac crest

— median arcuate ligament

— aorta (cut)

— psoas minor

— sympathetic trunk

— genitofemoral nerve

— psoas major

S

l ←→ m

I

Fig. 4.88 *Quadratus lumborum, psoas minor and the medial and lateral arcuate ligaments of the diaphragm, from beneath which emerge the sympathetic trunk and subcostal nerve respectively.*

MUSCLES
Psoas major
This long fusiform muscle (Fig. 4.86) attaches to the sides of the last thoracic and all five lumbar vertebral bodies, to the intervening discs and to the fronts of the lumbar transverse processes. At the side of each lumbar vertebral body, psoas major attaches to a fascial tunnel conveying a lumbar artery and vein (see Fig. 4.91). The muscle inclines downwards, passing behind the inguinal ligament to enter the anterior compartment of the thigh (Fig. 4.87). The psoas major tendon, which also receives most of the fibres of iliacus, passes in front of the hip joint capsule, from which it is separated by a bursa, and attaches to the lesser trochanter of the femur.

Psoas major is innervated by the anterior rami of the upper lumbar nerves and its principal actions are flexion and medial rotation of the hip joint. In addition, the muscle flexes the lumbar spine both anteriorly and laterally. Within the substance of psoas major the anterior rami of the lumbar nerves form the lumbar plexus, whose branches emerge from the lateral, anterior and medial surfaces of the muscle.

Psoas minor
When present, this small muscle lies on the anterior surface of psoas major and gives way to a long narrow tendon (Fig. 4.87) which attaches to the iliopubic eminence of the hip bone.

Iliacus
This fan-shaped muscle attaches to the upper portion of the abdominal surface of the ilium and adjacent part of the sacrum (Fig. 4.87). Most of its fibres attach to the tendon of psoas major although some reach the femur below the lesser trochanter. The muscle is innervated by the femoral nerve (see Fig. 4.91) and assists psoas major in flexing the hip joint.

Quadratus lumborum
Quadratus lumborum is anchored inferiorly to the iliolumbar ligament and adjacent part of the iliac crest (Fig. 4.88). Superiorly it reaches the medial part of the lower border of the twelfth rib. There are intermediate attachments to the transverse processes of the upper four lumbar vertebrae. This muscle is innervated by the subcostal nerve and anterior rami of the upper three lumbar nerves, and is a lateral flexor of the lumbar spine. When the diaphragm contracts during inspiration, quadratus lumborum stabilizes the twelfth rib.

FASCIAE
The psoas and iliac fasciae form a continuous layer covering the anterior surfaces of their respective muscles (Fig. 4.87). The psoas fascia fuses superiorly with the diaphragmatic fascia, and laterally and inferiorly with the transversalis fascia. Fascial thickenings over the upper parts of psoas major and quadratus lumborum form the medial and lateral arcuate ligaments (lumbocostal arches) which provide attachment for the diaphragm (Fig. 4.88). Fascial layers covering the anterior and posterior surfaces of quadratus lumborum constitute part of the lumbar (thoracolumbar) fascia (see page 4.60). These layers fuse at the lateral border of the muscle and give attachment to transversus abdominis.

NERVES
On each side of the midline the sympathetic trunk enters the abdomen behind the medial arcuate ligament of the diaphragm and descends on the medial border of psoas major (Figs. 4.86 & 4.88). The anterior rami of the subcostal and lumbar nerves emerge through their respective intervertebral foramina and enter the substance of psoas major. All spinal nerves within psoas receive grey rami communicantes from the sympathetic trunk, but only the last thoracic and upper two lumbar nerves supply white rami to the trunk.

Subcostal (T12) nerve
This nerve follows the lower border of the twelfth rib and enters the abdomen behind the lateral arcuate ligament of the diaphragm (Fig. 4.88). It crosses the anterior surface of quadratus lumborum and continues on the deep surface of transversus abdominis. The nerve pierces transversus to enter the neurovascular plane of the abdominal wall, and its subsequent course is similar to that of the lower intercostal nerves (see page 4.6).

4.53

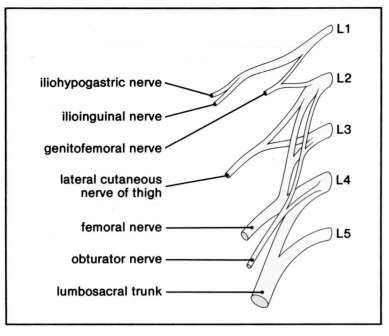

Fig. 4.89 *Diagrammatic representation of the lumbar plexus to show the origins of each of its branches.*

Lumbar plexus

Within psoas major the anterior rami of the upper four lumbar nerves form the lumbar plexus whose branches are distributed to the lower part of the abdominal wall, the lower limb and the sacral plexus in the pelvic cavity (Figs. 4.89 & 4.91).

First lumbar nerve

Although a few first lumbar (L1) fibres contribute to the genitofemoral nerve (Fig. 4.89), most form a nerve that emerges from the lateral border of psoas major and crosses the anterior surface of quadratus lumborum (Fig. 4.90).

After a variable distance this nerve divides into iliohypogastric and ilioinguinal branches (see Fig. 4.86) which continue into the anterolateral abdominal wall. Their paths and distribution are considered on page 4.7.

Genitofemoral (L1 & L2) nerve

This nerve emerges through the anterior surface of psoas major on which it descends, dividing into two branches (Fig. 4.90). The genital branch enters the deep inguinal ring and innervates the cremaster muscle while the femoral branch passes behind the inguinal ligament to reach the subcutaneous tissue covering the femoral triangle (see page 6.50).

Fig. 4.90 *Branches of the lumbar plexus emerge from the substance of psoas major.*

Lateral cutaneous (L2 & L3) nerve of thigh

Emerging from the lateral side of psoas major, this nerve inclines across the anterior surface of iliacus (Fig. 4.90). It passes behind or through the inguinal ligament close to the anterior superior iliac spine (a site of possible entrapment) and enters the superficial fascia on the anterolateral aspect of the thigh (see page 6.3).

Femoral (L2, L3 & L4) nerve

This large nerve appears at the lateral border of psoas major and descends in the gutter between this muscle and iliacus (Fig. 4.90). It innervates iliacus (Fig. 4.91), passes behind the inguinal ligament lateral to the femoral artery and enters the anterior compartment of the thigh (see page 6.6).

Obturator (L2, L3 & L4) nerve

Descending vertically within psoas major, this nerve emerges from the medial border of the muscle near the pelvic brim (Figs. 4.90 & 4.91). It passes behind the common iliac vessels and runs downwards and forwards on the lateral pelvic wall as far as the obturator canal (see page 5.19). Within the canal it divides into anterior and posterior branches which enter the medial compartment of the thigh (see page 6.10).

Lumbosacral trunk

Fibres from the fourth lumbar anterior ramus join those of the fifth to form the lumbosacral trunk (Fig. 4.91). The trunk emerges from the medial side of psoas major (Fig. 4.90) and crosses the sacroiliac joint to enter the pelvis where it contributes to the formation of the sacral plexus (see page 5.19).

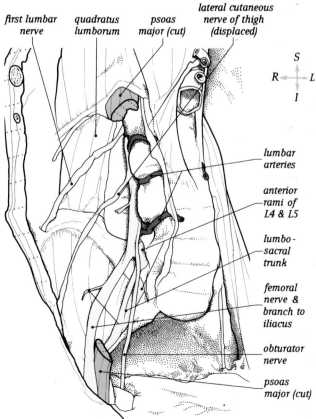

Fig. 4.91 *Removal of most of psoas major and the genitofemoral nerve exposes the lumbar plexus.*

4.55

DIAPHRAGM

The diaphragm is a musculotendinous partition separating the thoracic and abdominal cavities. Its periphery consists of skeletal muscle fibres which merge centrally with an aponeurotic tendon (Fig. 4.92). The diaphragm has a pronounced convexity towards the thorax and has two domes or cupolas, the right usually lying at a higher level than the left (Figs. 4.93 & 4.94).

MUSCULATURE
Peripherally the diaphragmatic muscle is attached to the sternum, the costal margin and the vertebral column. The sternal attachment is by two small slips to the posterior surface of the xiphisternum. The costal attachment is to the inner surfaces of the lower six ribs and costal cartilages (Fig. 4.93) by slips that interdigitate with those of transversus abdominis.

The diaphragm attaches to the vertebral column by two crura (pillars), one on each side of the abdominal aorta (Fig. 4.92). Both crura are anchored to the sides of the upper two lumbar vertebral bodies while the longer right crus is also attached to the third lumbar vertebra. The crura are linked in front of the aorta by the median arcuate ligament, the fibres interdigitating as they ascend towards the central tendon. Lateral to each crus the diaphragm attaches to the transverse process of the first lumbar vertebra by the medial arcuate ligament (lumbocostal arch) and to the twelfth rib by the lateral arcuate ligament (see Fig. 4.88).

A triangular gap, the vertebrocostal trigone (Fig. 4.92), often exists between the fibres attaching to the last rib and those arising from the vertebral column.

Fig. 4.92 *Abdominal surface of the diaphragm after removal of peritoneum. The xiphisternum and anterior costal margin have been excised, including part of the anterior periphery of the diaphragm.*

CENTRAL TENDON
The muscle fibres of the diaphragm converge on the margins of the central tendon, a V-shaped area of dense fibrous tissue with its apex directed towards the xiphisternum and its lateral parts running backwards into the domes (Fig. 4.92). The central tendon gives attachment to the fibrous pericardium and is pierced by the inferior vena cava (Figs. 4.92 & 4.94).

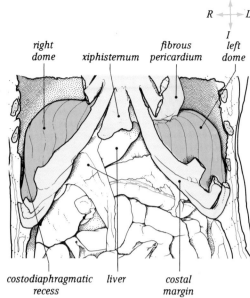

Fig. **4.93** *The anterior chest and abdominal walls have been removed (except for the costal margins) to reveal the diaphragm. The abdominal organs are undisturbed but both lungs and the diaphragmatic pleura have been removed.*

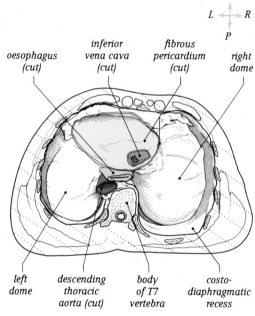

Fig. **4.94** *Thoracic surface of the diaphragm. The parietal pleura remains* in situ *and the base of the fibrous pericardium has been retained.*

STRUCTURES PASSING BETWEEN THORAX AND ABDOMEN

Apertures in the diaphragm transmit the inferior vena cava and the oesophagus. The opening for the inferior vena cava (caval opening) lies to the right of the midline, and the oesophageal opening (hiatus) is slightly to the left (Fig. 4.92). During quiet breathing these openings lie respectively at the levels of the eighth and tenth thoracic vertebrae. The caval opening pierces the central tendon and transmits the right phrenic nerve as well as the vena cava. The oesophageal opening, which also transmits the vagal trunks and branches of the left gastric vessels, is surrounded by muscle fibres of the right crus (Fig. 4.92). The left phrenic nerve pierces the left dome adjacent to the apex of the heart while on each side the thoracic splanchnic nerves pass through the crura to reach the coeliac plexus. The left crus may also be pierced by the hemiazygos vein.

DIAPHRAGM

The aorta enters the abdomen by descending behind rather than through the diaphragm and is accompanied by the thoracic duct and azygos vein (Fig. 4.95). The three vessels pass behind the median arcuate ligament and in front of the twelfth thoracic vertebral body. The subcostal nerves and vessels enter the abdomen behind the lateral arcuate ligaments anterior to quadratus lumborum while the sympathetic trunks descend behind the medial arcuate ligaments anterior to psoas major (see Figs. 4.88 & 4.92). Close to the xiphisternum the superior epigastric vessels (branches of the internal thoracic vessels) pass between the sternal and costal slips of the diaphragm to enter the rectus sheath. Around the periphery of the diaphragm, intercostal nerves and vessels pass between the muscular slips to leave the lower intercostal spaces and reach the abdominal wall.

MOVEMENTS

The diaphragm is an important muscle of inspiration and also assists the muscles of the abdominal walls and pelvic floor in raising the pressure within the abdomen and pelvis. Thus, the diaphragm contracts during acts of lifting and straining (for example, defecation and childbirth).

The shape and position of the diaphragm vary according to body position and the phase of ventilation. During full inspiration the diaphragm contracts, pulling its central tendon downwards to approximately the level of the tenth thoracic vertebra. The descent of the diaphragm, which is enhanced by an upright body posture, enlarges the thoracic cavity. When the diaphragm relaxes during expiration, its central tendon is pushed superiorly by intra-abdominal pressure, compressing the thoracic contents. With the body recumbent or head downwards, this upwards displacement is accentuated by the weight of the abdominal organs.

NERVE SUPPLY

The right and left phrenic nerves provide the main motor and sensory supply to the diaphragm. The phrenic nerves arise in the neck, from the third, fourth and fifth cervical nerves (see page 7.9). Each nerve descends through the thorax (see page 2.32) and divides into terminal branches which pierce the diaphragm and innervate it from the abdominal surface.

Each phrenic nerve provides the motor supply to its own half of the diaphragm except the crus, which is innervated by the lower intercostal nerves. In addition, each phrenic nerve carries sensory fibres from the pericardium and from pleura and peritoneum covering the central portion of the diaphragm. Irritation of these sensory fibres may produce pain referred to the shoulder, since the skin covering this area is also supplied by the fourth cervical segment of the spinal cord. Sensory fibres from the peritoneum and pleura covering the periphery of the diaphragm are conveyed by the lower intercostal nerves.

BLOOD SUPPLY

The major blood supply is provided by the inferior phrenic arteries (see Fig. 4.92) which are usually direct branches of the aorta (see Fig. 4.79). The corresponding veins drain into the inferior vena cava. Also, the musculophrenic vessels (terminal branches of the internal thoracic vessels) supply the periphery of the diaphragm.

RELATIONS

The inferior surface of the diaphragm is in contact with abdominal organs including the liver, kidneys, spleen and stomach. Its thoracic surface is related to the heart and lungs and their associated pericardium and pleura (see Figs. 4.93 & 4.94). Upward and downward excursions of the diaphragm cause corresponding movements of all the organs related to it. During the later stages of expiration the periphery of the diaphragm comes into contact with the chest wall as the costodiaphragmatic recesses deepen (see Fig. 4.93).

Fig. 4.95 *The aortic opening of the diaphragm has been opened by division of the median arcuate ligament and removal of parts of both crura. The aorta is accompanied by the azygos vein and thoracic duct.*

Fig. 4.96 *Lateral and superior views of a typical (third) lumbar vertebra.*

VERTEBRAE

The upper four lumbar vertebrae are very similar. Each has a large body with concave sides and a comparatively small vertebral foramen (Fig. 4.96). The tapering transverse processes are directed laterally and backwards and bear small accessory processes on their posterior surfaces. The spinous process is deep and rectangular. Facets on the superior articular processes face medially to 'grasp' the laterally directed inferior facets of the vertebra above.

The fifth lumbar vertebra has shorter transverse processes and a less angular spinous process. Its inferior articular facets are widely separated and face anteriorly. They articulate with the sacrum (Fig. 4.97) and prevent forward displacement of the vertebra. One or both transverse processes may be fused with the upper part of the sacrum (sacralization of the fifth lumbar vertebra), which can cause difficulty in the interpretation of radiographs.

JOINTS

In the anatomical position the lumbar intervertebral discs are thicker anteriorly than posteriorly; this wedging is especially noticeable in the lumbosacral disc (between the fifth vertebra and the sacrum). Synovial joints similar to those in other regions of the spine occur between the facets on the articular processes of the lumbar vertebrae and also between facets on the fifth vertebra and the sacrum.

Adjacent laminae are joined by ligamenta flava and neighbouring spines by interspinous and supraspinous ligaments. It is through these ligaments that a needle is inserted when a lumbar puncture is performed. From the transverse process of the fifth vertebra, the iliolumbar ligament radiates laterally to reach the iliac crest and the front of the sacroiliac joint.

MOVEMENTS

The lumbar spine possesses considerable mobility in extension, flexion and lateral flexion. However, only a small amount of rotation is possible because of the orientation of the articular processes. Extension is produced by the erector spinae muscles while flexion, often gravity-assisted and accompanied by flexion at the hip joints, is brought about by contraction of the rectus abdominis muscles. Lateral flexion is produced by the external and internal oblique muscles of the abdomen and by psoas major and erector spinae.

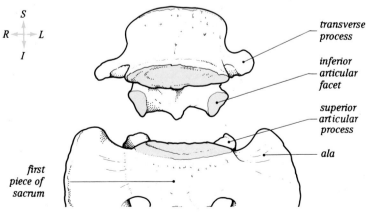

Fig. 4.97 *Anterior view of fifth lumbar vertebra and upper part of sacrum. The inferior articular facets are widely separated and articulate with facets on the superior processes of the sacrum.*

LUMBAR FASCIA

The lumbar (thoracolumbar) fascia comprises the deep fascia and intermuscular septa of the lumbar region. On each side the three layers, anterior, middle and posterior (Fig. 4.98), merge near the lateral borders of erector spinae and quadratus lumborum, continuing laterally as a single fibrous sheet that provides attachment for the transversus abdominis and internal oblique muscles of the abdominal wall.

The posterior layer is the deep fascia of the loin overlying erector spinae and gives attachment to latissimus dorsi. It is thickest inferiorly where it attaches to the iliac crest but fades out superiorly. Medially the posterior layer attaches to the lumbar spinous processes. The middle layer lies in between erector spinae and quadratus lumborum and attaches to the tips of the lumbar transverse processes. This layer extends from the iliac crest to the twelfth rib. The anterior layer lies in front of quadratus lumborum, attaching medially to the anterior aspects of the lumbar transverse processes and blending inferiorly with the iliolumbar ligament.

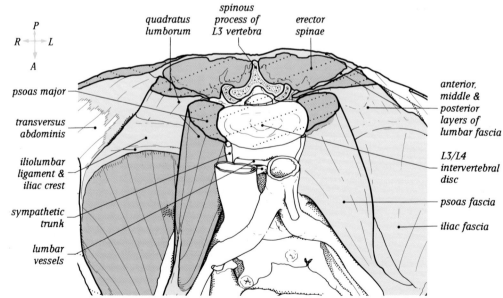

Fig. 4.98 *Transverse section at the level of the disc between the third and fourth lumbar vertebrae. Most of the psoas and lumbar fasciae has been preserved.*

ERECTOR SPINAE

The erector spinae (postvertebral) group of muscles occupies the groove between the spinous and transverse processes of the vertebrae (Fig. 4.98). More substantial in the lumbar region than elsewhere, these muscles are important in maintaining the upright position of the trunk. Bilateral contraction of erector spinae produces extension of the lumbar spine while unilateral contraction assists in lateral flexion. Erector spinae is innervated by the posterior rami of the lumbar spinal nerves.

5
PELVIS AND PERINEUM

PELVIC CAVITY

lumbo-sacral trunk (cut)   *L5 vertebra*   *promontory & ala of sacrum*

obturator internus   *anterior rami of S1 & S2*   *piriformis*   *pelvic inlet*   *iliopectineal line*

Fig. 5.1 *Pelvis and lower abdomen after removal of all the organs and most of the vessels to demonstrate the pelvic inlet and cavity.*

The pelvic cavity is continuous superiorly with the abdominal cavity; but by convention an arbitrary plane, the pelvic inlet (pelvic brim), is used to delineate the two regions (Fig. 5.1). The inlet lies at approximately 45 degrees to the horizontal and is bounded posteriorly by the sacral promontory, laterally by the arcuate and iliopectineal lines, and anteriorly by the pubic crests and the upper margin of the pubic symphysis (Fig. 5.2).

The lateral walls of the pelvis are formed principally by the hip bones and the obturator internus muscles. Above each of these muscles is the obturator

canal which transmits the obturator nerve and artery into the thigh. The posterior wall of the pelvis comprises the sacrum and the piriformis muscles. On each side piriformis leaves the pelvis through the greater sciatic foramen and enters the gluteal region, accompanied by several nerves and vessels.

The pelvic floor (pelvic diaphragm), formed by the left and right levator ani muscles (see Figs. 5.6 & 5.16), is pierced in the midline by structures that continue into the perineum.

The pelvis contains the bladder, the rectum, parts of the sigmoid colon and ileum, and sometimes the appendix. In the male the pelvis also contains the prostate gland (Fig. 5.3) and seminal vesicles while in the female pelvis (Fig. 5.4) lie the ovaries, uterine tubes, uterus and upper part of the vagina. However, in the infant the pelvic cavity is comparatively shallow and therefore parts of the bladder and uterus may lie above the pelvic brim.

PERITONEUM

Peritoneum lines the lateral and posterior pelvic walls and covers most of the pelvic organs (Figs. 5.3 & 5.4). In both sexes peritoneum passes from the anterior abdominal wall onto the upper surface of the bladder. In the male it descends on the posterior surface of the bladder and then passes onto the rectum forming a recess, the rectovesical pouch (Fig. 5.3). In the female, peritoneum is reflected from the bladder onto the anterior surface of the body of the uterus, forming the vesicouterine pouch (Fig. 5.4). It covers the fundus of the uterus and on each side passes over the uterine tube, forming the broad ligament. From the posterior surface of the uterus, peritoneum passes over the vault of the vagina onto the anterior wall of the rectum, forming the rectouterine pouch (of Douglas). Fluid may collect in the rectovesical pouch of the male or the rectouterine pouch of the female and, if infected, may form a pelvic abscess.

pelvic inlet   promontory & ala of sacrum

greater sciatic foramen

sacrospinous ligament

sacrotuberous ligament

obturator canal

pubic crest & tubercle   pubic symphysis

sacroiliac joint

iliopectineal line

obturator membrane

  Fig. 5.2 *Bony pelvis to show the pelvic inlet, greater sciatic foramen and obturator canal.*

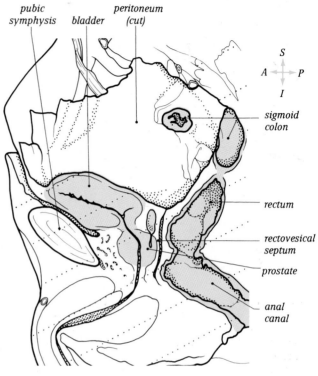

Fig. 5.3 *Median sagittal section through the male pelvis to show the peritoneum and the principal pelvic viscera.*

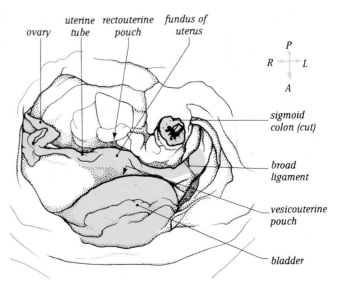

Fig. 5.4 *Superior view of peritoneum and organs within the female pelvis. The small intestine and most of the sigmoid colon have been removed.*

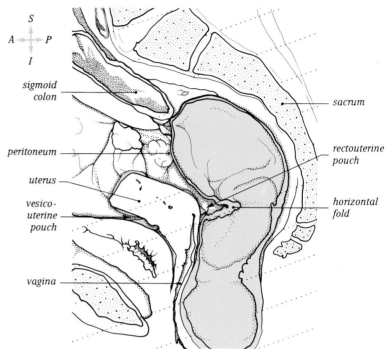

Fig. 5.5 *Median sagittal section through the female pelvis to show the rectum and its anterior and posterior relations.*

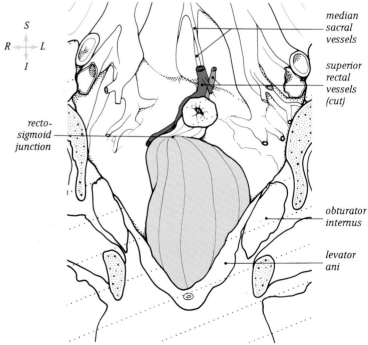

Fig. 5.6 *Coronal section through the male pelvis. The anterior aspect of the rectum has been stripped of its peritoneum.*

The rectum is the distal portion of the large intestine and lies in the posterior part of the pelvic cavity (Fig. 5.5). It is continuous with the sigmoid colon at the rectosigmoid junction in front of the third piece of the sacrum (Fig. 5.6), where there is often an acute angulation in the intestine which may hamper the passage of a colonoscope. The rectum curves downwards and forwards lying first on the anterior surface of the sacrum and then on the upper surface of the pelvic floor. It deviates to either side of the midline and these lateral flexures become pronounced when the organ is distended. The lowest part of the rectum, the ampulla, is its most dilatable portion. Turning abruptly downwards and backwards, the rectum pierces the pelvic floor and terminates at the anorectal junction where it is continuous with the anal canal (see Fig. 5.3).

Unlike the colon, the rectum is devoid of appendices epiploicae and has no taeniae, the longitudinal muscle being distributed uniformly around its circumference. The mucous membrane projects into the rectal lumen as three shelves which form the horizontal folds.

RELATIONS
The upper two-thirds of the rectum are related to the most inferior portion of the peritoneal cavity. The upper third of the organ is covered anteriorly and on both sides by peritoneum while the middle third, lying behind the rectouterine or rectovesical pouch, has peritoneum only on its anterior surface (Fig. 5.5).

Posterior to the upper part of the rectum are the sacrum, coccyx and the piriformis muscles while its lower part rests on the levator ani muscles. Descending behind the organ are the superior rectal vessels (Fig. 5.6), the hypogastric plexus of autonomic nerves and, on each side of the midline, the sympathetic trunk and sacral plexus. Lateral to the rectum lie the pelvic plexuses of autonomic nerves and the ureters.

Anterior to the upper portion of the rectum lie those parts of the sigmoid colon and ileum that descend into the pelvic cavity. The anterior relations of the rectal ampulla are of clinical interest since they may be palpated on rectal examination. In the male these are the prostate gland (see Fig. 5.3), the base of the bladder, the seminal vesicles and ampullae of the vasa. These structures are separated from the rectum by the rectovesical septum. In the female, since the rectal ampulla lies adjacent to the posterior wall of the vagina, rectal examination permits palpation of the cervix of the uterus (Fig. 5.5).

BLOOD SUPPLY
The arterial supply to the rectum is derived principally from the superior rectal artery (Fig. 5.6), the continuation of the inferior mesenteric artery (see page 4.38). This supply may be supplemented by middle rectal branches from the internal iliac arteries. Venous blood drains into the portal venous system via the superior rectal vein and its continuation, the inferior mesenteric vein. In addition, middle rectal veins drain into the internal iliac veins. Since the superior and middle rectal veins interconnect, the wall of the rectum is a site of portacaval anastomosis (see page 4.38).

The female internal organs of reproduction include the uterus and vagina and the paired ovaries and uterine (Fallopian) tubes. The uterus and ovaries are particularly affected by atrophy (shrinkage) after the menopause.

UTERUS
The uterus is a pear-shaped organ approximately 8cm in length. Its major component is the body (or corpus) which remains somewhat enlarged after pregnancy. Inferiorly the uterus tapers into the cylindrical neck or cervix which protrudes into the upper part of the vagina (Fig. 5.7).

The uterus is most commonly positioned with its body lying on the superior surface of the bladder (see Fig. 5.8). As the bladder fills and empties, the uterine body moves on the relatively immobile cervix. Thus, when the bladder is empty the uterine body is anteflexed (bent forwards on the cervix), but when the bladder is distended the uterus may become retroflexed.

Fig. 5.7 *Median sagittal section to show the right ovary, uterine tube and broad ligament.*

Body

The uterine body possesses anteroinferior and posterosuperior surfaces. The right and left borders give attachment to the broad ligaments and superiorly give origin to the uterine tubes (Figs. 5.7 & 5.9). The rounded upper end of the organ between the attachments of the tubes is called the fundus.

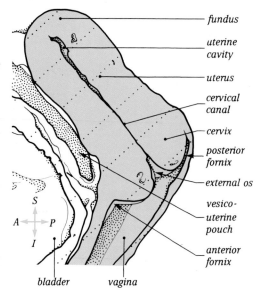

Fig. 5.8 *Uterus and vagina in sagittal section.*

On the posterosuperior surface of the uterus lie the sigmoid colon or coils of ileum. Both surfaces are covered with peritoneum which continues laterally as the broad ligament (Fig. 5.9). Adjacent to the uterus within each broad ligament is the uterine artery and its associated plexus of veins. On each side the round ligaments of the ovary and the uterus attach to the uterine body close to the origin of the uterine tube. These ligaments, remnants of the fetal gubernaculum, run laterally within the broad ligament, often raising ridges in the peritoneum. The round ligament of the ovary attaches to the medial pole of the ovary while the round ligament of the uterus runs to the lateral pelvic wall and turns forwards in the extraperitoneal tissues. Crossing the external iliac vessels the round ligament of the uterus enters the deep inguinal ring, traverses the inguinal canal and terminates in the subcutaneous tissues of the labium majus (see Fig. 4.14).

The wall of the uterine body comprises a thick layer of smooth muscle (myometrium) lined by a vascular mucosa (endometrium) whose thickness varies with the phases of the menstrual cycle. The uterine cavity is narrow in sagittal section but triangular in coronal section, being widest where the uterine tubes enter (Fig. 5.9). Tapering inferiorly, the cavity communicates via the internal os with the cervical canal.

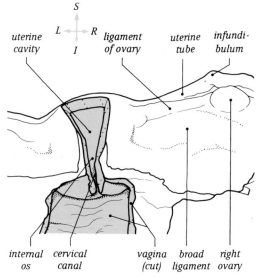

Fig. 5.9 *Uterine cavity and cervical canal exposed by removal of parts of their posterior walls.*

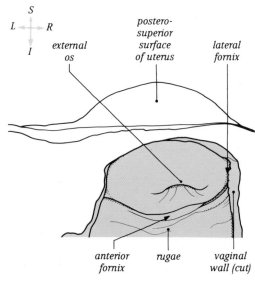

Fig. 5.10 *Intravaginal part of the cervix revealed by removal of the posterior wall of the vagina.*

Cervix

The uterine cervix is thick-walled and has a narrow lumen, the cervical canal (Figs. 5.8 & 5.9). The canal communicates superiorly with the uterine cavity via the internal os and opens inferiorly into the vagina at the external os. The external os is circular before the first vaginal delivery but thereafter presents an oval aperture. Although approximately in line with the body of the uterus, the cervix lies roughly at right angles to the long axis of the vagina (a position called anteversion). Approximately half of the cervix lies above the vagina (the supravaginal part) and is covered posteriorly by peritoneum passing from the uterine body onto the vault of the vagina. The root of the broad ligament is attached to this part of the cervix and contains the uterine artery (Fig. 5.11). The vessel runs medially above the ureter before turning upwards at the side of the cervix. Anteriorly the supravaginal part of the cervix is related to the posterior surface of the bladder.

The uterine body and cervix are supplied by branches of the uterine artery, a branch of the internal iliac artery. Venous blood passes into the uterine venous plexus which drains into the internal iliac vein (Fig. 5.11).

UTERINE TUBES

The paired uterine tubes, each approximately 10cm long, run in the free upper borders of the broad ligaments (Figs. 5.7 & 5.9) and convey ova from the ovaries to the uterine cavity. Near the ovary the lumen of each tube communicates with the peritoneal cavity via its pelvic aperture. This minute opening leads into the funnel-shaped infundibulum which bears a series of finger-like processes, the fimbriae, one of which attaches to the ovary. The infundibulum leads into the ampulla which forms the comparatively wide lateral part of the uterine tube. The medial part of the tube, the isthmus, is narrower and continues through the uterine wall as the intramural part of the tube.

The blood supply to the medial part of the uterine tube is provided by terminal branches of the uterine artery. This vessel runs laterally in the upper part of the broad ligament and anastomoses with the ovarian artery which supplies the lateral portion of the tube. Venous blood drains into veins which accompany the arteries.

Fertilization of ova normally occurs in the uterine tube, usually within its ampulla. Blockage of the tubes is a common cause of infertility.

OVARIES

The ovaries lie close to the lateral pelvic walls suspended from the posterior surfaces of the broad ligaments (Fig. 5.7). Each ovary is ovoid, approximately 4cm long and 2cm broad, with one pole directed medially towards the uterus and the other laterally towards the fimbriated end of the uterine tube. Each ovary is attached to the broad ligament by a sleeve of peritoneum, the mesovarium, which conveys the ovarian vessels. However, most of the ovarian surface is devoid of peritoneum. The round ligament of the ovary attaches to the medial pole of the organ and runs within the broad ligament to reach the side of the uterine body. The ovary often lies in a hollow, the ovarian fossa, on the lateral pelvic wall between the external and internal iliac vessels. The ureter descends in the posterior boundary of the fossa while the obturator nerve and vessels cross its floor (Fig. 5.11). Therefore, ovarian disease which involves the parietal peritoneum at this site may produce pain referred via the nerve to the medial side of the thigh.

The ovary is supplied by the ovarian artery (Fig. 5.11), a direct branch of the abdominal aorta (see page 4.46). After crossing the pelvic brim this vessel enters the broad ligament and divides into terminal branches within the mesovarium. The ovary is drained by numerous veins (the pampiniform plexus) which unite to form the ovarian vein. On the right the ovarian vein terminates in the inferior vena cava while the left ovarian vein usually joins the renal vein (see page 4.47).

VAGINA

The vagina is a midline tubular organ approximately 8cm to 10cm long which slopes downwards and forwards (Figs. 5.7 & 5.8). Its upper two-thirds, including the blind-ending vault, lie in the pelvic cavity. The vagina pierces the pelvic floor and terminates inferiorly by opening into the vestibule between the labia minora (see page 5.26). The anterior and posterior vaginal walls lie in mutual contact so that the lumen forms a transverse cleft. The lining possesses numerous transverse ridges (rugae; Fig. 5.10).

The uterine cervix pierces the upper part of the anterior vaginal wall and an annular groove surrounds the intravaginal part of the cervix. This groove is deepest superiorly where it is termed the posterior fornix (Fig. 5.8). On either

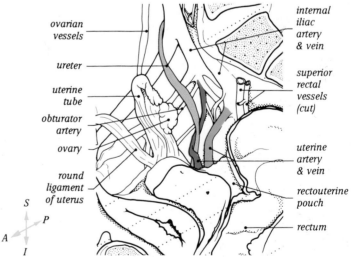

Fig. 5.11 *Uterine vessels and the ureter after removal of peritoneum from the lateral pelvic wall.*

side are the lateral fornices whilst below the cervix is the comparatively shallow anterior fornix (Fig. 5.10).

Anteriorly the vagina is closely applied to the posterior wall of the bladder and urethra. Posteriorly lie the rectouterine pouch of peritoneum and the ampulla of the rectum (Fig. 5.11). Lateral to its inferior third are the medial borders of the levator ani muscles which provide important support to the vagina and uterus. Weakness of the pelvic floor musculature may lead to prolapse (descent of the uterus into the vagina).

The blood supply to the vagina is provided by branches of the uterine arteries and occasionally by vessels arising directly from the internal iliac arteries (see Fig. 5.31). Venous blood passes into an extensive venous plexus surrounding the upper vagina and eventually reaches the internal iliac veins.

PELVIC URETERS

Each ureter enters the pelvis by crossing in front of the common iliac vessels or the commencement of the external iliac vessels (Fig. 5.12). The ureter passes downwards and backwards before curving forwards to reach the posterior surface of the bladder. The ureter crosses the medial aspect of the obturator nerve and vessels and the superior vesical vessels before running forwards along the levator ani muscle. The pelvic peritoneum covers the medial aspect of the ureter and separates it from the rectum, sigmoid colon or coils of ileum.

Fig. 5.12 Coronal section through the male pelvis to show the interior of the bladder and some of its relations.

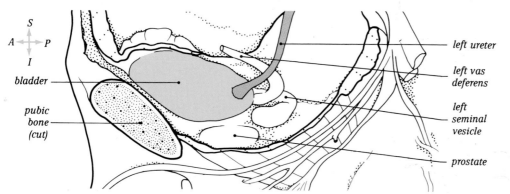

In the male the ureter passes under the vas deferens and terminates near the seminal vesicle (Fig. 5.13). In the female the ureter descends close to the posterior aspect of the ovary (see Fig. 5.11) and is covered with peritoneum as far as the root of the broad ligament. Here the ureter crosses under the uterine artery and is closely related to the lateral aspect of the uterine cervix.

5.8   Fig. 5.13 Lateral view of the male bladder after removal of the left pelvic wall.

BLADDER

The urinary bladder lies in the anterior part of the pelvic cavity. When distended the organ has an approximately spherical shape but, when empty, assumes the form of a tetrahedron with four angles and four surfaces. The two posterolateral angles receive the ureters while the inferior angle, the bladder neck, is continuous with the urethra. The anterior angle gives attachment to a fibrous cord, the urachus (Fig. 5.14). This remnant of the fetal allantois ascends in the extraperitoneal tissues of the anterior abdominal wall to the umbilicus.

The superior surface and the two inferolateral surfaces expand considerably as urine accumulates but the comparatively small posterior surface or base expands only a little. This surface lies between the entrances of the ureters and the bladder neck.

The wall of the bladder consists of smooth muscle (detrusor) whose thickness gradually decreases as the organ fills. Although the interior of the distended bladder is smooth, the mucosa becomes rugose when the organ empties (Fig. 5.14), except in the region of the trigone. This is the triangular area between the ureteric orifices and the internal urethral meatus (Fig. 5.12). The ureters pierce the musculature of the bladder wall obliquely and open at slit-like orifices.

RELATIONS

The superior surface of the bladder is covered with peritoneum (Fig. 5.13) on which rest coils of ileum and sigmoid colon. In both sexes the inferolateral surfaces lie against the obturator internus and levator ani muscles and their associated fascial coverings. Between the bladder and these muscles run the obturator nerve and vessels and the superior vesical vessels (see Fig. 5.15). Anterior to the bladder is the retropubic space, filled with adipose tissue and veins (Fig. 5.14). The empty bladder lies behind the pubic bones but as it fills it rises above the level of the pubic crests and comes into contact with the lower part of the anterior abdominal wall. The distended bladder intervenes between the parietal peritoneum and the abdominal wall (see Fig. 4.20); surgical access to the organ can be made through an abdominal incision without opening the peritoneum.

In the male the seminal vesicle and the ampulla of the vas deferens are applied to each side of the posterior surface. Peritoneum descends a short distance on this surface before being reflected onto the anterior surface of the rectum to form the rectovesical pouch (Fig. 5.12). Below the level of this pouch the bladder is related to the rectovesical septum and the ampulla of the rectum. Inferior to the male bladder lie the prostate gland and the prostatic plexus of veins.

In the female the posterior part of the superior surface of the bladder is related to the body of the uterus (Fig. 5.14). Peritoneum passes from the superior surface of the bladder onto the uterine body, forming the vesico-uterine pouch. Against the posterior surface of the female bladder lie the cervix of the uterus and the anterior wall of the vagina. The inferior angle of the bladder in the female lies at a lower level than in the male and is closely related to the two levator ani muscles.

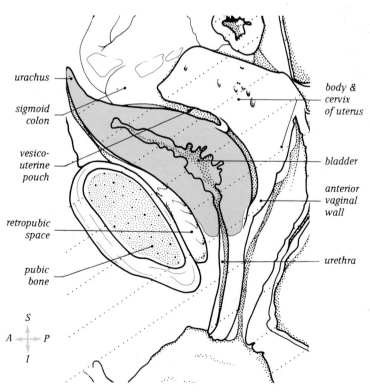

Fig. 5.14 *Median sagittal section through the female pelvis to show the bladder and some of its relations.*

BLADDER

BLOOD SUPPLY

The bladder is supplied by branches of the internal iliac arteries. On each side the superior vesical artery runs anteriorly along the lateral wall of the pelvis before turning medially to reach the bladder (Fig. 5.15). Anteriorly each superior vesical artery is continuous with a fibrous cord, the medial umbilical ligament (remnant of the fetal umbilical artery), which continues upwards in the extraperitoneal tissues of the abdominal wall to the umbilicus (see Fig. 4.20). The bladder receives additional supply from the inferior vesical and obturator arteries. In the female the uterine and vaginal arteries also contribute to the vascular supply of the bladder.

Venous blood passes into an extensive network of veins, the vesical plexus, which communicates with the prostatic or vaginal venous plexus and drains into the internal iliac veins.

NERVE SUPPLY

The motor innervation to the detrusor muscle is by parasympathetic nerves conveyed in the pelvic splanchnic nerves and the pelvic plexus of autonomic nerves (see Fig. 5.29). In the male the smooth muscle surrounding the bladder neck (preprostatic sphincter) is innervated by sympathetic nerves derived from the hypogastric plexus. The parasympathetic motor innervation stimulates contraction of the bladder at the time of micturition while the sympathetic supply to the male bladder neck prevents reflux ejaculation.

FEMALE URETHRA

The female urethra is a fibromuscular tube 3–4cm long and begins at the internal urethral meatus of the bladder. Embedded in the anterior wall of the vagina it inclines downwards and forwards through the pelvic floor (Fig. 5.16) and terminates in the vestibule at the external meatus between the clitoris and the vaginal opening.

The urethra passes close to the posterior aspect of the pubic symphysis (see Fig. 5.14) to which it is attached by the pubourethral ligaments. The middle third of the urethra is encircled by striated muscle fibres of the external urethral sphincter, whose tone is the principal factor in maintaining continence of urine. Occlusive force on the urethra is also provided by contractions of the levator ani muscles (Fig. 5.16). Micturition occurs when bladder pressure is higher than urethral pressure and is produced by contraction of the detrusor muscle of the bladder wall accompanied by relaxation of the external urethral sphincter.

The arterial supply to the urethra is provided by the inferior vesical arteries, and venous drainage is to the vesical plexus of veins. The mucosa receives its sensory nerve supply from the pudendal nerve, derived from the second, third and fourth sacral segments which also innervate the external urethral sphincter by way of the pelvic splanchnic nerves.

Fig. 5.15 *The arterial supply and relations of the bladder in a female pelvis.*

Fig. 5.16 *The female urethra pierces the pelvic floor embedded in the anterior wall of the vagina. The fibres of levator ani pass close to the urethra and attach to the vagina.*

MALE URETHRA

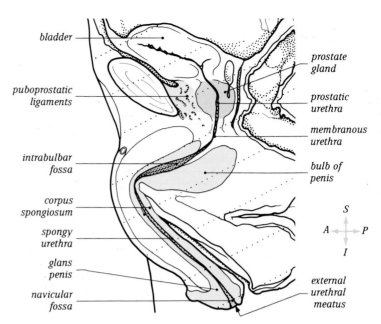

Fig. 5.17 *Male urethra in sagittal section showing its course and its prostatic, membranous and spongy parts.*

The male urethra is a fibromuscular tube approximately 20cm long. Beginning at the internal urethral meatus of the bladder, it descends through the prostate gland and the pelvic floor and enters the bulb of the penis (Fig. 5.17). It then traverses the corpus spongiosum and glans of the penis and terminates at the external urethral meatus. In the male the urethra not only drains urine from the bladder but also receives secretions from the prostatic ducts, the ejaculatory ducts and the ducts of the bulbourethral glands.

The male urethra is described in three parts: prostatic, membranous and spongy. The prostatic and membranous parts pass downwards while the spongy part turns forwards in the bulb of the penis (Fig. 5.17). This abrupt angulation is of considerable importance when catheters or cystoscopes are being introduced. Furthermore, although the spongy and prostatic parts can be readily dilated, the external meatus and the membranous urethra are comparatively narrow.

PROSTATIC URETHRA

Passing downwards and forwards through the prostate gland, the prostatic urethra is approximately 3cm long. A midline ridge, the urethral crest, projects from the posterior wall producing bilateral grooves, the prostatic sinuses (Fig. 5.18). Opening into each sinus are numerous prostatic ducts. The urethral crest is most prominent near its midpoint where it presents a rounded elevation, the seminal colliculus. A midline orifice on the colliculus leads into a blind-ending sac, the prostatic utricle, which is a remnant of the ducts that give rise to the uterus in the female embryo. On each side of the utricle is the opening of the ejaculatory duct.

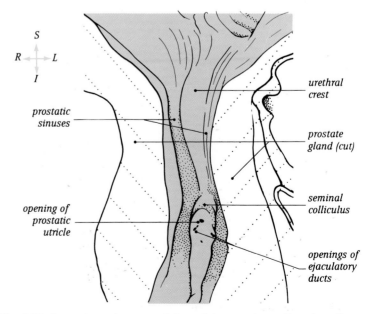

Fig. 5.18 *Prostatic urethra opened through its anterior wall to show the urethral crest and seminal colliculus.*

MALE URETHRA

MEMBRANOUS URETHRA
Emerging from the anterior aspect of the apex of
the prostate, the membranous urethra descends
through the pelvic floor and pierces the perineal
membrane. It is approximately 2cm long and its
mucosa is folded, giving the lumen a stellate
appearance on cross-section. Encircling the
membranous urethra is the striated muscle of the
external urethral sphincter (Fig. 5.19), the main
structure responsible for urinary continence.
Lateral to the sphincter are the medial borders of
the levatores ani.

Posterolateral to the membranous urethra are the
paired bulbourethral glands, each about 1cm in
diameter (Fig. 5.19). Their ducts pierce the perineal
membrane and open into the spongy urethra. An
additional posterior relation of the membranous
urethra is the ampulla of the rectum while
anteriorly lies the lower border of the pubic
symphysis to which the urethra is anchored by the
pubourethral ligaments.

SPONGY URETHRA
The spongy (or penile) urethra is approximately
15cm in length, commencing in the bulb of the
penis and traversing the erectile tissue of the
corpus spongiosum and glans (see Fig. 5.17). The
mucosa presents numerous small recesses or
lacunae and most of its lumen forms a transverse
slit. Within the bulb the urethra is wider, forming
the intrabulbar fossa. The lumen is also expanded
within the glans to form the navicular fossa which
opens at the surface as a vertical slit, the external
meatus.

BLOOD SUPPLY
The prostatic and membranous parts of the
urethra receive blood from the inferior vesical
arteries. The spongy part is supplied by the
internal pudendal artery via the dorsal arteries of
the penis and the arteries to the bulb. Venous
blood passes into the prostatic venous plexus and
the internal pudendal veins.

NERVE SUPPLY
The principal sensory innervation of the mucosa is
provided by the pudendal (S2, S3 & S4) nerve, a
branch of the sacral plexus. The same spinal cord
segments innervate the external sphincter via the
pelvic splanchnic nerves.

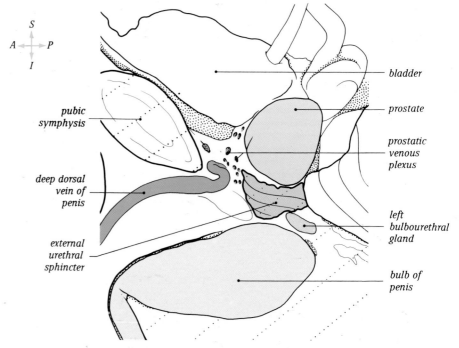

Fig. 5.19 *The left pelvic wall and levator ani have been removed to show the prostate gland, external
urethral sphincter, left bulbourethral gland and bulb of the penis.*

MALE INTERNAL ORGANS OF REPRODUCTION

The organs of reproduction in the male comprise the paired testes, epididymides, **vasa deferentia**, seminal vesicles, ejaculatory ducts and bulbo-urethral glands as well as the prostate gland and penis. The superficial organs (the external genitalia) include the penis (see page 5.24), and the testes and epididymides within the scrotum (see pages 4.11 & 4.12).

The reproductive organs described here are those that lie within the pelvis, namely the prostate, the seminal vesicles, the intrapelvic parts of the vasa deferentia (Fig. 5.20) and the ejaculatory ducts.

PROSTATE GLAND

The prostate gland is an approximately spherical organ lying immediately below the bladder (Fig. 5.21). The flattened superior surface (base) is applied to the neck of the bladder and is pierced by the urethra, which descends through the gland and emerges near the blunt apex. The prostate is divided into two lateral lobes which meet anteriorly, and a single posterior lobe. The part of the posterior lobe which lies above and between the ejaculatory ducts (see below) is sometimes described as the median lobe (see Fig. 5.22).

Fig. 5.20 *Lateral view of the prostate gland, left seminal vesicle and vasa deferentia.*

Anteriorly the prostate is anchored by the puboprostatic ligaments (see Fig. 5.17) to the inferior border of the pubic symphysis. Inferior to the organ lies the membranous urethra (Fig. 5.21) surrounded by the external urethral sphincter, and posteriorly are the rectovesical septum and the ampulla of the rectum. On each side of the prostate is the medial border of levator ani.

With advancing age the gland often enlarges (benign prostatic hypertrophy) and may obstruct the prostatic part of the urethra, thus interfering with micturition.

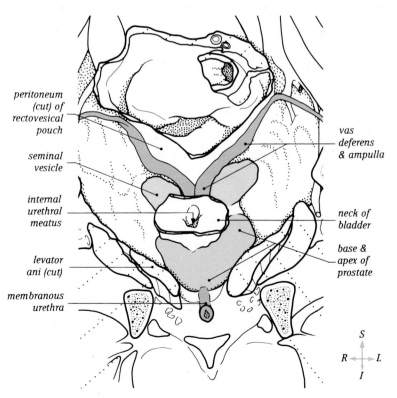

Fig. 5.21 *Coronal section of the pelvic walls and floor. Most of the bladder has been removed to reveal the prostate, the seminal vesicles and the vasa deferentia.*

MALE INTERNAL ORGANS OF REPRODUCTION

SEMINAL VESICLES

Each seminal vesicle is a sacculated gland approximately 3cm long, lying lateral to the ampulla of the vas deferens (Figs. 5.22 & 5.23). The seminal vesicles lie in front of the rectum and rectovesical pouch of peritoneum (Fig. 5.21) and extend up the posterior wall of the bladder as far as the terminal parts of the ureters (Fig. 5.23).

VASA DEFERENTIA

Each vas (ductus) deferens begins at the tail of the epididymis in the scrotum, ascends within the spermatic cord and traverses the inguinal canal (see pages 4.9–4.12). After emerging from the deep inguinal ring the vas runs along the lateral pelvic wall, covered by peritoneum, and passes medial to the superior vesical vessels and obturator nerve and vessels. The vas then crosses above the ureter (Fig. 5.23) and turns downwards and medially posterior to the bladder (Fig. 5.21). The terminal part of the vas is dilated to form the ampulla

which lies medial to the seminal vesicle. The ampulla is related posteriorly to the peritoneum of the rectovesical pouch and to the rectovesical septum and rectum.

EJACULATORY DUCTS

The duct of each seminal vesicle joins the terminal part of the corresponding vas deferens to form the ejaculatory duct (Fig. 5.22). The right and left ducts pierce the prostate gland and run downwards, forwards and medially through its substance to open into the prostatic urethra at slit-like orifices on the summit of the seminal colliculus.

BULBOURETHRAL GLANDS

The bulbourethral glands lie adjacent to the membranous urethra and are described on page 5.12.

BLOOD SUPPLY

The artery to the vas deferens is usually a small vessel which arises from the superior vesical artery and accompanies the vas as far as the epididymis. The ampulla of the vas, the seminal vesicle and prostate gland are supplied by the inferior vesical artery. From the internal reproductive organs, blood passes into the venous plexus (see Fig. 5.19) surrounding the prostate to drain into the internal iliac veins.

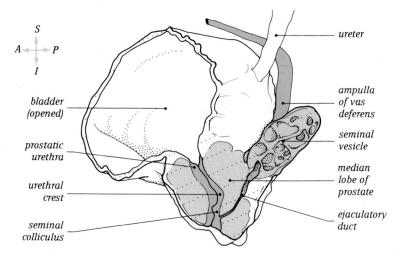

Fig. 5.22 *Prostate gland and left seminal vesicle dissected to reveal the ejaculatory duct and interior of the seminal vesicle.*

EJACULATION

Semen contains spermatozoa from the testes and secretions from the ampullae of the vasa, the seminal vesicles and prostate. Under the control of the sympathetic nervous system, contraction of smooth muscle in the vasa, seminal vesicles and prostate propels secretions into the prostatic urethra. Semen is then expelled from the urethra by contractions of the bulbo-spongiosus muscles which compress the bulb of the penis (see page 5.25). Reflux of semen into the bladder is prevented by contraction of the smooth muscle in the wall of the bladder neck, the 'preprostatic sphincter'.

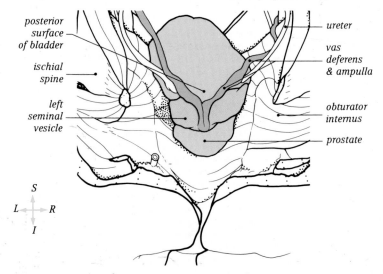

Fig. 5.23 *Removal of the rectum and the posterior wall of the pelvis exposes the bladder, prostate, seminal vesicles and vasa deferentia.*

PELVIC WALL

The pelvic wall is formed by the bones of the pelvic girdle and their associated ligaments, muscles and fascia. The bony component comprises the right and left hip (innominate) bones anterolaterally and the sacrum and coccyx posteriorly. The pelvic cavity is usually wider and shallower in females because of differences in the shapes of the surrounding bones.

HIP BONE

Only the medial or pelvic surface of the hip bone is considered here; the lateral surface is described on page 6.14. Each hip bone is formed by the fusion of three components: ilium; ischium; and pubis (Fig. 5.24). The anterosuperior part of the ilium contributes to the posterior abdominal wall and gives attachment to iliacus. The lower portion of the ilium extends below the pelvic inlet and contributes to the lateral wall of the pelvis. On the posterior part of the bone is the auricular surface which articulates with the corresponding surface of the sacrum at the sacroiliac joint.

The ischium has a rounded tuberosity inferiorly which bears body weight in the sitting position. Posteriorly is the pointed spine which separates the greater and lesser sciatic notches while anteriorly the ramus of the ischium ascends to fuse with the inferior pubic ramus.

The pubic bone has a superior ramus which merges with the ilium near the iliopubic eminence, and an inferior ramus which is continuous below the obturator foramen with the ramus of the ischium. The bodies of the right and left pubic bones articulate at the pubic symphysis.

The obturator foramen is a large aperture which is almost completely occluded by the obturator membrane (Fig. 5.26). Superiorly the membrane leaves a small gap, the obturator canal, which provides access between the pelvis and the medial compartment of the thigh.

SACRUM AND COCCYX

The sacrum is a triangular bone formed by the fusion of five vertebrae (Figs. 5.24 & 5.25). It slopes backwards and downwards and is concave anteriorly. The fused pedicles and laminae enclose the sacral canal, triangular in cross-section, which opens inferiorly at the V-shaped sacral hiatus. The canal contains the lower part of the cauda equina, comprising the roots of the sacral and coccygeal nerves. The anterior rami of the upper four sacral nerves pass into the pelvis via the anterior sacral foramina and contribute to the sacral plexus. The posterior rami traverse the posterior sacral foramina and are distributed to the erector spinae muscles and the overlying skin (see Fig. 1.24). Lateral to the foramina are the lateral masses, each of which bears an auricular process directed laterally for articulation with the ilium.

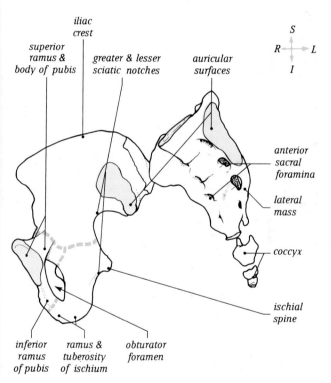

Fig. 5.24 Oblique view of the right hip bone showing its three compartments, the sacrum and coccyx.

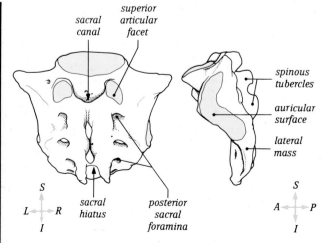

Fig. 5.25 Posterosuperior (left) and lateral (right) views of the sacrum.

PELVIC WALL

The upper surface of the sacrum resembles that of a lumbar vertebra and carries the lumbosacral disc. The two superior articular processes of the sacrum face backwards and articulate with the inferior processes of the fifth lumbar vertebra. The dorsal surface of the sacrum gives attachment to the lowest fibres of erector spinae (Fig. 5.26) and to the posterior ligaments of the sacroiliac joint and the sacrotuberous ligament. The anterior and posterior longitudinal ligaments of the vertebral column terminate inferiorly by attaching to the sacrum.

Below the apex of the sacrum lies the coccyx (see Fig.5.24), which may be a small single bone or up to four rudimentary vertebrae. The coccyx and sacrum usually articulate via a small intervertebral disc or they may be fused.

JOINTS

The pelvic girdle forms a stable ring because its constituent bones are bound together at the two sacroiliac joints and the pubic symphysis.

The symphysis is a secondary cartilaginous joint containing a pad of fibrocartilage (Fig. 5.26) that separates the bodies of the right and left pubic bones. The joint is stabilized by ligaments attached around the articular margins.

The sacroiliac joints allow very little movement since the articulating surfaces of their synovial cavities are irregular and behind each cavity is the thick posterior interosseous ligament. Each joint is further supported by the anterior and posterior sacroiliac ligaments and the iliolumbar, sacrospinous and sacrotuberous ligaments. Body weight acting downwards through the lumbosacral disc tends to rotate the sacrum, tipping its lower part backwards, a movement prevented by the sacrospinous and sacrotuberous ligaments (Fig. 5.26).

The iliolumbar ligament attaches medially to the transverse process of the fifth lumbar vertebra and laterally to the iliac crest and front of the sacroiliac joint (see Fig. 4.98). The sacrospinous ligament passes from the lateral margins of the sacrum and coccyx to the ischial spine. The larger sacrotuberous ligament passes from the side and dorsum of the sacrum and the posterior surface of the ilium to the ischial tuberosity. These two ligaments convert the greater and lesser sciatic notches into the greater and lesser sciatic foramina (Fig. 5.26).

Fig. 5.26 *Right hemipelvis showing the pubic symphysis, the obturator membrane, the ligaments and the foramina.*

MUSCLES

Piriformis is a flat muscle attached to the pelvic surfaces of the second, third and fourth pieces of the sacrum (Fig. 5.26). Running laterally through the greater sciatic foramen, it enters the buttock and attaches to the upper part of the greater trochanter of the femur (see Fig. 6.14). Piriformis rotates the hip joint laterally and is innervated by the first and second sacral nerves. Numerous vessels and nerves accompany the muscle through the greater sciatic foramen (Fig. 5.27).

Obturator internus is a fan-shaped muscle with an extensive attachment to the margins of the obturator foramen and the pelvic surface of the obturator membrane (Fig. 5.27). The muscle fibres converge on the lesser sciatic foramen to form a tendon which turns laterally to enter the gluteal region. The tendon is attached to the medial aspect of the greater trochanter (see page 6.14). The muscle laterally rotates the hip joint. The nerve to obturator internus (L5, S1 & S2) enters the muscle within the perineum, having traversed the greater and lesser sciatic foramina.

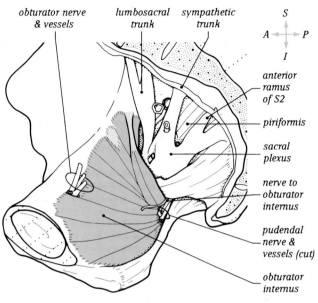

Fig. 5.27 *Right hemipelvis showing the pelvic attachment of obturator internus.*

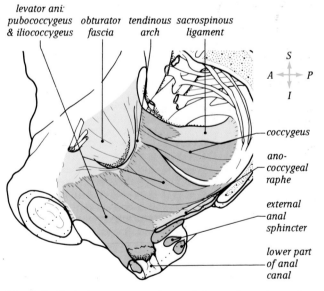

Fig. 5.28 *Right levator ani and part of the anal canal seen in a median sagittal section of the pelvis.*

PELVIC FASCIA

This term includes the fascial lining of the pelvic walls and the extraperitoneal connective tissue surrounding the pelvic viscera. The pelvic surfaces of oburator internus (Fig. 5.28), piriformis and levator ani are covered by fascia which is continuous superiorly with the transversalis and iliac fasciae. Between the pelvic organs, the pelvic fascia mostly comprises a loose meshwork of connective tissue. However, it is condensed anterior to the rectum to form the rectovesical septum; and some of the arteries to the pelvic organs, notably the uterine and vaginal vessels, are accompanied by thickened bands of fascia termed 'ligaments'. Radiating from the uterine cervix to the pelvic walls are the lateral sacral and uterosacral ligaments which provide support to the uterus.

PELVIC FLOOR

The pelvic floor (or diaphragm) is a muscular partition separating the cavity of the pelvis above from the perineum below. It slopes downwards towards the midline, forming a trough which inclines downwards and forwards (see Fig. 5.28). In the midline anteriorly, a narrow triangular gap between the muscle fibres transmits the urethra in both sexes and also the vagina in the female (see Fig. 5.16). Posteriorly the pelvic floor is pierced by the anal canal.

The pelvic floor is formed principally by the right and left levator ani muscles which are supplemented posteriorly by the coccygeus muscles (see insignificant muscle applied to the medial surface of the sacrospinous ligament. Medially it attaches to the lateral border of the sacrum and coccyx, and laterally to the ischial spine.

Each levator ani muscle has a linear attachment to the pelvic wall. The attachment commences anteriorly on the pelvic surface of the body of the pubis and continues backwards as the tendinous arch along the obturator fascia as far as the ischial spine (Fig. 5.28). The levator ani muscle has two parts; the anterior part comprises pubococcygeus and the posterior part is iliococcygeus.

Pubococcygeus runs backwards and downwards. Its most anterior fibres lies near the midline and pass close to the urethra. In the male they support the prostate (see Fig. 5.21) while in the female they attach to the vagina (see Fig. 5.16). The intermediate fibres of pubococcygeus reach the anal canal and either attach to its wall or loop behind the anorectal junction. The posterior fibres attach to the coccyx or fuse in the midline with fibres from the other side at the anococcygeal raphe.

The fibres of iliococcygeus pass downwards and medially below those of pubococcygeus and attach to the coccyx and to the anococcygeal raphe.

The levator ani muscles support the pelvic contents, actively maintaining the positions of the pelvic viscera. In particular, the pubococcygeus muscles compress the urethra and vagina and provide support for the bladder and uterus. The levator ani fibres that loop behind the anal canal help to maintain the angulation of the anorectal junction and play an important role in the continence of faeces. During defecation, the fibres attaching to the wall of the anal canal pull the organ upwards. Levator ani and coccygeus are innervated by the fourth sacral nerve. Weakening of these muscles is a common gynaecological problem and may result in the descent (prolapse) of the pelvic organs.

PELVIC NERVES

AUTONOMIC NERVES
The pelvic organs receive their autonomic innervation via the right and left pelvic plexuses which lie adjacent to the internal iliac arteries and their branches (Fig. 5.29). Nerves pass from the plexuses to the bladder, reproductive organs and the rectum by accompanying the arteries to these organs. The plexuses and their branches contain efferent fibres from both the parasympathetic and sympathetic systems which reach the pelvis from different parts of the spinal cord.

Parasympathetic nerves
The parasympathetic component of the pelvic plexuses is provided by the pelvic splanchnic nerves ('nervi erigentes'), which leave the spinal cord in the second, third and fourth sacral nerves. The parasympathetic fibres control micturition, dilation of the erectile tissues in both sexes, and defecation. The pelvic plexuses also provide the parasympathetic innervation of the descending and sigmoid parts of the colon. These fibres ascend into the abdomen in the hypogastric plexus and are distributed with the branches of the inferior mesenteric artery.

Fig. 5.29 *Right pelvic plexus of autonomic nerves and its relations. The obturator nerve descends on the pelvic wall. This specimen has an abnormal obturator artery.*

Sympathetic nerves

The sympathetic fibres destined for the pelvic autonomic plexuses arise from the lower thoracic and upper lumbar segments of the spinal cord and pass through the lumbar portions of the sympathetic trunks on the posterior abdominal wall. From here they descend in the hypogastric plexus (see Fig. 4.86) to reach the pelvis. Sympathetic fibres innervate the smooth muscle of the reproductive organs in both sexes and in the male are responsible for coordinating ejaculation (see page 5.14).

The two sympathetic trunks pass from the posterior abdominal wall (see page 4.50) into the pelvis by crossing behind the common iliac vessels. Descending in front of the sacrum and piriformis muscles (Fig. 5.30), they incline towards the midline and fuse on the anterior surface of the coccyx. Each trunk bears three or four ganglia and provides grey rami communicantes, consisting of postganglionic fibres, to the sacral nerves. These fibres supply blood vessels and sweat glands in the areas innervated by the appropriate sacral nerves.

SPINAL NERVES

The lower lumbar and upper sacral spinal nerves are predominantly concerned with the innervation of the lower limb. However, a few fibres derived from these spinal nerves are distributed to the pelvic walls and floor and to the perineum.

Obturator nerve

This branch of the lumbar plexus (see page 4.54) emerges from the medial border of psoas major and enters the pelvis by crossing in front of the ala of the sacrum. It descends lateral to the common and internal iliac vessels and the ureter (Fig. 5.29) and reaches the medial surface of obturator internus. The nerve approaches the obturator vessels from above and continues with them through the obturator canal (Fig. 5.30) into the medial compartment of the thigh (see page 6.10).

Sacral and coccygeal nerves

The anterior rami of the first four sacral nerves emerge through the anterior sacral foramina and merge to form the sacral plexus (Fig. 5.30). The fifth sacral nerve and the coccygeal nerves are small and do not contribute to the plexus. All the sacral and coccygeal nerves receive grey rami communicantes from the sympathetic trunk.

Sacral plexus

This plexus lies on the posterior pelvic wall in front of piriformis (Fig. 5.30), covered anteriorly by the pelvic fascia. The plexus is formed by the anterior rami of the upper four sacral nerves and is supplemented by the lumbosacral trunk which carries fibres from the fourth and fifth lumbar nerves (see page 4.55). The branches of the sacral plexus are distributed to the lower limb, pelvic walls and floor, and perineum as indicated in the following table.

Fig. 5.30 *Right hemipelvis showing the sacral plexus and pelvic portion of the sympathetic trunk.*

To lower limb:
superior gluteal nerve
inferior gluteal nerve
tibial nerve (sciatic nerve)
common peroneal nerve (sciatic nerve)
posterior cutaneous nerve of thigh
nerve to quadratus femoris
To pelvic walls and floor:
nerve to levator ani (and to coccygeus)
nerve to piriformis
nerve to obturator internus
To perineum:
pudendal nerve

Those branches which leave the pelvis accompany the piriformis through the greater sciatic foramen to enter the buttock (see page 6.14). The nerve to obturator internus and the pudendal nerve then pass forwards through the lesser sciatic foramen to gain the perineum (Fig. 5.30).

PELVIC BLOOD VESSELS AND LYMPHATICS

The pelvic walls and floor and the pelvic organs receive most of their arterial supply from branches of the internal iliac artery, which also provides branches to the perineum and lower limb. The rectum, however, receives its principal supply from the superior rectal artery (see pages 4.38 & 5.5) while the posterior wall of the pelvis is supplied by the median sacral artery (see Fig. 5.30). The ovaries are supplied by the ovarian branches of the abdominal aorta (see pages 4.46 & 5.7).

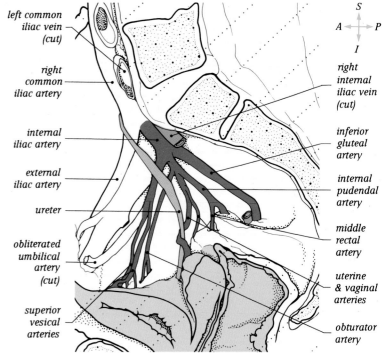

Fig. 5.31 *Right internal iliac artery and some of its branches.*

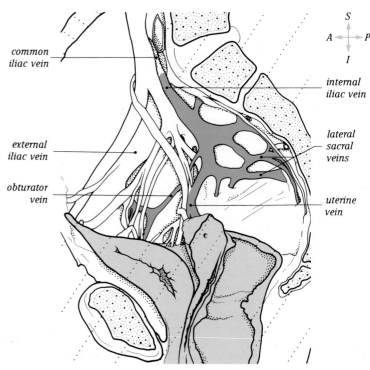

Fig. 5.32 *Right internal iliac vein and tributaries.*

INTERNAL ILIAC ARTERY AND BRANCHES

The internal iliac artery arises in front of the sacroiliac joint as one of the terminal branches of the common iliac artery (Fig. 5.31). The internal iliac artery runs downwards and backwards on the lateral pelvic wall, giving rise to visceral and parietal branches.

Visceral branches

The superior vesical artery runs forwards adjacent to the bladder to which it gives one or more branches (see Fig. 5.15). The artery usually gives rise to the slender artery to the vas deferens and then continues forwards as the obliterated umbilical artery to the umbilicus (see page 4.6).

The inferior vesical artery occurs only in the male and supplies the lower part of the bladder, the prostate gland, the seminal vesicle and the pelvic ureter.

The uterine artery runs medially in the root of the broad ligament, crosses above the ureter (see Fig. 5.11) and supplies the vagina and the uterine cervix, body and tube. The artery follows the lateral border of the body of the uterus, then runs laterally in the broad ligament, close to the uterine tube, and terminates by anastomosing with the ovarian artery.

The vagina is supplied by branches of the uterine artery together with one or two small vaginal arteries from the internal iliac artery.

The middle rectal artery (Fig. 5.31) supplies the muscle coat of the rectum and in the male may give additional branches to the prostate and seminal vesicles.

Parietal branches

The obturator artery runs downwards and forwards, with the corresponding vein and nerve, to enter the obturator canal. It supplies the medial compartment of the thigh and the hip joint (see page 6.10). Occasionally the obturator artery takes origin from the inferior epigastric artery and descends into the pelvis to reach the obturator canal. Such a vessel (an 'abnormal obturator artery'; see Fig. 5.29) passes close to the femoral ring and may be damaged during femoral hernia operations.

The superior and inferior gluteal arteries pass through the greater sciatic foramen into the buttock, the superior artery running above piriformis (see Fig. 5.30) and the inferior below (see page 6.14).

The internal pudendal artery provides the principal arterial supply to the perineum. The artery passes through the greater sciatic foramen into the gluteal region, curves round the ischial spine and then passes forwards through the lesser sciatic foramen into the perineum (see page 5.23).

The iliolumbar artery ascends the posterior abdominal wall to anastomose with the lower lumbar arteries.

The lateral sacral artery supplies the posterior wall of the pelvis and anatomoses with the median sacral artery.

INTERNAL ILIAC VEIN AND TRIBUTARIES

The branches of the internal iliac artery are accompanied by veins which drain the buttock and perineum, the pelvic walls and most of the pelvic organs. These veins unite to form the internal iliac vein,(Fig. 5.32). which ascends on the lateral pelvic wall posterior to the artery. The vein terminates by joining the external iliac vein to form the common iliac vein (see page 4.46).

Most of the veins emerging from the pelvic organs anastomose freely, forming extensive venous plexuses (the vesical, prostatic, uterine and vaginal plexuses). While most blood from these plexuses passes into the internal iliac vein, some enters either the superior rectal vein via portacaval anastomoses or the vertebral veins via the anterior sacral foramina.

PELVIC LYMPHATICS

Lymph from the pelvis is drained by lymphatic vessels that accompany the arteries. Most of the lymph drains into nodes adjacent to the internal iliac artery and then into efferent vessels which pass to the common iliac nodes (see page 4.49). However, lymphatic vessels from the ovaries and the rectum pass directly to the aortic nodes, and some vessels from the body of the uterus accompany the round ligament through the inguinal canal to terminate in the superficial inguinal nodes.

Below the pelvic floor lies the perineum, a superficial region traversed by the anal canal and the lower parts of the genital and urinary tracts. It is a diamond-shaped area, extending anteriorly to the pubic symphysis, posteriorly to the coccyx and laterally to the ischial tuberosities (Fig. 5.33). On each side the region is bounded by the conjoined rami of the ischium and pubis and by the sacrotuberous ligament, which is overlapped by the inferior border of gluteus maximus. Inferiorly the perineum is bounded by skin. By convention, the perineum is divided into two triangles by a line joining the ischial tuberosities. Posteriorly is the anal triangle, containing the anal canal and the ischiorectal fossae, and anteriorly lies the urogenital triangle, containing the external genitalia.

Fig. 5.33 *Deep dissection of the male perineum to show its boundaries. The bulb of the penis has been removed to expose the perineal membrane and gluteus maximus on one side has been resected to reveal the sacrotuberous ligament.*

ANAL CANAL

The anal canal is the terminal part of the intestine and is approximately 4cm long. Beginning at the anorectal junction, it passes downwards and backwards as far as the anus (see Fig. 5.3). Its upper part is lined by mucous membrane bearing several longitudinal ridges, the anal columns; while the lower part is lined by skin. The smooth muscle coat of the rectum continues into the wall of the anal canal and thickens to form the internal anal sphincter. Striated fibres from the levator ani muscles (Fig. 5.34) blend with the outer layers of the wall and continue as far as the perianal skin.

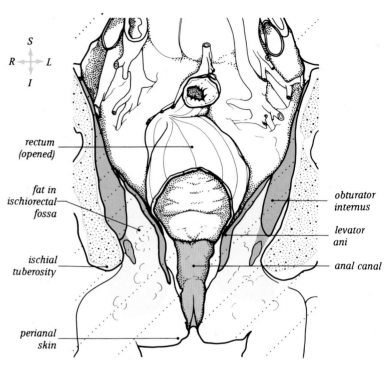

Fig. 5.34 *Coronal section through the pelvis to show the anal canal and ischiorectal fossae.*

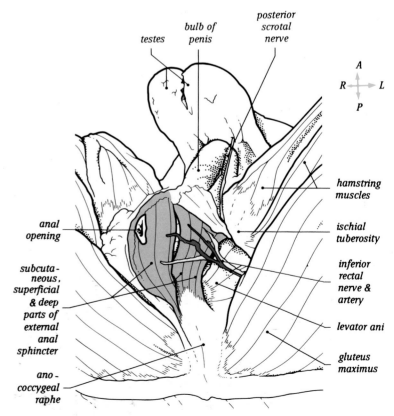

Fig. 5.35 *Oblique view of the anal triangle to show the parts of the external anal sphincter and the inferior rectal nerve and vessels.*

In addition, the lower two-thirds of the anal canal are encircled by the external anal sphincter (Fig. 5.35), composed of striated muscle fibres. This sphincter comprises three parts of which the uppermost, the deep part, blends with the levator ani muscles. Inferior to this lies the superficial part, attached posteriorly to the coccyx and anococcygeal raphe and anteriorly to the posterior border of the perineal membrane. The most inferior component of the sphincter, the subcutaneous part, encircles the anal opening. Continence of faeces is not dependent on the external sphincter alone, since the fibres of the levator ani muscles that maintain the anorectal angulation play a major role.

The anal canal is supplied by inferior rectal branches (Fig. 5.35) from the pudendal nerve which innervate the external sphincter and the cutaneous lining. The internal sphincter and the mucous membrane lining the upper part are innervated, like the rectum, by autonomic nerves (see page 5.18). The blood supply is provided by inferior rectal branches of the internal pudendal artery. The anal canal is a site of portacaval anastomosis since venous blood passes not only via inferior rectal veins to the internal iliac vein but also into the superior rectal vein, a tributary of the portal venous system (see page 4.39). Lymph drains from the upper part of the canal to the internal iliac nodes, but from the lower part it passes to the superficial inguinal nodes.

The cutaneous lining of the lower part of the anal canal has a rich nerve supply. Tears (fissures) in this skin are painful and produce reflex spasm of the external sphincter.

ISCHIORECTAL FOSSA

On each side of the anal canal is a fat-filled space extending laterally as far as obturator internus, upwards to the levator ani muscles and downwards to the perianal skin (Fig. 5.34). Anteriorly each fossa tapers and continues above the perineal membrane and external urethral sphincter almost as far as the pubic symphysis. Entering each fossa from the gluteal region via the lesser sciatic foramen are the nerve to obturator internus, the pudendal nerve (Fig. 5.36) and the internal pudendal artery with its venae comitantes.

The nerve to obturator internus arises from the sacral plexus and supplies the muscle from within the ischiorectal fossa (see Fig. 5.27).

The pudendal nerve and the internal pudendal vessels pass along the lateral wall of the fossa in a fascial tunnel, the pudendal canal. Branches from the nerve and artery traverse the upper part of the fossa to supply the anal canal and the posterior part of the scrotum or labium majus (Fig. 5.35).

INTERNAL PUDENDAL ARTERY

This vessel provides most of the arterial blood to the perineum. Arising from the internal iliac artery within the pelvis (see Fig. 5.31), it enters the buttock through the greater sciatic foramen and then traverses the lesser sciatic foramen to enter the ischiorectal fossa. The artery runs forwards along the lateral wall of the fossa in the pudendal canal and gives off inferior rectal branches and posterior scrotal or labial branches. The artery continues above the perineal membrane, where it provides branches to the bulb of the penis (or vestibule) and crus of the penis (or clitoris), and terminates by dividing into deep and dorsal arteries of the penis (or clitoris). In the male the dorsal artery passes below the pubic symphysis and continues along the dorsum of the penile shaft (Fig. 5.36), lateral to the deep dorsal vein, and gives branches to the erectile tissue of the corpus cavernosum. The deep artery pierces the perineal membrane and supplies the erectile tissue of the corpus cavernosum. In the female there are comparable but smaller branches to the clitoris. The internal pudendal artery and its branches are accompanied by venae comitantes which drain into the internal iliac vein.

PUDENDAL NERVE

The pudendal nerve provides the principal innervation to the perineum. It arises from the sacral plexus (S2, S3 & S4) and accompanies the internal pudendal artery into the perineum. In the ischiorectal fossa the nerve divides into the dorsal nerve of penis (or clitoris) and the perineal nerve (Fig. 5.36).

The perineal nerve supplies an inferior rectal branch to the anal canal and posterior scrotal (or labial) branches to the skin of the genitalia (Fig. 5.35). On reaching the anterior part of the perineum, the perineal nerve gives branches to all muscles in the superficial perineal pouch as well as sensory branches to the urethra.

The dorsal nerve of the penis continues forwards with the internal pudendal artery above the perineal membrane and below the pubic symphysis. It runs along the dorsum of the penis, lateral to the dorsal artery (Fig. 5.36), and innervates the skin of the distal two-thirds of the organ. The dorsal nerve of the clitoris has a similar course and distribution.

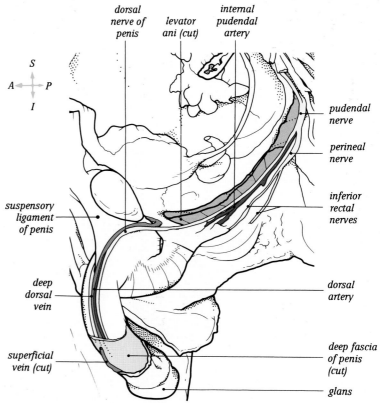

Fig. 5.36 *Left pudendal nerve exposed by removal of the lateral wall of the pelvis.*

MALE EXTERNAL GENITALIA

The male external genitalia comprise the scrotum and the penis. An account of the scrotum and its contents is given on pages 4.11 and 4.12. The penis consists of a shaft which is free and a root which lies in the superficial perineal pouch, attached to the inferior surface of the perineal membrane.

PERINEAL MEMBRANE AND POUCHES

The perineal membrane is a shelf of dense fascia spanning the triangular interval between the right and left ischial and pubic rami (see Fig. 5.33). The membrane has a long free posterior margin and a short anterior margin which is separated from the pubic symphysis by a small gap transmitting the deep dorsal vein of the penis. The central part of the membrane is pierced by the urethra and bulbourethral ducts.

At the root of the penis and around the neck of the scrotum the superficial fascia attaches laterally to the ischial and pubic rami. Posteriorly the fascia is anchored to the free edge of the perineal membrane. The space contained by the superficial fascia of the penis and scrotum is called the superficial perineal pouch. This pouch communicates with the subcutaneous tissues of the anterior abdominal wall but not with the ischiorectal fossae, the thighs or pelvic cavity. If the spongy part of the urethra is ruptured, urine may escape into the superficial pouch (superficial extravasation of urine).

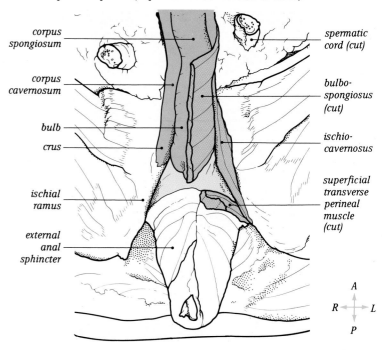

Fig. 5.37 *Root of penis. On one side, ischiocavernosus has been excised to reveal the crus, and bulbospongiosus removed to expose half of the bulb.*

On the pelvic aspect of the perineal membrane lie the external urethral sphincter and bulbourethral glands in a space often called the deep perineal pouch. This pouch is limited superiorly by a layer of fascia covering the upper surface of the sphincter at the level of the apex of the prostate. The term 'urogenital diaphragm' is sometimes applied to the muscular structures contained within the deep perineal pouch.

Fig. 5.38 *'Step' dissection of the shaft of the penis to show the three corpora and the dorsal vessels.*

PENIS

The erectile tissue of the shaft of the penis consists of the paired corpora cavernosa lying in apposition and the midline corpus spongiosum.

The corpus spongiosum is uniform in diameter except at its extremity where it expands into the glans (see Fig. 5.36) whose prominent margin forms the corona of the penis. Proximally the corpus spongiosum continues into the root of the penis to form the bulb which is attached to the inferior surface of the perineal membrane (Fig. 5.37). The spongy (penile) part of the urethra enters the bulb from above, pierces the perineal membrane and curves downwards and forwards. It traverses the corpus spongiosum and glans (see Fig. 5.17) and terminates at the external urethral meatus near the apex of the glans.

Dorsal to the corpus spongiosum are the paired corpora cavernosa (Fig. 5.38) which extend distally as far as the concave proximal surface of the glans. Proximally the corpora cavernosa continue inferior to the pubic symphysis and diverge as the crura. Each crus tapers posteriorly and is attached to the inferior surface of the perineal membrane and the adjacent rami of the pubis and ischium (Fig. 5.37; see Fig. 5.33).

Fascial layers and skin

The three corpora of the penis are enveloped by a sleeve of deep fascia which also covers the dorsal vessels and nerves of the organ (Fig. 5.38). Proximally the deep fascia is anchored to the front of the pubic symphysis by the suspensory ligament of the penis (see Fig. 5.36) while distally it terminates at the corona by fusing with the corpora. Covering the deep fascia is the superficial fascia.

The superficial fascia of the penis is membranous, devoid of fat and traversed by superficial nerves and vessels (see Fig. 5.36). Proximally it is continuous with the superficial fascia of the anterior abdominal wall and can also be traced around the scrotum where it contains smooth muscle, the dartos.

The cutaneous covering of the penis is freely mobile except over the glans to which it is adherent. The skin is reflected distally beyond the corona over the glans to form the hood-like prepuce or foreskin. This is attached to the undersurface of the glans by a vascular fold, the frenulum.

Muscles

Surrounding the bulb of the penis are the paired bulbospongiosus muscles (Fig. 5.37). Their fibres attach to the perineal membrane and pass downwards and backwards to meet at a midline raphe and blend posteriorly with the external anal sphincter. The bulbospongiosus muscles contract during ejaculation and the terminal stages of micturition to compress the urethra and expel its contents.

Covering each crus is the ischiocavernosus muscle (Fig. 5.37). From the posterior end of each crus a small superficial transverse perineal muscle runs medially to the penile bulb. All the penile muscles are innervated by the perineal branch of the pudendal nerve.

Vessels

The erectile tissues of the penis have a rich blood supply. Each internal pudendal artery (see Fig. 5.36) provides branches to the bulb and to the corresponding crus before terminating as the dorsal and deep arteries. The deep artery traverses the length of the corpus cavernosum while the artery to the bulb continues along the corpus spongiosum to reach the glans. The principal venous drainage is via the midline deep dorsal vein which runs beneath the deep fascia (Fig. 5.38). This vein is accompanied by the dorsal arteries and passes inferior to the pubic symphysis into the pelvic cavity where it terminates in the prostatic venous plexus. From this plexus, blood drains either into the internal iliac veins or the internal pudendal veins.

Erection of the penis is controlled by parasympathetic nerves (the nervi erigentes) from the sacral segments of the spinal cord. Stimulation of these nerves causes arterial dilatation and simultaneous venous constriction. This results in engorgement of the erectile tissues leading to enlargement and stiffening of the penis.

The skin of the penis and the front of the scrotum are supplied by the external pudendal branches of the femoral arteries. The superficial veins of the penis and the anterior part of the scrotum drain via the external pudendal veins which are tributaries of the long saphenous vein (see Fig. 6.5). The posterior part of the scrotum is supplied by posterior scrotal branches from the internal pudendal artery and venous blood passes into the internal pudendal veins.

CUTANEOUS INNERVATION

The pudendal nerve supplies most of the penis and scrotum via its dorsal and posterior scrotal branches. However, the anterior part of the scrotum and the proximal part of the shaft of the penis are innervated by the ilioinguinal nerve which descends from the superficial inguinal ring (see page 4.7).

LYMPHATIC DRAINAGE

Lymph from the superficial tissues of the penis and scrotum passes to the superficial inguinal nodes while that from the deeper tissues is conveyed via lymphatic vessels accompanying the internal pudendal artery and passes to the internal iliac nodes.

FEMALE EXTERNAL GENITALIA

CLITORIS AND BULBS OF VESTIBULE

The perineal membrane is thinner in the female than in the male and is pierced by both the vagina and the urethra. Attached to the inferior surface of the membrane is erectile tissue similar to that in the male, namely the crura of the clitoris and the bulbs of the vestibule covered by the thin ischiocavernosus and bulbospongiosus muscles respectively (Figs. 5.39 & 5.40). The right and left crura attach to the medial margins of the ischial and pubic rami. Passing forwards and medially they merge beneath the pubic symphysis to form the shaft of the clitoris. This turns downwards and backwards towards the urethral opening and its tip is capped by the glans of the clitoris.

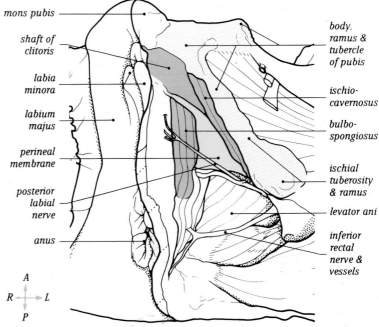

Fig. 5.39 *Superficial dissection of one side of the female perineum showing the muscles and cutaneous nerves.*

FEMALE EXTERNAL GENITALIA

The paired bulbs of the vestibule surround the urethral and vaginal openings (Fig. 5.40). Anteriorly they taper and fuse into a midline venous plexus that continues forwards to terminate as the glans of the clitoris. The posterior end of each bulb is expanded and covers the greater vestibular (Bartholin's) gland. This gland is approximately one centimetre in diameter and drains into a minute duct which opens into the vestibule lateral to the vaginal opening. Superficial transverse perineal muscles pass laterally from the bulbs of the vestibule to the ischial tuberosities.

LABIA

The most superficial parts of the female external genitalia are the skin folds, the labia majora (see Fig. 5.39). These meet at the posterior commissure (fourchette) and anteriorly at the mons pubis. The mons is a pad of fat overlying the pubic symphysis and covering most of the clitoris. Between the labia majora lie the two labia minora which become more prominent anteriorly. The labia minora fuse in the midline, forming two folds of skin around the glans of the clitoris. The hood-like anterior fold comprises the prepuce of the clitoris and the smaller posterior fold forms the frenulum.

VESTIBULE

The labia minora enclose a cleft, the vestibule, into which the vagina and urethra open (Fig. 5.40). The vaginal opening (introitus) is an anteroposterior slit, usually surrounded by a fringe of skin, the hymen. The external urethral meatus lies approximately 1 cm anterior to the vaginal opening.

The term 'vulva' is used to describe the mons pubis, the labia majora and minora, the clitoris and the vestibule.

CUTANEOUS INNERVATION AND BLOOD SUPPLY

The mons pubis and the anterior parts of the labia are innervated by the ilioinguinal nerves (see page 4.7). The posterior part of the vulva receives cutaneous innervation from the labial branches of the pudendal nerves, supplemented by branches of the posterior cutaneous nerves of the thighs and the perineal branches of the fourth sacral nerves.

The skin and subcutaneous tissues are supplied by the internal pudendal artery (see page 5.23) and the superficial and deep external pudendal branches of the femoral artery. Most of the venous blood passes into the venae comitantes of the internal pudendal artery, but anteriorly some blood drains by external pudendal veins into the long saphenous vein. Lymph from the skin and superficial tissues passes to the superficial inguinal nodes (see page 6.3) while lymphatics from deeper structures follow the course of the arteries to reach the internal iliac nodes.

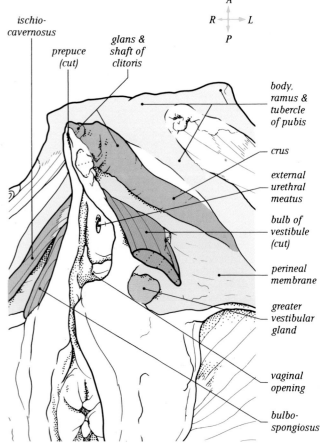

Fig. 5.40 *Deeper dissection of the female perineum. The glans, shaft and left crus of the clitoris have been exposed. The left bulb of the vestibule has been cut to reveal the greater vestibular gland.*

6

LOWER LIMB

INTRODUCTION

Fig. 6.1 *'Step' dissection through the midthigh showing the relationships of the compartments.*

Fig. 6.2 *'Step dissection through the midcalf showing the relationships of the compartments.*

The lower limb, which supports the body during standing and locomotion, consists of three parts linked by hinge joints at the knee and ankle. The buttock and thigh, with the enclosed femur, articulate with the pelvic girdle at the multiaxial hip joint; the leg, including the tibia and fibula, lies in an intermediate position; and the foot, with its tarsals, metatarsals and phalanges, forms the most distal part.

The thigh has anterior, posterior and medial compartments (Fig. 6.1) whilst the leg has anterior, posterior and lateral compartments (Fig. 6.2). Each compartment contains muscle groups with common actions and is traversed by a neurovascular bundle providing its innervation and blood supply. The whole limb is covered by skin, superficial fascia and deep fascia which invests the muscles and forms intermuscular septa (Fig. 6.2).

Principal nerves and vessels enter the lower limb from the abdomen and pelvis via different routes (Fig. 6.3).

The femoral vessels enter the limb from the iliac fossa, passing beneath the inguinal ligament into the anterior compartment of the thigh. The vessels traverse the popliteal fossa, and in the upper part of the leg the vessels divide. The anterior vessels enter the anterior compartment and continue onto the dorsum of the foot; the posterior vessels descend through the posterior compartment to the sole.

In the foot, most of the short (intrinsic) muscles and most of the blood and nerve supply are located in the sole. Attaching to the tarsals, metatarsals and phalanges are tendons from muscles which originate in the leg.

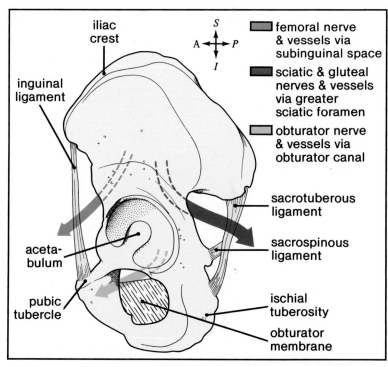

Fig. 6.3 *Sites of access of the principal nerves and vessels from the abdomen and pelvis into the root of the lower limb.*

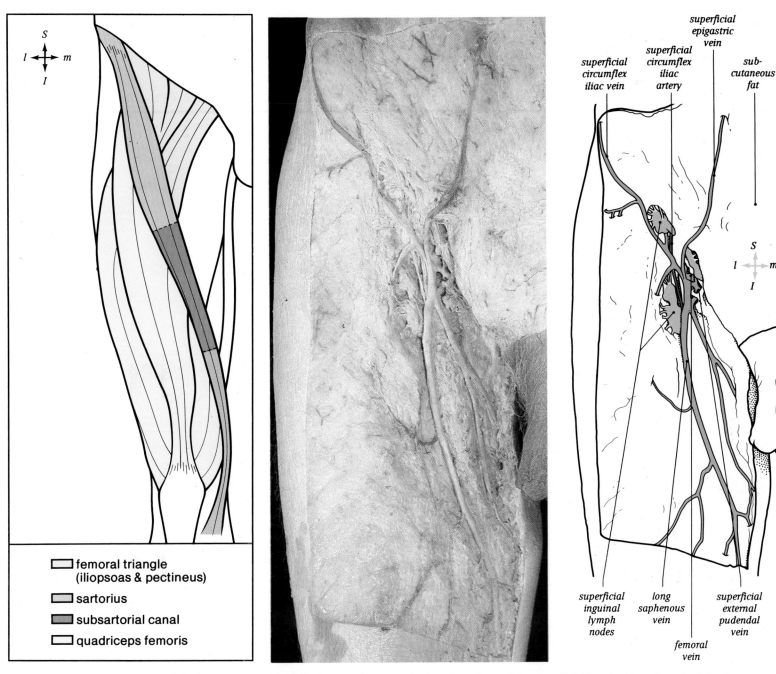

Fig. 6.4 *Anterior compartment of thigh.*

Fig. 6.5 *Long saphenous vein, its tributaries and the superficial inguinal lymph nodes lying in superficial fascia.*

The anterior compartment is the largest in the thigh, occupying the region between the inguinal ligament and the knee. Lateral and anteromedial intermuscular septa separate the contents from the posterior (hamstring) and medial (adductor) compartments respectively (see Fig. 6.1). The anterior compartment (Fig. 6.4) contains quadriceps femoris, sartorius and the tendon of iliopsoas, and is innervated by the femoral nerve. The femoral artery and vein, the principal vessels of the lower limb, traverse the compartment and leave via the opening in adductor magnus to gain the popliteal fossa.

SUPERFICIAL FASCIA
The superficial fascia contains the long saphenous vein and its tributaries with their accompanying arteries, superficial inguinal lymph nodes and cutaneous nerves. The long saphenous vein ascends on the medial side of the thigh (Fig. 6.5) and passes through the saphenous opening in the fascia lata to empty into the femoral vein. The saphenous vein drains the superficial tissues of the entire limb except the lateral side of the leg and foot. Near its termination the vein receives tributaries which drain the buttock, the perineum and the abdominal wall below the umbilicus. These tributaries are accompanied by corresponding branches of the femoral artery.

The superficial inguinal lymph nodes, often palpable in the living, lie just distal and parallel to the inguinal ligament and adjacent to the termination of the long saphenous vein (Fig. 6.5). These nodes receive lymph from the same superficial tissues as those drained by the long saphenous vein and its tributaries. Efferent lymphatics from the superficial nodes pass through the fascia lata and drain into the deep inguinal nodes within the femoral triangle (see page 6.6).

The lateral cutaneous nerve of the thigh (L2 & L3) pierces the inguinal ligament close to the anterior superior iliac spine (see Fig. 6.11) and supplies skin as far as the knee. The intermediate and medial cutaneous nerves of the thigh arise from the femoral nerve and supply the anterior and medial surfaces of the thigh. Sometimes the obturator nerve gives a cutaneous branch to the medial side of the thigh. The femoral branch of the genitofemoral nerve (L1 & L2) passes beneath the inguinal ligament to supply skin over the femoral triangle, and the ilioinguinal nerve emerges through the superficial inguinal ring to supply the adjacent medial aspect of the thigh.

FASCIA LATA
The fascia lata (deep fascia) completely invests the thigh, providing attachment for muscles and associated intermuscular septa in the anterior compartment. It attaches superiorly to the inguinal ligament and iliac crest and inferiorly is continuous with the deep fascia of the leg. Below and lateral to the pubic tubercle is the saphenous opening which transmits the terminal part of the long saphenous vein.

Over the lateral aspect of the thigh the fascia lata is particularly thick, forming the iliotibial tract. Gluteus maximus and tensor fasciae latae are attached to its upper part (see Fig. 6.25).

MUSCLES
Quadriceps femoris

The four parts of quadriceps femoris, namely rectus femoris, vastus lateralis, vastus intermedius and vastus medialis, cover the front and sides of the femur (Figs. 6.6–6.8). Rectus femoris is attached by a straight head to the anterior inferior iliac spine and by a reflected head to the ilium above the acetabulum.

Vastus lateralis attaches to the intertrochanteric line, the lateral lip of the linea aspera and the lateral supracondylar ridge of the femur (see Figs. 6.9 & 6.10). Vastus intermedius attaches to the upper two-thirds of the anterior and lateral surfaces of the femoral shaft whilst vastus medialis anchors to the spiral line and medial lip of the linea aspera. Distally these four muscles form a common tendon which attaches to the upper border (base) of the patella. From the lower border (apex) of the patella the tendon continues

Fig. 6.6 *Muscles of the anterior compartment of thigh after removal of the skin and fascia lata.*

iliopsoas
tensor fasciae latae
pectineus
sartorius
adductor longus
rectus femoris
gracilis
vastus lateralis & medialis
iliotibial tract

S
l — m
I

Fig. 6.7 *Muscles comprising quadriceps femoris. Sartorius and tensor fasciae latae have been cut.*

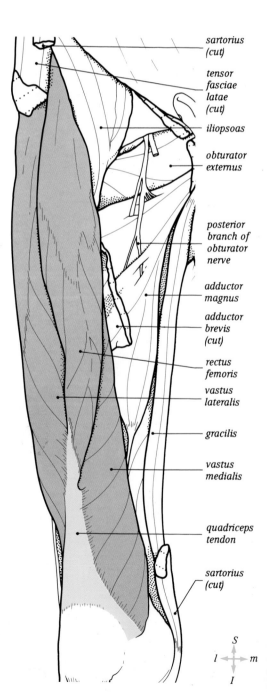

sartorius (cut)
tensor fasciae latae (cut)
iliopsoas
obturator externus
posterior branch of obturator nerve
adductor magnus
adductor brevis (cut)
rectus femoris
vastus lateralis
gracilis
vastus medialis
quadriceps tendon
sartorius (cut)

S
l — m
I

as the ligamentum patellae (see Fig. 6.67) to attach to the tibial tubercle.

Quadriceps femoris is a powerful extensor of the knee joint during standing, walking and running. In addition, rectus femoris flexes the hip. The lower fibres of vastus medialis stabilize the position of the patella (see page 6.40). Quadriceps femoris is supplied by branches of the femoral nerve.

Sartorius

This strap-like muscle is attached proximally to the anterior superior iliac spine and descends obliquely across the thigh (Fig. 6.6), crosses the posteromedial side of the knee and, with gracilis and semitendinosus, attaches to the upper end of the subcutaneous surface of the tibia (see Fig. 6.71). Sartorius flexes and laterally rotates the hip and flexes the knee. It is supplied by the femoral nerve.

Fig. 6.8 *Quadriceps femoris. Vastus intermedius is partially revealed by removal of rectus femoris.*

Fig. 6.9 *Femoral attachments (posterior view) of the vasti muscles.*

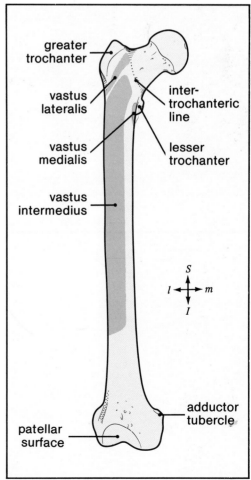

Fig. 6.10 *Femoral attachments (anterior view) of the vasti muscles.*

ANTERIOR COMPARTMENT OF THIGH

FEMORAL TRIANGLE

The femoral triangle occupies the upper medial part of the anterior compartment of the thigh (see Fig. 6.4). Its upper boundary is the inguinal ligament; its lateral limit is the medial border of sartorius and its medial boundary is the lateral border of adductor longus. The roof is fascia lata and the floor comprises iliopsoas and pectineus (Fig. 6.12). The triangle contains the femoral vessels and nerve, and the deep inguinal lymph nodes.

SUBSARTORIAL (ADDUCTOR) CANAL

This canal is an intermuscular space linking the apex of the femoral triangle with the popliteal fossa. Triangular in cross-section, it lies beneath sartorius, occupying the groove between adductors longus and magnus and vastus medialis. Through the canal run the femoral artery and vein, the nerve to vastus medialis and the saphenous nerve (Fig. 6.13).

FEMORAL VESSELS

The femoral artery, a continuation of the external iliac, is the main artery of the lower limb. It enters the anterior compartment behind the midpoint of the inguinal ligament where it is relatively superficial and easily palpable, descends through the femoral triangle (Fig. 6.11) and the subsartorial canal, and continues through the opening in adductor magnus as the popliteal artery (see page 6.16).

The femoral artery or its main branches supply all three compartments of the thigh. Subcutaneous branches of the artery traverse the saphenous opening or pierce the fascia lata to accompany the superficial veins in the groin (see Fig. 6.5). The largest deep branch is the profunda femoris artery (Fig. 6.14), which arises from the posterolateral aspect of the femoral artery about 4cm below the inguinal ligament and runs distally behind the femoral artery, leaving the triangle by passing between pectineus and adductor longus. The profunda femoris and its perforating branches pass through the adductor muscles and contribute to the anastomosis in the posterior

compartment of the thigh. One of the perforating arteries gives a large nutrient branch to the femur. Close to its origin the profunda femoris artery usually gives medial and lateral circumflex femoral branches (Fig. 6.14). The medial circumflex artery winds round the medial aspect of the femur between iliopsoas and pectineus to join the cruciate anastomosis (see page 6.14) and the lateral circumflex artery encircles the femur, passing laterally deep to sartorius and rectus femoris.

The femoral vein is the continuation of the popliteal vein at the opening in adductor magnus. In the subsartorial canal it lies behind the femoral artery and continues through the femoral triangle lying medial to the artery (Fig. 6.11). Passing deep to the inguinal ligament the femoral vein becomes the external iliac vein. Tributaries of the femoral vein, except the long saphenous vein, correspond to the branches of the femoral artery.

Femoral sheath

The femoral artery and vein are invested in a thick fascial sleeve, the femoral sheath, derived from the transversalis and iliac fasciae. The sheath passes deep to the inguinal ligament and tapers inferiorly, blending with the adventitia of the vessels about 2.5cm distal to the ligament.

Two vertical septa divide the sheath into three compartments. The femoral artery lies laterally while the femoral vein occupies the intermediate compartment. The medial compartment is called the femoral canal (Fig. 6.14) and contains fat and lymph nodes. The upper limit of the femoral canal is the femoral ring (see Fig. 4.13), an aperture bounded in front by the inguinal ligament and behind by the superior ramus of the pubis whilst laterally lies the femoral vein and medially the lacunar ligament. A femoral hernia descends through the femoral ring to enter the femoral canal.

FEMORAL NERVE

The femoral nerve (L2, L3 & L4) enters the thigh beneath the inguinal ligament lying on iliopsoas lateral to the femoral sheath (Fig. 6.11). After a brief course in the femoral triangle, it divides into several superficial and deep branches. The superficial branches are the intermediate and medial cutaneous nerves of the thigh and the nerves to sartorius and pectineus. The deep branches include the nerves supplying rectus femoris and the vasti, and the saphenous nerve which enters the subsartorial canal.

DEEP INGUINAL LYMPH NODES

The deep inguinal lymph nodes lie in the femoral triangle medial to the femoral vein. They receive lymph from the superficial inguinal nodes and from all parts of the limb deep to the investing fascia. They also drain the glans of the penis or clitoris. Efferent vessels pass proximally through the femoral canal to reach the external iliac nodes.

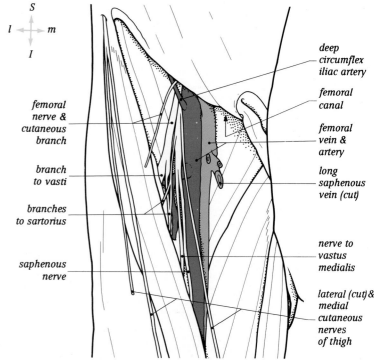

Fig. 6.11 *Contents of the femoral triangle exposed by removal of its roof (fascia lata). The deep inguinal lymph nodes lie within the femoral canal.*

inguinal
ligament

superficial
inguinal
ring

spermatic
cord

iliopsoas

pectineus

lateral
cutaneous
nerve of
thigh

sartorius

adductor
longus

gracilis

adductor
magnus

S
l ←→ m
I

femoral
nerve

lateral
circumflex
femoral
artery

sartorius

nerve to
vastus
medialis

adductor
longus

femoral
vein

saphenous
nerve

femoral
artery

S
l ←→ m
I

femoral
canal

femoral
nerve (cut)

medial &
lateral
circumflex
femoral
arteries

femoral
artery
& vein (cut)

profunda
femoris
artery
& vein

vastus
medialis

adductor
longus

saphenous
nerve (cut)

Fig. 6.12 *Floor of the femoral triangle after removal of its roof and contents.*

Fig. 6.13 *Contents and boundaries of the subsartorial canal exposed by displacement of sartorius laterally.*

Fig. 6.14 *Profunda femoris vessels seen after removal of segments of the femoral artery and vein.*

MEDIAL COMPARTMENT OF THIGH

The medial compartment of the thigh is wedge-shaped and lies between the anterior and posterior compartments. It contains pectineus, adductors longus, brevis and magnus, gracilis and obturator externus. The obturator nerve and vessels and the profunda femoris vessels, together with their perforating branches, supply the compartment.

MUSCLES
The muscles are arranged in three layers. The anterior layer consists of pectineus, adductor longus and gracilis from lateral to medial

Fig. 6.15 *Anterior layer of muscles of the medial compartment of thigh revealed by removal of the fascia lata.*

Fig. 6.16 *Adductor brevis and branches of the anterior division of the obturator nerve revealed by removal of part of adductor longus.*

(Fig. 6.15). Deep to these, forming the intermediate layer, is adductor brevis (Figs. 6.16 & 6.17). The posterior layer consists of obturator externus and adductor magnus (Figs. 6.18 & 6.19). The proximal attachments of these muscles lie on the outer surface of the bony pelvis between the superior pubic and ischial rami. In addition, obturator externus is attached to the obturator membrane.

pectineus (cut)

superior pubic ramus

obturator externus

posterior & anterior divisions of obturator nerve

adductor brevis

pectineus (cut)

adductor magnus

quadriceps femoris

gracilis

S
l ←→ m
I

Fig. 6.17 *Divisions of the obturator nerve revealed by removal of adductor longus and part of pectineus. In this specimen the posterior division lies in front of obturator externus.*

anterior division (cut)

obturator externus

posterior division of obturator nerve

adductor magnus

pectineus (cut)

adductors longus & brevis (cut)

femoral vein & artery (cut) traversing adductor opening

S
l ←→ m
I

Fig. 6.18 *Adductor magnus and the posterior division of the obturator nerve. Adductor brevis has been removed.*

iliopsoas (cut)

psoas bursa

capsule of hip joint

anterior & posterior divisions of obturator nerve (cut)

obturator externus

adductor magnus (cut)

iliopsoas (cut)

sciatic nerve

hamstrings

adductor magnus (cut)

S
l ←→ m
I

Fig. 6.19 *Obturator externus completely revealed by removal of parts of iliopsoas and adductor magnus.*

MEDIAL COMPARTMENT OF THIGH

The more anterior muscles have higher attachments than those of the deeper layers (Fig. 6.20). Distally the muscles attach to the femur, except for gracilis (see Fig. 6.71) which descends below the knee to gain the proximal end of the subcutaneous surface of the tibia in company with sartorius and semitendinosus. Obturator externus passes laterally below and behind the capsule of the hip joint (see Fig. 6.62) to the trochanteric fossa on the medial aspect of the greater trochanter. Pectineus and adductors longus, brevis and magnus slope downwards and laterally to attach in the region of the linea aspera, the sequence being related to the layer in which the muscle lies (Fig. 6.21). Adductor magnus has the longest attachment, extending from the gluteal tuberosity above to the adductor tubercle below.

All the muscles in the compartment except obturator externus adduct the hip joint. During walking they stabilize the femur whilst the abductors of the hip prevent tilting of the pelvis (see page 6.12). In addition, pectineus and adductor longus are medial rotators and obturator externus a lateral rotator. Pectineus assists flexion at the hip joint and gracilis flexes and medially rotates the knee joint.

All the muscles in the medial compartment are innervated by the obturator nerve. Pectineus usually has an additional supply from the femoral nerve, and the ischial part of adductor magnus receives fibres from the sciatic nerve.

OBTURATOR NERVE

The obturator nerve gains the compartment through the obturator canal and promptly divides into anterior and posterior divisions (see Fig. 6.17). The former passes anterior to obturator externus whilst the posterior division usually pierces and supplies the muscle before emerging onto its surface. The two divisions then descend respectively anterior and posterior to adductor brevis. The anterior division supplies adductors longus and brevis, pectineus and gracilis (see Fig. 6.16), and gives sensory branches to the hip joint and to skin on the medial side of the thigh. The posterior division lies on and supplies adductor magnus (see Fig. 6.18) and gives sensory branches which accompany the femoral artery through the opening in adductor magnus to supply the knee joint. Since the obturator nerve innervates the hip and knee joints, disease in one joint may cause referred pain in the other.

VESSELS

The blood supply is derived from the profunda femoris artery and its perforating branches, supplemented by the obturator artery and other branches of the femoral artery. The obturator artery is small and forms an arterial circle around the margins of the obturator membrane, supplying the proximal parts of the muscles. An acetabular branch passes beneath the transverse acetabular ligament and accompanies the round ligament to the head of the femur. Venae comitantes accompanying the arteries in the compartment drain into the profunda femoris or internal iliac veins.

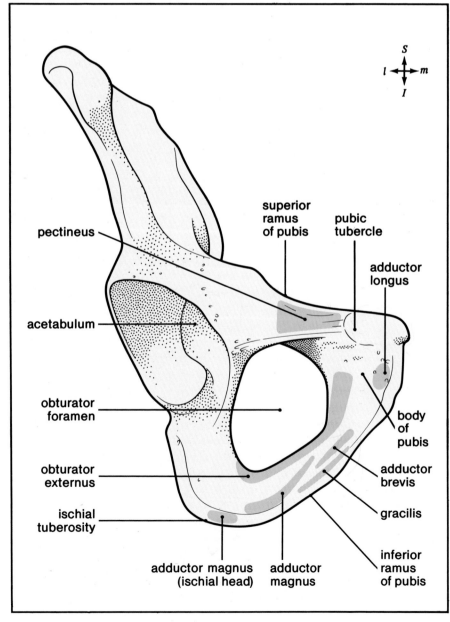

Fig. 6.20 *Attachments of the muscles of the medial compartment of the thigh to the hip bone.*

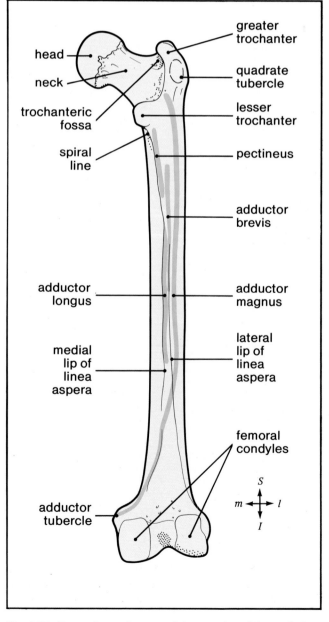

Fig. 6.21 *Femoral attachments of the muscles of the medial compartment of the thigh.*

GLUTEAL COMPARTMENT

The gluteal region or buttock forms part of the root of the limb. It overlies the dorsum of the ilium, ischium and sacrum and is continuous proximally with the lower trunk and distally with the posterior compartment of the thigh. Three substantial muscles (gluteus maximus, medius and minimus) covered by deep fascia and a thick layer of subcutaneous fat form the bulk of the buttock and account for its surface contour. The gluteal fold, a prominent surface feature, lies at the junction of the buttock and thigh.

GLUTEUS MAXIMUS

This very large trapezoidal muscle is the most superficial in the buttock. Its fibres slope downwards and laterally (Fig. 6.22) and its lower edge passes obliquely across the gluteal fold. Some of the sensory nerves to the skin of the buttock penetrate the medial part of the muscle whilst others emerge around its upper and lower borders (Fig. 6.23). Proximally the muscle has an extensive attachment: to the ilium behind the posterior gluteal line; to the

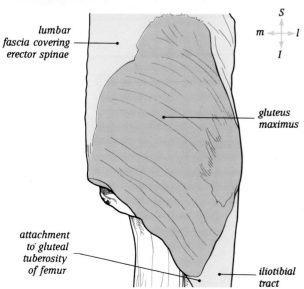

Fig. 6.22 *The attachments of gluteus maximus include the lumbar fascia and the iliotibial tract.*

Fig. 6.23 *Removal of the skin and subcutaneous fat reveals superficial nerves and vessels.*

lower part of the sacrum; to the coccyx; to the sacrotuberous ligament; and to the lumbar (thoracolumbar) and gluteal fasciae. A synovial bursa is usually present where it crosses the ischial tuberosity. Distally some of the deeper fibres are attached to the gluteal tuberosity of the femur (Fig. 6.24), but most of the muscle is attached through the iliotibial tract (Fig. 6.25) to the anterior surface of the lateral tibial condyle. The nerve supply is from the inferior gluteal nerve (L5, S1 & S2).

Gluteus maximus is a strong extensor of the thigh, especially during running and climbing, and also produces abduction at the hip joint. As an antigravity muscle it extends the trunk on the hip and through the iliotibial tract it stabilizes the knee joint and the supporting limb during walking and standing.

Fig. 6.24 *Reflection of gluteus maximus exposes gluteus medius and neurovascular structures.*

Fig. 6.25 *Attachment of gluteus maximus and tensor fasciae latae to the iliotibial tract.*

TENSOR FASCIAE LATAE

This small muscle is attached proximally to the ilium between the anterior superior iliac spine and iliac tubercle (Fig. 6.26) and distally to the anterior border of the iliotibial tract (Fig. 6.25) which it tenses. It is supplied by the superior gluteal nerve.

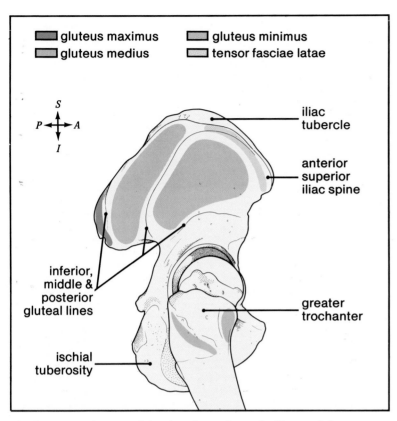

Fig. 6.26 *Attachments of the gluteal muscles to the ilium and the greater trochanter.*

STRUCTURES DEEP TO GLUTEUS MAXIMUS

The arrangement of these structures is clarified by noting whether they enter the buttock above or below the piriformis muscle (Fig. 6.24).

Structures entering above piriformis

The superior gluteal nerve (L4, L5 & S1) arises within the pelvis from the sacral plexus and enters the buttock through the greater sciatic foramen, running laterally between gluteus medius and gluteus minimus (Fig. 6.27). It supplies both muscles and terminates in tensor fasciae latae.

The superior gluteal artery arises from the posterior aspect of the internal iliac artery. It enters the buttock accompanying the corresponding nerve and divides into a superficial branch which supplies the overlying gluteus maximus (Fig. 6.24) and two deep branches, an upper and lower, which supply gluteus medius and minimus (Fig. 6.27). The deep branches also contribute to anastomoses around the greater trochanter and anterior superior iliac spine. The accompanying veins form an extensive plexus between the muscles and drain into the internal iliac vein.

Gluteus medius and minimus

These fan-shaped muscles lie superior to piriformis. Gluteus medius (Fig. 6.24) is attached proximally to the dorsum of the ilium between the posterior and middle gluteal lines and to the gluteal fascia which separates it from gluteus maximus. Distally it is attached to the lateral surface of the greater trochanter. Gluteus minimus lies immediately deep to gluteus medius and attaches proximally to the dorsum of the ilium between the middle and inferior gluteal lines (Fig. 6.26) and distally to the anterior surface of the greater trochanter (Fig. 6.27). Both are supplied by the superior gluteal nerve.

Although gluteus medius extends the hip and minimus medially rotates it, their importance is in abduction of the hip. During walking, gluteus medius and minimus of the supporting limb contract to prevent tilting of the pelvis towards the unsupported side. Failure of this mechanism is the basis of Trendelenburg's sign of hip instability.

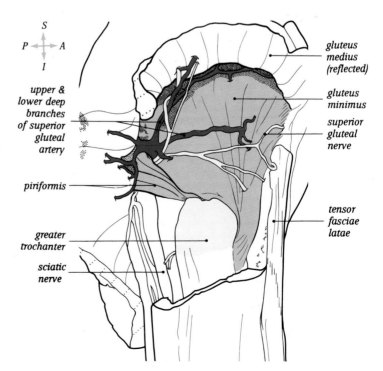

Fig. 6.27 *Reflection of gluteus medius reveals gluteus minimus and the superior gluteal artery and nerve entering the buttock above piriformis.*

GLUTEAL COMPARTMENT

Structures entering below piriformis

These are: three nerves laterally, the sciatic nerve, nerve to quadratus femoris and posterior cutaneous nerve of thigh; medially the internal pudendal artery, pudendal nerve and nerve to obturator internus; and in intermediate position, the inferior gluteal nerve and vessels.

The sciatic nerve (Fig. 6.28), the largest nerve in the lower limb, arises from the spinal nerves L4, L5, S1, S2 & S3 and supplies the entire limb except for the gluteal structures and the medial and anterior compartments of the thigh. It leaves the greater sciatic foramen about half-way between the posterior superior iliac spine and ischial tuberosity and curves laterally and downwards, crossing the midpoint between the ischial tuberosity and greater trochanter. The nerve is separated from the capsule of the hip joint by obturator internus and the gemelli, quadratus femoris and the upper border of adductor magnus (Fig. 6.28). A branch of the inferior gluteal artery accompanies the nerve.

The nerve to quadratus femoris (L4, L5 & S1) lies deep to the sciatic nerve, obturator internus and the gemelli and supplies the inferior gemellus, quadratus femoris and the hip joint.

Superficial and medial to the sciatic nerve is the posterior cutaneous nerve of thigh (Fig. 6.28) which arises from spinal nerves S1, S2 & S3. Within the buttock its perineal branch runs forwards to supply the skin on the posterior part of the scrotum or labium majus. Other branches curl round the lower border of gluteus maximus to supply the skin over the buttock.

The inferior gluteal nerve and vessels occupy an intermediate position. The nerve turns immediately posteriorly to supply gluteus maximus.

The inferior gluteal artery, a branch of the internal iliac artery, accompanies the nerve and supplies gluteus maximus (see Fig. 6.24) and the short lateral rotators of the hip joint and contributes to the trochanteric and cruciate anastomoses. Venae comitantes accompany the artery and drain into the internal iliac system.

The pudendal nerve (S2, S3 & S4), internal pudendal vessels, and nerve to obturator internus (L5, S1 & S2), also supplying the superior gemellus, enter beneath the medial part of piriformis (Fig. 6.28). Their course is brief in the buttock before turning forwards into the lesser sciatic foramen, crossing the sacrospinous ligament or ischial spine to enter the pudendal canal (see page 5.23).

SHORT MUSCLES OF BUTTOCK

The short muscles of the buttock are, from above downwards, piriformis, obturator internus with the gemelli, and quadratus femoris (Fig. 6.28). Piriformis arises from the ventral surface of the sacrum (see page 5.16) and runs laterally through the greater sciatic foramen to converge on the medial border of the greater trochanter. It is innervated within the pelvis by the first and second sacral (S1 & S2) nerves. Obturator internus attaches to the lateral wall of the pelvic cavity (see Fig. 6.64), including the obturator membrane, and runs backwards towards the lesser sciatic foramen where its tendon makes a right-angled turn to run laterally across the buttock to the medial aspect of the greater trochanter above the trochanteric fossa. The superior and inferior gemelli are small muscles that arise from the upper and lower margins of the lesser sciatic notch and fuse with the obturator internus tendon.

Quadratus femoris attaches to the lateral margin of the ischial tuberosity and to the quadrate tubercle of the femur and the subjacent shaft. Being behind the hip joint, all the short muscles laterally rotate the hip.

CRUCIATE ARTERIAL ANASTOMOSIS

The cruciate anastomosis lies at the lower border of quadratus femoris and receives contributions from: above, the inferior gluteal artery; below, the first perforating artery; and on each side, the medial and lateral circumflex femoral arteries.

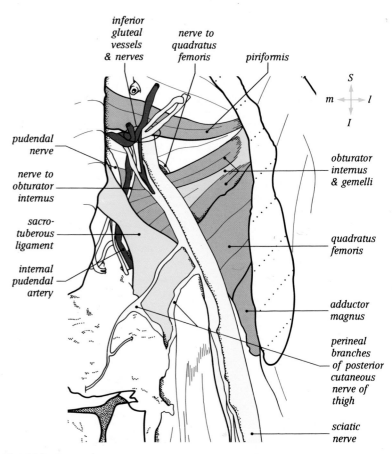

Fig. 6.28 *Structures emerging below piriformis and the course and relations of the sciatic nerve.*

POSTERIOR COMPARTMENT OF THIGH

The posterior compartment is enclosed within deep fascia, the fascia lata (Fig. 6.29), and extends from the gluteal region above to the popliteal fossa below. It contains the posterior cutaneous nerve of thigh, 'hamstring' muscles, sciatic nerve and terminal branches of the profunda femoris artery.

'HAMSTRING' MUSCLES

These three muscles, semimembranosus, semitendinosus and biceps femoris (long head) (Fig. 6.30), attach proximally to the ischial tuberosity and distally to the upper end of the tibia or fibula and are innervated by the sciatic nerve.

They span the entire length of the femur and act on two joints, the hip for extension and the knee for flexion. After flexion of the trunk, the hamstrings act as antigravity muscles by pulling on the ischial tuberosities, thus extending the trunk into an upright position at the hip.

cutaneous branch (cut)

S

m ← → l

I

posterior cutaneous nerve of thigh

perforating vein

'window' cut in fascia lata

anomalous short saphenous vein

long saphenous vein

Fig. 6.29 *Nerves and veins of the posterior compartment of thigh seen through a 'window' cut in the investing layer of deep fascia. This short saphenous vein continues proximally (above the level of the popliteal fossa) to terminate in the long saphenous vein.*

sciatic nerve

attachment of gluteus maximus to gluteal tuberosity

ischial tuberosity

branches to hamstrings

long head of biceps femoris

semi membranosus

short head of biceps femoris

branch to short head

semi-tendinosus

S

m ← → l

I

Fig. 6.30 *Principal contents of the posterior compartment of thigh seen after removal of deep fascia.*

Semimembranosus

This muscle is attached to the upper and lateral parts of the ischial tuberosity by a wide flat tendon, which is overlapped by the tendons of biceps and semitendinosus close to the tuberosity, and descends on the medial side of the popliteal fossa to its main attachment into a horizontal groove on the posteromedial aspect of the medial tibial condyle. Some of its fibres pass upwards and laterally behind the knee joint to form the oblique posterior ligament; others descend to reinforce the fascia over popliteus (see Fig. 6.34).

Semitendinosus

Proximally, semitendinosus is attached to the medial part of the ischial tuberosity. It descends on the medial side of the popliteal fossa, forming a narrow tendon which overlies semimembranosus, and attaches to the medial surface of the upper end of the tibial shaft close to the attachments of sartorius and gracilis (see Fig. 6.71). Besides contributing to the common actions of the hamstring group, semitendinosus and semimembranosus produce medial rotation of the leg at the knee.

Biceps femoris

This muscle has two heads. Proximally, the long head is attached to the medial part of the ischial tuberosity close to the semitendinosus and descends to the lateral side of the popliteal fossa where it fuses with the short head, which originates from the lateral lip of the linea aspera and lateral supracondylar ridge of femur (see Fig. 6.30). Inferiorly, the tendon of biceps is attached to the head of the fibula. In addition to the general actions of the hamstrings, biceps produces lateral rotation of the leg at the knee.

SCIATIC NERVE

The sciatic nerve emerges at the lower border of gluteus maximus lying just beneath the deep fascia, passes deep to the long head of biceps and descends in the midline of the limb. In the distal third of the thigh it usually divides into two terminal branches, the tibial and common peroneal nerves, which continue into the popliteal fossa (Fig. 6.33). Division may occur more proximally in the thigh, within the buttock or even the pelvis. Proximally, fibres from the medial (tibial) part of the sciatic nerve supply the hamstrings (see Fig. 6.30) and the ischial head of adductor magnus. More distally, a branch from the lateral (common peroneal) part of the nerve supplies the short head of biceps.

POSTERIOR CUTANEOUS NERVE OF THIGH

The nerve enters the thigh superficial and slightly medial to the sciatic nerve and descends beneath the fascia lata to the upper part of the popliteal fossa (Fig. 6.31). Apart from branches arising near the lower border of gluteus maximus (see Fig. 6.23), the nerve gives sensory fibres to the skin on the back of the thigh.

PROFUNDA FEMORIS ARTERY

Perforating branches of the profunda femoris artery penetrate adductor magnus and terminate in the posterior compartment. They anastomose with branches from the inferior gluteal artery above and the popliteal artery below.

POPLITEAL FOSSA

The popliteal fossa is a diamond-shaped space behind the knee joint. It contains the principal blood vessels and nerves passing between the thigh and the posterior and lateral compartments of the leg. It has a roof, four walls and a floor.

ROOF

The roof is formed by the investing layer of deep fascia. In the superficial fascia overlying the roof are the posterior cutaneous nerve of the thigh, which continues into the proximal part of the leg, and the short saphenous vein (Fig. 6.31). The vein usually penetrates the roof to drain into the popliteal vein but occasionally continues proximally to drain into the long saphenous vein (see Fig. 6.29).

superficial branches of posterior cutaneous nerve of thigh

long saphenous vein

investing layer of deep fascia

posterior cutaneous nerve of thigh

short saphenous vein

Fig. 6.31 *Removal of skin and superficial fascia reveals the cutaneous nerves. The short saphenous vein and accompanying nerve pierce the roof of the popliteal fossa.*

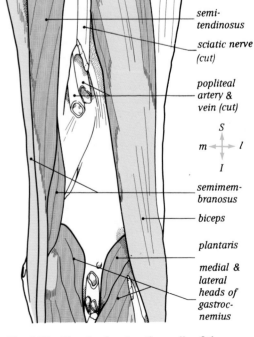

semitendinosus

sciatic nerve (cut)

popliteal artery & vein (cut)

semimembranosus

biceps

plantaris

medial & lateral heads of gastrocnemius

Fig. 6.32 *Muscles forming the walls of the popliteal fossa.*

WALLS

The walls overhang the fossa. Superiorly they are formed by the diverging tendons of the hamstrings, namely semitendinosus and semimembranosus lying medially and biceps laterally. Inferiorly are the medial and lateral heads of gastrocnemius which converge at the inferior angle (Fig. 6.32). Adjacent to the lateral head of gastrocnemius is the small plantaris muscle. On each side of the popliteal fossa the hamstring tendons overlap the heads of gastrocnemius and between the medial head of gastrocnemius and semimembranosus there is frequently a bursa (Fig. 6.34).

CONTENTS

The principal contents of the fossa are embedded in fat and comprise the popliteal artery and vein together with the two terminal branches of the sciatic nerve, the common peroneal and tibial nerves (Fig. 6.33). These vessels and nerves are responsible for the blood and nerve supply of most of the leg and foot.

The popliteal artery lies deepest and is the continuation of the femoral artery from the thigh. It enters through the opening in adductor magnus and descends vertically on the floor of the fossa to the inferior angle where it leaves beneath the fused heads of gastrocnemius. The artery is so deep that it is difficult to palpate unless the knee is flexed to relax the boundaries and roof of the fossa. The artery supplies the surrounding muscles and also forms a substantial plexus of articular branches anastomosing symmetrically around the knee joint.

The popliteal vein lies superficial to the artery and is formed at the inferior angle of the fossa by the union of the venae comitantes which accompany the tibial arteries in the leg. It continues proximally with the artery through the opening in adductor magnus to enter the subsartorial canal and become the femoral vein.

The tibial and common peroneal nerves (Fig. 6.33), entering the fossa from the posterior compartment of the thigh, lie just beneath the roof, superficial to the popliteal vessels. The tibial nerve enters from beneath the hamstrings and descends vertically, bisecting the fossa, and leaves beneath the gastrocnemius at the inferior angle of the fossa where it enters the posterior compartment of the leg. The tibial nerve is mainly motor in its distribution, supplying gastrocnemius, plantaris, popliteus and soleus. All these branches arise within the fossa. The nerve also gives sensory branches to the knee joint and a large cutaneous branch which passes into the calf to form the sural nerve. The common peroneal nerve descends under cover of the tendon of biceps to reach the lateral angle of the fossa where it enters the lateral (peroneal) compartment of the leg by winding around the neck of the fibula. The common peroneal nerve supplies sensory branches to the knee joint and two cutaneous nerves, one to the lateral side of the calf and the other, the lateral sural cutaneous nerve, joining the sural nerve in the calf.

The remaining contents of the popliteal fossa are the deeply placed popliteal lymph nodes which lie close to the popliteal artery. They drain the deep structures of the leg and foot and the knee joint, and receive superficial lymphatics which accompany the short saphenous vein from the lateral side of the foot and leg.

FLOOR

The floor of the fossa is formed, from above downwards, by the popliteal surface of the femur, the capsule of the knee joint reinforced by the oblique posterior ligament, and popliteus (Fig. 6.34).

POPLITEUS

This muscle is attached to a triangular area on the posterior surface of the proximal end of the tibia above the soleal line. The tendon passes upwards and laterally, penetrating the capsule of the knee joint (see Fig. 6.69) to become attached to a pit below the lateral epicondyle of the femur. Its action is to 'unlock' the knee joint by producing lateral rotation of the femur on the tibia during flexion of the joint from the fully extended position. Popliteus is supplied by the tibial nerve.

S
m ← → l
I

opening in adductor magnus

popliteal vein

popliteal artery

tibial nerve

common peroneal nerve

muscular branches

lateral head of gastrocnemius

medial head of gastrocnemius

Fig. 6.33 *Principal vessels and nerves of the popliteal fossa revealed by removal of fat.*

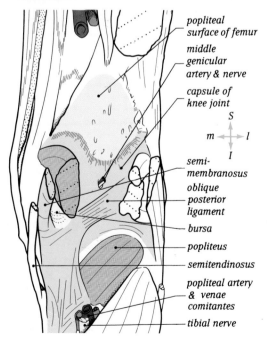

popliteal surface of femur

middle genicular artery & nerve

capsule of knee joint

S
m ← → l
I

semi-membranosus

oblique posterior ligament

bursa

popliteus

semitendinosus

popliteal artery & venae comitantes

tibial nerve

Fig. 6.34 *Floor seen after removal of walls and contents of the fossa.*

POSTERIOR COMPARTMENT OF LEG

The compartment extends from the popliteal fossa above to the ankle below. Gastrocnemius and soleus account for its bulk (Fig. 6.35) and the characteristic contour of the calf. Their common tendon is conspicuous as it passes towards the ankle. Deeper are tibialis posterior and the two long flexors of the toes, flexor hallucis longus and flexor digitorum longus, whose tendons pass distally into the foot. The posterior tibial artery and its venae comitantes and the tibial nerve pass distally between soleus and the long flexors to enter the foot where they supply structures in the sole.

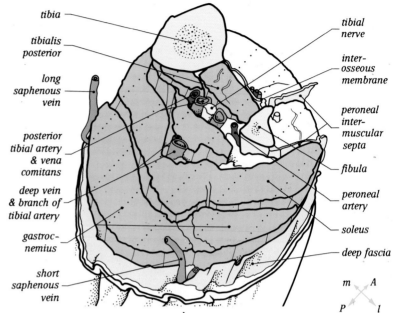

Fig. 6.35 *Step dissection showing the muscle layers in the upper third of the leg and the location of principal nerves and vessels.*

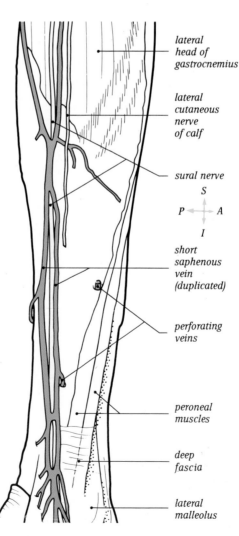

Fig. 6.36 *Short saphenous vein and sural nerve. Perforating veins pierce the deep fascia to connect with deep veins in the calf muscles.*

SUPERFICIAL STRUCTURES AND DEEP FASCIA

The short saphenous vein begins on the lateral side of the foot as a continuation of the dorsal venous arch. Passing behind the lateral malleolus (Fig. 6.36) it ascends in the midline of the calf and usually terminates by piercing the fascial roof of the popliteal fossa (see Fig. 6.31). The vein has frequent communications with the long saphenous vein and important communicating (perforating) veins which pierce the investing deep fascia to link up with the deep veins of the calf particularly just above the ankle.

The sural nerve is formed principally from the cutaneous branch of the tibial nerve and descends from the popliteal fossa to pierce the deep fascia in the proximal part of the calf. Here it is joined by the sural communicating branch of the common peroneal nerve and continues distally with the short saphenous vein posteroinferior to the lateral malleolus to reach the foot (Fig. 6.36). The nerve supplies skin over the lower two-thirds of the calf and on the lateral side of the ankle and foot.

The investing deep fascia is continuous proximally with the popliteal fascia and distally near the heel is thickened in two places. The first forms a thick band stretching between the tibia and fibula over which the tendo calcaneus passes, separated by a bursa. The second thickening, the flexor retinaculum, bridges the gap between the medial malleolus and the medial surface of the calcaneum, completing a fibro-osseous tunnel similar to the carpal tunnel of the wrist. It is the gateway into the sole of the foot for the tendons of the deep muscles of the compartment and the neurovascular bundle.

SUPERFICIAL MUSCLES

Gastrocnemius

The muscle has medial and lateral heads attached to the respective femoral condyles. The medial head is the larger and its fibres extend more distally. The two heads share a common aponeurosis which overlies that of the subjacent soleus (Fig. 6.37). The long parallel fibres of gastrocnemius provide a large range of movement and are used especially during walking and running. Because of its femoral attachments it is a weak flexor of the knee joint.

Soleus

This muscle attaches to the soleal line on the posterior border of the tibia, from where it arches across to the posterior aspect of the head and upper shaft of the fibula (Figs. 6.38 & 6.39). Its short multipennate fibres are continually in action during standing.

The aponeuroses of gastrocnemius and soleus form the tendo calcaneus (Achillis) which is attached to the middle third of the posterior surface of the calcaneum, separated from the upper part of the bone by a bursa. The two muscles are the principal plantar flexors of the foot at the ankle joint.

Plantaris

This muscle attaches to the lower end of the femur close to the lateral head of gastrocnemius. Its long thin tendon passes deep to the medial head of gastrocnemius (see Fig. 6.39) between the aponeuroses of gastrocnemius and soleus to insert into the posterior surface of the calcaneum medial to the tendo calcaneus. It is a weak flexor of the knee and ankle joints.

Gastrocnemius, soleus and plantaris are supplied by the tibial nerve in the popliteal fossa (see Fig. 6.33). Soleus is further supplied by the tibial nerve as it passes beneath the soleal arch.

NEUROVASCULAR STRUCTURES

Posterior tibial artery

At the lower border of popliteus the popliteal artery divides into two terminal branches, the anterior tibial artery (see page 6.31) and the larger posterior tibial artery. The latter, accompanied by its venae comitantes, passes deep to the soleal arch and descends on the fascia of tibialis posterior (Fig. 6.35) between flexor digitorum longus and flexor hallucis longus. Near the ankle the artery lies on the distal end of the tibia and the capsule of the ankle joint. Passing beneath the flexor retinaculum it gives calcaneal branches to the superficial tissues of the heel and then divides into medial and lateral plantar arteries. It provides branches to the muscles in the calf and also a large nutrient artery to the tibial shaft.

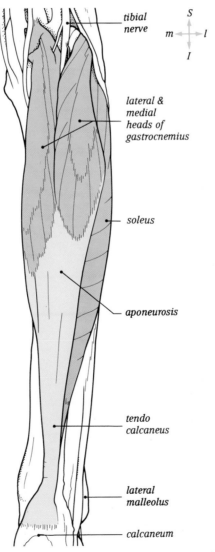

Fig. 6.37 *Removal of the deep fascia reveals the superficial flexor muscles, gastrocnemius and soleus.*

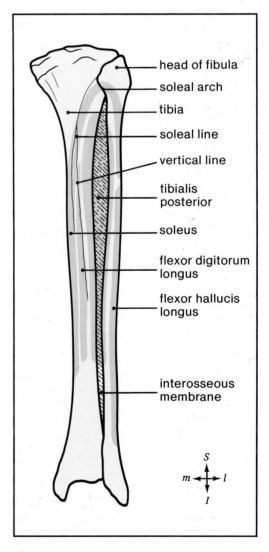

Fig. 6.38 *Skeleton of the leg showing attachments of soleus and deep muscles of the calf to the tibia and fibula.*

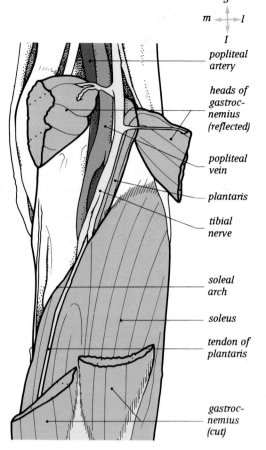

S
m ← → l
I

popliteal
artery

heads of
gastroc-
nemius
(reflected)

popliteal
vein

plantaris

tibial
nerve

soleal
arch

soleus

tendon of
plantaris

gastroc-
nemius
(cut)

Fig. 6.39 *Partial removal of the two heads of gastrocnemius reveals soleus and the neurovascular bundle passing beneath the soleal arch to enter the calf.*

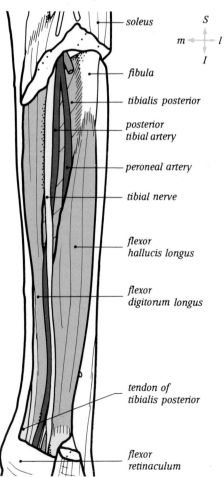

soleus

S
m ← → l
I

fibula

tibialis posterior

posterior
tibial artery

peroneal artery

tibial nerve

flexor
hallucis longus

flexor
digitorum longus

tendon of
tibialis posterior

flexor
retinaculum

Fig. 6.40 *Removal of the superficial flexor group shows the deep muscles of the compartment and the main neurovascular bundle.*

The most conspicuous branch, the peroneal artery, arises just beyond the soleal arch (Fig. 6.40) and passes distally and laterally deep to flexor hallucis longus and upon the fascia of tibialis posterior. It gives muscular branches and a nutrient branch to the fibula. The peroneal artery terminates behind the lateral malleolus as lateral calcaneal branches supplying the tissues of the heel. In the lower leg a communicating artery links the peroneal and posterior tibial arteries.

A perforating branch of the peroneal artery passes forwards through the interosseous membrane into the anterior compartment of the leg. When the anterior tibial artery is small, this perforating artery may substitute for it distally, continuing into the foot as the dorsalis pedis artery.

Tibial nerve
The tibial nerve enters the compartment from the popliteal fossa by passing beneath the soleal arch. Usually the posterior tibial artery lies medially as it descends through the calf on the fascia of tibialis posterior and on the distal end of the tibia (Fig. 6.40). Like the artery, as it enters the foot it often terminates beneath the flexor retinaculum as two branches, the medial and lateral plantar nerves. It supplies soleus and the deep leg muscles and gives sensory branches to skin over the ball of the heel.

DEEP MUSCLES
Lying deep to soleus are flexor digitorum longus, flexor hallucis longus and tibialis posterior (Figs. 6.35 & 6.40). Proximally their attachments are limited by the origin of soleus from the tibia and fibula. Their tendons enter the foot beneath the flexor retinaculum.

Flexor digitorum longus arises from the posterior surface of the tibia (see Fig. 6.38) and from the fascia covering tibialis posterior. In the foot the tendon divides into four slips which are attached to the bases of the terminal phalanges of the lateral toes. The muscle flexes the toes and assists in plantar flexion of the ankle joint.

Flexor hallucis longus has extensive attachments to the posterior surface of the shaft of the fibula (see Fig. 6.38), the posterior peroneal intermuscular septum and the fascia covering tibialis posterior. Its muscle fibres characteristically extend almost as far as the ankle (Fig. 6.40) and give way to a tendon which passes beneath the flexor retinaculum to insert into the base of the distal phalanx of the great toe. It is a powerful flexor of the hallux, especially in forward propulsion of the foot at the take-off point during walking. Plantar flexion at the ankle joint is also assisted.

Tibialis posterior is the deepest muscle in the compartment and attaches to the posterior surface of the tibia (see Fig. 6.38), to the medial surface of the fibula and to the upper two-thirds of the interosseous membrane. Passing under the flexor retinaculum the tendon enters the foot to attach principally to the tuberosity of the navicular and by small slips to the other tarsal bones. Together with tibialis anterior its action is to invert the foot. It is also a weak plantar flexor of the ankle joint.

All three deep muscles of the calf are supplied by the tibial nerve. Further details of their tendons in the sole of the foot are given on page 6.23.

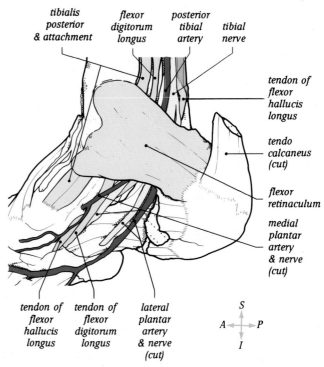

Fig. 6.41 *Long tendons and the principal vessels and nerves from the posterior compartment of the leg pass deep to the flexor retinaculum to enter the sole of the foot.*

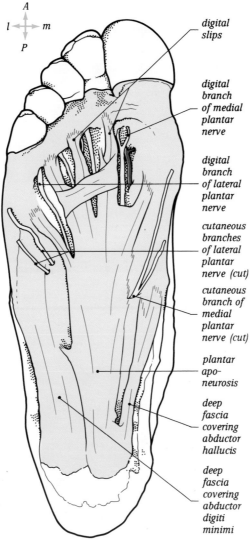

The sole of the foot contains the plantar aponeurosis, intrinsic muscles, tendons originating from muscles in the leg, and plantar vessels and nerves. The tendons, accompanied by the vessels and nerves, enter the sole deep to the flexor retinaculum (Fig. 6.41), between the medial aspect of the calcaneum and the medial malleolus. The skin of the sole is thick and heavily keratinized and is firmly attached to the deep fascia by fibrous septa which traverse and loculate the subcutaneous fat.

PLANTAR APONEUROSIS

The plantar aponeurosis, the deep fascia of the sole covering the superficial layer of muscles, is especially thick in its central portion. Posteriorly the aponeurosis is attached to the medial and lateral calcaneal tubercles. Anteriorly it widens and diverges into five digital slips (Fig. 6.42) which attach to the fibrous flexor sheaths and plantar metatarsal plates (see Fig. 6.87). These plates give the aponeurosis indirect attachment to the bases of all the proximal phalanges, providing an important support for the longitudinal arches of the foot (see Figs. 6.89–6.91).

Fig. 6.42 *Plantar aponeurosis, deep fascia and cutaneous nerves revealed by removal of the skin of the sole.*

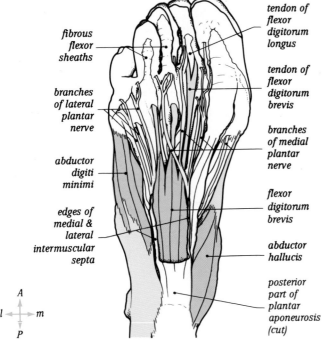

fibrous
flexor
sheaths

tendon of
flexor
digitorum
longus

branches
of lateral
plantar
nerve

tendon of
flexor
digitorum
brevis

branches
of medial
plantar
nerve

abductor
digiti
minimi

flexor
digitorum
brevis

edges of
medial &
lateral
intermuscular
septa

abductor
hallucis

posterior
part of
plantar
aponeurosis
(cut)

A
l — m
P

Fig. 6.43 *Superficial intrinsic muscles and plantar nerves after removal of deep fascia, part of the plantar aponeurosis and second fibrous tendon sheath. In this specimen, flexor digitorum brevis has only three tendons.*

fibrous
flexor
sheath

digital
branches of
medial
plantar
nerve

tendon
of flexor
hallucis
longus

lumbricals

tendon
of flexor
digitorum
brevis (cut)

abductor
digiti
minimi

flexor
digitorum
longus

lateral
plantar
nerve & artery

medial
plantar
artery & nerve

flexor
digitorum
brevis
(cut)

flexor
accessorius

abductor
hallucis

A
l — m
P

Fig. 6.44 *Removal of flexor digitorum brevis has revealed the plantar nerves and arteries, which enter the sole deep to abductor hallucis.*

MUSCLES AND TENDONS
The muscles and tendons in the sole of the foot are arranged in four layers.

Superficial intrinsic muscles
This layer comprises three muscles which span the length of most of the foot and attach to the deep surface of the plantar aponeurosis. Abductor hallucis (Fig. 6.43) lies on the medial side of the foot and arises from the medial calcaneal tubercle and the adjacent flexor retinaculum. Its tendon passes to the great toe with the medial tendon of flexor hallucis brevis and attaches to the medial side of the base of the proximal phalanx. It is supplied by the medial plantar nerve.

Flexor digitorum brevis lies centrally (Fig. 6.43) and attaches to the medial calcaneal tubercle. It has four tendons which pass forwards to enter the fibrous flexor sheaths of the lateral four toes. Each tendon splits to allow the passage of the long flexor tendon (Figs. 6.43 & 6.44), then reunites to attach to the flexor surface of the middle phalanx. Flexor digitorum brevis aids flexion of the proximal parts of the toes and is supplied by the medial plantar nerve.

Abductor digiti minimi traverses the lateral border of the sole (Fig. 6.43) and is attached posteriorly to the medial and lateral calcaneal tubercles. Entering the little toe, its tendon attaches to the lateral side of the proximal phalanx. The muscle is supplied by the lateral plantar nerve.

Long flexor tendons and associated intrinsic muscles
This layer includes the tendons of two long flexor muscles which arise in the leg, namely flexor hallucis longus and flexor digitorum longus. Attached to the tendon of flexor digitorum longus (Fig. 6.45) are flexor accessorius and the four lumbricals.

The tendon of flexor hallucis longus grooves the posterior surface of the talus and curves forwards inferior to the sustentaculum tali and the 'spring' ligament. It passes deep to the tendon of flexor digitorum longus to which it is usually attached. The tendon of flexor hallucis longus continues forwards inferior to the head of the first metatarsal, where it passes between the sesamoid bones in the two tendons of the flexor hallucis brevis (see below), and enters the fibrous flexor sheath of the great toe to reach its attachment to the base of the distal phalanx (Fig. 6.45). The actions and innervation of flexor hallucis longus are described on page 6.20.

The tendon of flexor digitorum longus passes forwards medial to the sustentaculum tali and divides into four tendons, one for each of the lateral four toes (Figs. 6.44 & 6.45). Each tendon enters its fibrous flexor sheath and passes through the flexor digitorum brevis tendon before attaching to the base of the terminal phalanx. The actions and innervations of flexor digitorum longus are considered on page 6.20.

Flexor accessorius (Figs 6.44 & 6.45) is quadrangular and is anchored posteriorly to the medial and lateral tubercles of the calcaneum. Anteriorly the muscle attaches to the tendons of flexor digitorum longus. By pulling on these tendons it can flex the toes irrespective of the position of the ankle. Its nerve supply is from the lateral plantar nerve.

The lumbricals are four small muscles attached proximally to the tendons of flexor digitorum longus (Fig. 6.45). Distally, each slender tendon winds around the medial side of the appropriate digit to attach to the extensor expansion and base of the proximal phalanx. The lumbricals extend the lateral four toes but flex the metatarsophalangeal joints. The first lumbrical is supplied by the medial plantar nerve and the remainder by the lateral plantar nerve.

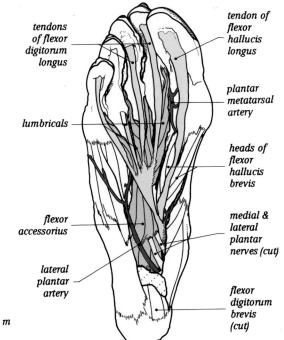

tendons of flexor digitorum longus

tendon of flexor hallucis longus

plantar metatarsal artery

lumbricals

heads of flexor hallucis brevis

flexor accessorius

medial & lateral plantar nerves (cut)

lateral plantar artery

flexor digitorum brevis (cut)

A
l — m
P

Fig. 6.45 *Tendons of flexor digitorum longus, flexor hallucis longus, flexor accessorius and the lumbricals, after removal of medial and lateral plantar nerves and the tendons of flexor digitorum brevis.*

Fig. 6.46 *Deep intrinsic muscles revealed by removal of long flexor tendons and abductors of the great and little toes.*

Deep intrinsic muscles

The three muscles in this layer are located in the anterior part of the foot (Fig. 6.46), adjacent to the metatarsals. Flexor hallucis brevis and adductor hallucis lie medially and are attached to the great toe whilst flexor digiti minimi brevis lies laterally and acts on the little toe.

Flexor hallucis brevis lies along the medial side of the foot and is attached posteriorly to the cuboid and the three cuneiforms. Passing forwards on either side of the flexor hallucis longus tendon (see Fig. 6.45), the muscle gives rise to two short tendons which lie inferior to the first metatarsophalangeal joint. Each tendon contains a sesamoid bone and enters the great toe to attach to the appropriate side of the base of the proximal phalanx. Flexor hallucis brevis flexes the proximal phalanx and is innervated by the medial plantar nerve.

Adductor hallucis (Fig. 6.46) consists of an oblique head which is attached to the bases of the second, third and fourth metatarsals, and a transverse head which lies across the anterior part of the sole, attached to the deep transverse metatarsal ligaments and the lateral three metatarsophalangeal joints. The two heads converge and attach to the lateral tendon and sesamoid of flexor hallucis brevis. Adductor hallucis assists flexor hallucis brevis and

may help to support the transverse arch of the foot. It is supplied by the lateral plantar nerve.

Flexor digiti minimi brevis lies along the plantar surface of the fifth metatarsal (Fig. 6.46), attaching posteriorly to the base of the bone and anteriorly to the lateral side of the base of the proximal phalanx of the little toe. The muscle flexes the proximal phalanx and is innervated by the lateral plantar nerve.

Interossei and tendons of peroneus longus and tibialis posterior

Lying deeply in the sole, attached to the metatarsals, the three plantar interosseous muscles (Fig. 6.47) attach by single heads to the plantar borders of the third, fourth and fifth metatarsals. The four dorsal interossei (Fig. 6.48) are bicipital and attach to contiguous surfaces of the shafts of the metatarsals. The tendons pass forwards dorsal to the deep transverse metatarsal ligaments and attach to the bases of the proximal phalanges and dorsal extensor expansions. These muscles assist extension of the phalanges and flexion of the metatarsophalangeal joints and are supplied by the lateral plantar nerve.

Fig. 6.47 *Interosseous muscles and the plantar arterial arch exposed by removing adductor hallucis.*

plantar metatarsal arteries

deep transverse metatarsal ligament

plantar interosseous muscles

dorsal interosseous muscles

plantar arch

adductor hallucis (cut)

lateral & medial plantar arteries

Fig. 6.48 *Dorsal aspect of the foot showing the dorsal interosseous muscles after partial removal of extensor digitorum brevis.*

capsules of interphalangeal joints

capsules of metatarsophalangeal joints

shafts of metatarsals

dorsalis pedis artery (cut)

dorsal interosseous muscles

extensor digitorum brevis (cut)

6.25

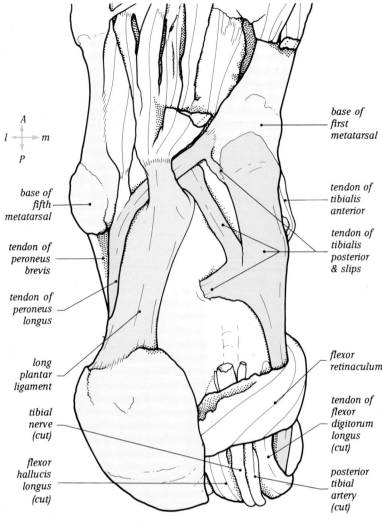

Fig. 6.49 *Tendons of peroneus longus and tibialis posterior lie deeply in the sole of the foot. The long plantar ligament has been preserved.*

The tendons of peroneus longus and tibialis posterior (Fig. 6.49) pass deeply into the sole to reach their attachments on tarsal and metatarsal bones. The peroneus longus tendon enters the lateral side of the sole and is retained in a groove inferior to the cuboid by the long plantar ligament. The tendon passes forwards and medially to reach the lateral aspect of the base of the first metatarsal and adjacent medial cuneiform (compare with tibialis anterior, page 6.28). The tendon of tibialis posterior enters the medial aspect of the foot deep to the flexor retinaculum (Figs. 6.41 & 6.49), attaches to the tuberosity of the navicular and sends additional slips to other tarsal bones and the metatarsal bases. These two tendons may help to support the medial longitudinal arch. The other actions of peroneus longus and tibialis posterior and their innervation are considered on pages 6.31 & 6.20.

BLOOD SUPPLY
Deep to the flexor retinaculum, the tibial artery divides into medial and lateral plantar branches (see Fig. 6.44). Passing forwards, the medial plantar artery runs deep to the superficial intrinsic muscles, gives off plantar cutaneous branches which pass between abductor hallucis and flexor digitorum brevis, and terminates by supplying digital branches to the medial (and occasionally lateral) side of the great toe. The larger lateral plantar artery passes forwards and laterally (see Fig. 6.47) deep to the superficial intrinsic muscles towards the base of the fifth metatarsal. Here the artery inclines medially and deeply to form the plantar arch, lying on the interossei and bases of the metatarsals.

A perforating branch between the first and second metatarsals usually links the arch with the dorsalis pedis artery (see page 6.31). From the arch, plantar metatarsal arteries (see Fig. 6.47) pass distally to the webs of the toes where they divide into digital branches. Venae comitantes accompany medial and lateral plantar arteries and their branches.

NERVE SUPPLY
Cutaneous branches of the tibial nerve supply the skin over the heel. Deep to the flexor retinaculum the tibial nerve divides into medial and lateral branches which supply their respective sides of the sole (see Figs. 6.41 & 6.44). The larger medial plantar nerve accompanies the corresponding artery and gives cutaneous branches to the medial three and one-half digits, including the nail beds. The nerve also supplies abductor hallucis, flexor hallucis brevis, flexor digitorum brevis and the first lumbrical.

The lateral plantar nerve accompanies the corresponding artery (see Fig. 6.44), supplying flexor accessorius and abductor digiti minimi and giving cutaneous branches to the sole. Near the base of the fifth metatarsal it divides into superficial and deep branches which supply the remaining muscles of the sole. The deep branch accompanies the plantar arch and terminates in adductor hallucis. In addition to muscular branches, the superficial branch also gives cutaneous branches to the lateral one and one-half toes.

ANTERIOR COMPARTMENT OF LEG AND DORSUM OF FOOT

The anterior compartment of the leg contains muscles which extend the ankle joint and toes and evert and invert the foot. Its neurovascular bundle comprises the anterior tibial artery and its venae comitantes and the deep peroneal nerve (see Fig. 6.52). The cutaneous branches of the superficial peroneal nerve are also present.

On the dorsum of the foot are the long extensor tendons, the dorsalis pedis artery, the dorsal venous arch and, more laterally, the belly of extensor digitorum brevis. The medial and lateral malleoli lie on each side of the ankle.

Superficial structures

The dorsal venous arch (Fig. 6.50) drains blood from the toes and sole of the foot. From its medial end the long saphenous vein passes in front of the medial malleolus and ascends to the posteromedial aspect of the knee. From the lateral side of the arch the short saphenous vein passes behind the lateral malleolus and ascends to the popliteal fossa (see page 6.16). The saphenous nerve accompanies the long saphenous vein (Fig. 6.51), supplying skin on the medial side of the leg and medial border of the foot as far as the ball (metatarsophalangeal joint) of the great toe. The sural nerve accompanies the short saphenous vein (Fig. 6.50) and supplies skin along the lateral border of the foot and little toe.

The superficial peroneal nerve enters the anterior compartment of the leg from the lateral (peroneal) compartment at the anterior border of peroneus longus (see Fig. 6.53). Shortly after piercing the deep fascia it divides into medial and lateral branches which supply the skin of the leg and dorsum of the foot (Fig. 6.50). On reaching the toes the medial branch supplies the medial side of the great toe and the contiguous aspects of the second and third toes while the lateral branch innervates the adjacent sides of the third, fourth, and fifth toes. Thus, all of the digital skin is innervated by the superficial peroneal nerve except for the cleft between the great and second toes (supplied by the deep peroneal nerve) and the lateral aspect of the little toe (supplied by the sural nerve).

The skin and subcutaneous tissues over the anteromedial surface of the tibia are comparatively thin and have a sparse blood supply. As a consequence, lacerations in this region may heal relatively slowly.

cutaneous branch of superficial peroneal nerve

saphenous nerve

medial malleolus

lateral malleolus

origin of long saphenous vein

origin of short saphenous vein

sural nerve

perforating vein

dorsal venous arch

terminal branch of deep peroneal nerve

digital veins

Fig. 6.50 *Superficial nerves and veins on the dorsum of the ankle and foot.*

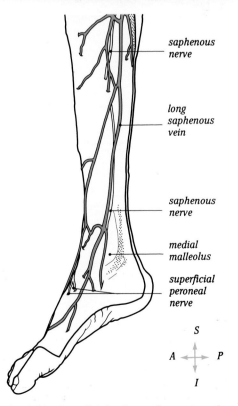

saphenous nerve

long saphenous vein

saphenous nerve

medial malleolus

superficial peroneal nerve

Fig. 6.51 *Superficial veins and nerves on the medial surface of the leg and foot.*

Deep fascia

In the region of the ankle and foot there are thickenings of the investing deep fascia forming retinacula (Fig. 6.53) which prevent bowstringing of the long extensor tendons during muscular contraction. As the tendons pass beneath the retinacula to reach the foot they are enveloped in synovial membrane. By convention, superior and inferior extensor retinacula are described (Fig. 6.54). The superior retinaculum forms a broad band passing between the anterior borders of the tibia and fibula. The inferior retinaculum is Y-shaped with its stem attached to the upper surface of the calcaneum.

Muscles

The muscles in the anterior compartment are tibialis anterior, extensor hallucis longus, extensor digitorum longus and peroneus tertius. All are supplied by the deep peroneal nerve. Tibialis anterior is the most medial (Figs. 6.52 & 6.53), attaching to the lateral condyle and anterolateral surface of the shaft of the tibia, the adjacent interosseous membrane and the deep fascia overlying the muscle. Distally its tendon crosses the anterior border of the lower end of the tibia and attaches to the base of the first metatarsal and adjacent part of the first cuneiform bone. The muscle inverts the foot and dorsiflexes the ankle joint.

The other three muscles all attach to the narrow anterior surface of the fibula and adjacent interosseous membrane. Extensor digitorum longus (Fig. 6.52) is attached to the proximal three-quarters of the bone, peroneus tertius (when present) to the distal quarter, and extensor hallucis longus overlaps them medially at midshaft level. In addition, extensor digitorum longus attaches to the anterior peroneal intermuscular septum and overlying deep fascia.

The proximal part of extensor hallucis longus is overlapped by adjacent muscles, but in the lower part of the leg its tendon emerges lateral to that of tibialis anterior. As it descends towards the ankle the tendon crosses from the lateral to the medial side of the neurovascular bundle. In the foot the tendon of extensor hallucis longus runs forwards to the great toe (see Fig. 6.55) where it attaches to the base of the distal phalanx. It is a powerful extensor of the toe, dorsiflexor (extensor) of the foot and assists inversion. Lateral to extensor hallucis longus, the muscle belly of extensor digitorum longus gives way distally to four tendons which pass to the dorsal aspects of the lateral four toes. Each tendon forms an extensor expansion which divides into three slips. The central slip attaches to the base of the middle phalanx whilst the two lateral slips combine to insert into the base of the distal phalanx (see Fig. 6.55). Extensor digitorum longus extends the lateral four toes and dorsiflexes the foot. Peroneus tertius is a continuation of the belly of extensor digitorum longus. It attaches to the lateral border of the fifth metatarsal (see Fig. 6.56) and everts the foot and dorsiflexes the ankle.

The muscles of the anterior compartment of the leg are active during walking in both the supporting and swing phases. In the weight-bearing limb they help to incline the leg forwards while the foot remains stationary on the ground. In the swinging limb the muscles maintain the ankle in dorsiflexion, thereby preventing the foot from dropping.

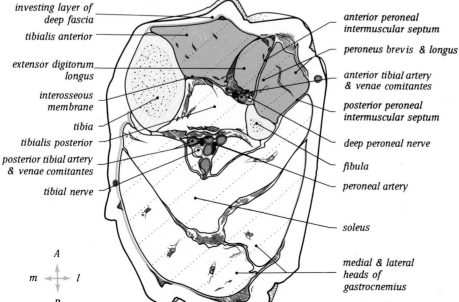

investing layer of deep fascia
tibialis anterior
extensor digitorum longus
interosseous membrane
tibia
tibialis posterior
posterior tibial artery & venae comitantes
tibial nerve

anterior peroneal intermuscular septum
peroneus brevis & longus
anterior tibial artery & venae comitantes
posterior peroneal intermuscular septum
deep peroneal nerve
fibula
peroneal artery
soleus
medial & lateral heads of gastrocnemius

A
m — l
P

Fig. 6.52 *Transverse section through the midcalf showing anterior and lateral compartments and their contents.*

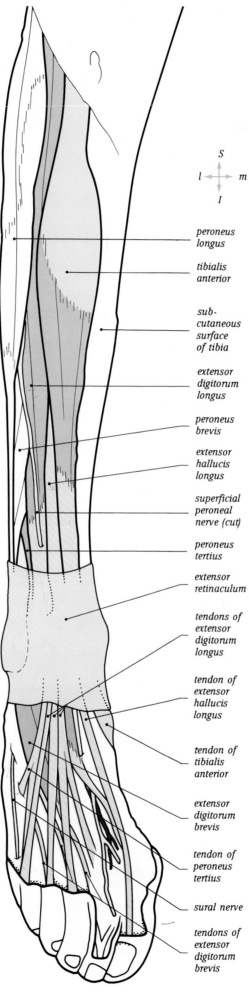

S
l — m
I

peroneus
longus

tibialis
anterior

sub-
cutaneous
surface
of tibia

extensor
digitorum
longus

peroneus
brevis

extensor
hallucis
longus

superficial
peroneal
nerve (cut)

peroneus
tertius

extensor
retinaculum

tendons of
extensor
digitorum
longus

tendon of
extensor
hallucis
longus

tendon of
tibialis
anterior

extensor
digitorum
brevis

tendon of
peroneus
tertius

sural nerve

tendons of
extensor
digitorum
brevis

Fig. 6.53 *Muscles of the anterior compartment of
the leg and tendons on the dorsum of the foot
seen after removal of deep fascia. The extensor
retinaculum has been retained.*

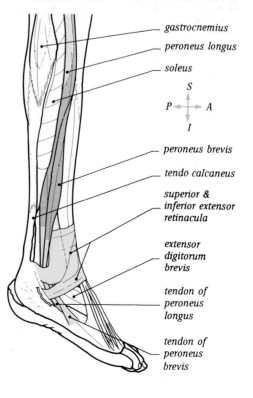

gastrocnemius

peroneus longus

soleus

S
P — A
I

peroneus brevis

tendo calcaneus

superior &
inferior extensor
retinacula

extensor
digitorum
brevis

tendon of
peroneus
longus

tendon of
peroneus
brevis

Fig. 6.54 *Lateral aspect of the leg and foot
showing peroneus longus and brevis.*

On the dorsum of the foot extensor digitorum brevis (Fig. 6.55) is attached to the upper surface of the calcaneum and overlying stem of the inferior extensor retinaculum. The muscle gives rise to four short tendons which pass deep to the long extensor tendons of the medial four toes (Fig. 6.55). The tendons to the second, third and fourth toes attach to the dorsal extensor expansions; the tendon to the great toe, extensor hallucis brevis, attaches to the base of the proximal phalanx. The muscle assists extension of the toes, particularly when the long extensors are flexing the leg forwards on the foot just before it is lifted from the ground during walking. The nerve supply is the deep peroneal nerve.

Fig. 6.55 *Principal structures on the dorsum of the ankle and foot seen after removal of the extensor retinaculum.*

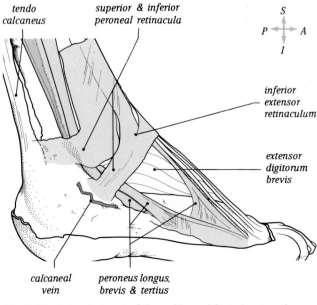

Fig. 6.56 *Lateral aspect of the ankle and foot showing the peroneal tendons and the retinacula.*

Neurovascular bundle

This comprises the deep peroneal nerve and the anterior tibial artery with its venae comitantes (see Fig. 6.52). The artery, a terminal branch of the popliteal artery (see page 6.17), reaches the anterior compartment after passing through the interosseous membrane. It then descends on the anterior surface of the membrane (Fig. 6.57) and at the ankle lies midway between the two malleoli. It continues distally as the dorsalis pedis artery on the lateral side of the extensor hallucis longus tendon (Fig. 6.55) where its pulsations are palpable in the living foot.

At the proximal end of the first intermetatarsal space the dorsalis pedis artery gives a deep branch which passes between the two heads of the first dorsal interosseous muscle to join the plantar arch (see page 6.26). This arrangement provides an anastomosis between the anterior and posterior tibial arteries. The dorsalis pedis artery terminates as the first dorsal metatarsal artery, supplying the great toe and adjacent border of the second toe, and the arcuate artery. It turns laterally beneath the extensor tendons across the bases of the metatarsals and gives metatarsal arteries which divide to supply adjacent borders of the remaining three digits.

The deep peroneal nerve, a terminal branch of the common peroneal nerve, winds around the neck of the fibula deep to peroneus longus (Fig. 6.57). The nerve accompanies the anterior tibial vessels into the foot and supplies all muscles in the anterior compartment. In the foot the nerve is close to the dorsalis pedis artery, usually lying lateral to the artery but sometimes medial to it (Fig. 6.55). It gives a branch to extensor digitorum brevis and the tarsal joints and terminates by supplying the skin between the great and second toes (Fig. 6.55).

LATERAL (PERONEAL) COMPARTMENT OF LEG

The lateral compartment of the leg extends from the head of the fibula above to the lateral malleolus below. Its principal contents are the peroneus longus and brevis muscles (see Fig. 6.54). Peroneus longus is attached to the upper two-thirds of the lateral surface of the fibula and peroneus brevis to the lower two-thirds, with brevis being the more anterior. Both muscles are attached to the two peroneal intermuscular septa and the overlying deep fascia. On reaching the ankle the tendons pass behind and then below the lateral malleolus, restrained by the superior and inferior peroneal retinacula and surrounded by synovial membrane (Fig. 6.56). The tendon of peroneus brevis passes forwards above the peroneal tubercle of the calcaneum to attach to the base of the fifth metatarsal. The peroneus longus tendon passes forwards below the peroneal tubercle and turns medially into the sole of the foot where it lies in a groove on the cuboid bone. It attaches to the lateral side of the base of the first metatarsal and the adjacent first cuneiform.

Peroneus longus and brevis are evertors of the foot and weak plantar flexors of the ankle joint. Their nerve supply is the superficial peroneal nerve, a terminal branch of

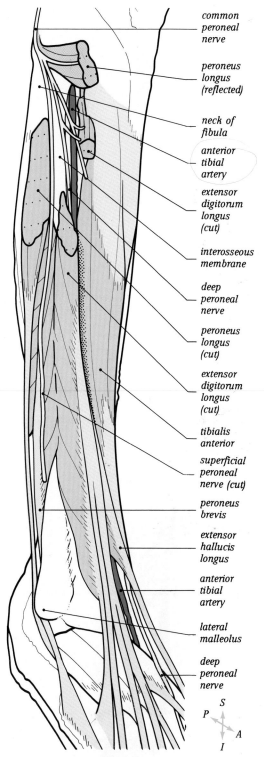

Fig. 6.57 *Common peroneal nerve and its branches and the anterior tibial artery seen after deep dissection of both compartments.*

the common peroneal nerve which enters the lateral (peroneal) compartment by winding around the neck of the fibula where it is palpable and may sometimes be compressed.

Branches of the peroneal artery, which arises from the posterior tibial artery (see page 6.19). pierce the posterior peroneal intermuscular septum to supply peroneus longus and brevis.

HIP JOINT

The hip joint is a synovial ball-and-socket joint between the head of the femur and the acetabulum of the hip bone (Fig. 6.58).

ARTICULAR SURFACES

The femoral head, covered by hyaline cartilage, forms two-thirds of a sphere and has a central pit (fovea; Fig. 6.58) giving attachment to the round ligament (ligamentum teres). The head surmounts the femoral neck whose base abuts the medial side of the greater trochanter. The acetabulum is a deep socket with a C-shaped articular area covered with hyaline cartilage, and a fat-filled non-articular area (acetabular fossa) whose margins give attachment to the base of the ligamentum teres (Fig. 6.59). The acetabulum is deficient inferiorly at the acetabular notch (Fig. 6.58) where blood vessels, bridged by the transverse acetabular ligament, enter the joint. A fibrocartilaginous labrum, attached to the margins of the acetabulum and the transverse ligament, helps to deepen the socket.

CAPSULE

Medially the fibrous capsule is attached to the outer margin of the labrum; laterally the capsule attaches to the intertrochanteric line (Figs. 6.58 & 6.60) at the root of the femoral neck and to the femoral shaft just above the lesser trochanter. From the femoral attachment of the capsule, retinacular fibres derived from the deep part of the capsule (Fig. 6.59) are reflected medially over the neck to the margins of the head. Posteriorly the line of attachment of the capsule is such that only the upper (medial) half of the femoral neck lies within the joint.

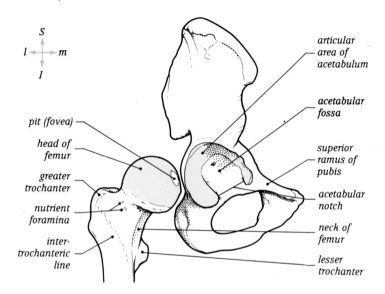

Fig. 6.58 *Articular surfaces of the hip joint comprise the acetabulum of the hip bone and the head of the femur.*

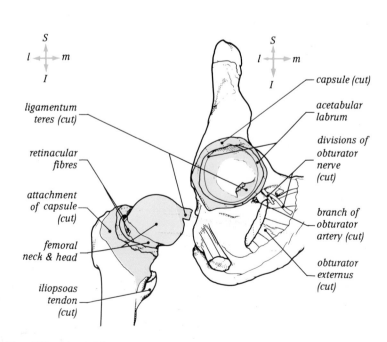

Fig. 6.59 *Internal features revealed by disarticulation of the joint after cutting the ligamentum teres and joint capsule.*

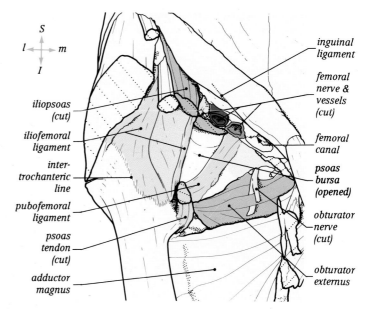

iliopsoas (cut)

iliofemoral ligament

inter-trochanteric line

pubofemoral ligament

psoas tendon (cut)

adductor magnus

inguinal ligament

femoral nerve & vessels (cut)

femoral canal

psoas bursa (opened)

obturator nerve (cut)

obturator externus

Fig. 6.60 *Anterior surface of the joint capsule, its associated ligaments and immediate relations.*

LIGAMENTS

The iliofemoral, pubofemoral and ischiofemoral ligaments are capsular thickenings which spiral downwards and laterally from the hip bone to the femur. The strong iliofemoral ligament (Fig. 6.60) is an inverted Y shape, the stem attaching to the anterior inferior iliac spine and the limbs to the upper and lower ends of the intertrochanteric line.

The pubofemoral ligament (Fig. 6.60) passes from the iliopectineal eminence to the femoral neck just above the lesser trochanter. The ischiofemoral ligament lies posteriorly (see Fig. 6.62) and reaches the root of the greater trochanter.

Within the joint is the ligamentum teres (Figs. 6.59 & 6.61) which has the form of a flattened cone, the base attaching to the margins of the acetabular fossa and transverse acetabular ligament, and the apex to the fovea on the femoral head.

femoral head

joint cavity

acetabular labrum

ligamentum teres

obturator canal

capsule (iliofemoral ligament)

obturator artery (cut)

obturator externus

divisions of obturator nerve (cut)

Fig. 6.61 *Joint capsule opened anteriorly and reflected to show the interior of the joint. The femur has been abducted and externally rotated.*

6.33

HIP JOINT

SYNOVIAL MEMBRANE AND BURSAE

Synovial membrane lines the interior of the capsule and the non-articular surfaces of the joint, clothes the ligamentum teres and is reflected over the retinacular fibres and the femoral neck as far as the head. The iliopsoas tendon and anterior aspect of the capsule are separated by a large bursa (see Fig. 6.60), which often is in communication with the joint cavity.

The tendon of obturator externus is separated from the capsule by a smaller bursa, which may also communicate with the joint.

MOVEMENTS

The hip joint is multiaxial and permits flexion, extension, abduction, adduction, medial and lateral rotation, and circumduction.

Flexion is produced by iliopsoas, assisted by sartorius, rectus femoris and pectineus. Gluteus maximus and the hamstrings are extensors. Abductors of the hip include gluteus medius and minimus while adduction is produced by adductors longus, brevis and magnus, pectineus and gracilis. Medial rotation is produced by iliopsoas, tensor fasciae latae and the anterior fibres of gluteus minimus and medius. Lateral rotation is produced by piriformis, quadratus femoris, obturator externus and internus, and the gemelli.

STABILITY

The hip joint is very stable, largely because of its bony morphology and the deep fit of the femoral head into the acetabulum. Other important factors include the ligaments and the tone of the muscles crossing the joint. The ilio-, pubo- and ischiofemoral ligaments all limit extension and medial rotation. The iliofemoral ligament, in particular, prevents hyperextension, especially in the upright posture when body weight acts behind the transverse axis of the hip joint and tilts the pelvis backwards. The ligamentum teres limits adduction of the hip.

RELATIONS

The joint is deeply placed behind the midpoint of the inguinal ligament. Laterally the greater trochanter covers the neck of the femur and is palpable on the lateral side of the thigh. Medially only the thin bone of the acetabular fossa (Figs. 6.63 & 6.64) separates the head of the femur from structures within the pelvis which are vulnerable following acetabular fracture accompanied by medial displacement of the femoral head. Posteriorly lie structures of the gluteal region (Fig. 6.62), including the sciatic nerve which may be damaged in posterior dislocation. Anteriorly the joint is covered by the iliopsoas and the femoral vessels and nerve. Obturator externus and the adductor muscles lie inferiorly (Fig. 6.64) whilst superiorly are gluteus medius and minimus.

BLOOD SUPPLY

The arterial supply of the hip joint, especially that of the head and neck of the femur, is of particular clinical importance. The joint receives branches from the obturator artery, superior and inferior gluteal arteries, and medial and lateral circumflex femoral arteries, either directly or from the trochanteric anastomosis which they form. From this anastomosis (Fig. 6.62), nutrient arteries travel in the retinacular fibres to enter foramina on the upper part of the femoral neck and terminate in the head. Since only the upper half of the neck is covered posteriorly by the joint capsule, fractures at this site may be classified as either intra- or extracapsular. Intracapsular fractures which tear the retinacula may deprive the head of the femur of much of its blood supply. Additional blood supply comes from a branch of the obturator artery conveyed in the ligamentum teres to the femoral head, and from one of the perforating branches of the profunda femoris artery via a nutrient artery which enters the shaft to supply the femoral neck and head.

NERVE SUPPLY

Nerves to the joint include the nerve to rectus femoris from the femoral nerve, branches from the anterior division of the obturator nerve, and the nerve to quadratus femoris from the sacral plexus.

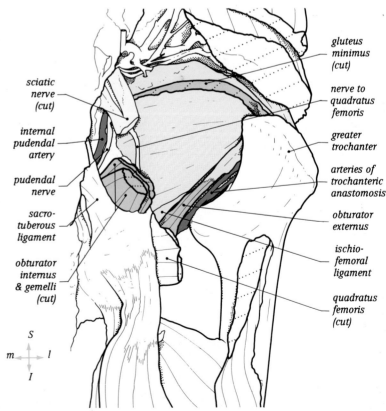

Fig. 6.62 *Posterior surface of the joint capsule, the ischiofemoral ligament and close relations.*

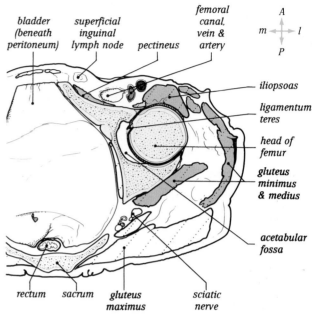

Fig. **6.63** *Transverse section through the hip joint showing its relations.*

Labels on Fig. 6.63:
- bladder (beneath peritoneum)
- superficial inguinal lymph node
- pectineus
- femoral canal, vein & artery
- iliopsoas
- ligamentum teres
- head of femur
- gluteus minimus & medius
- acetabular fossa
- rectum
- sacrum
- gluteus maximus
- sciatic nerve

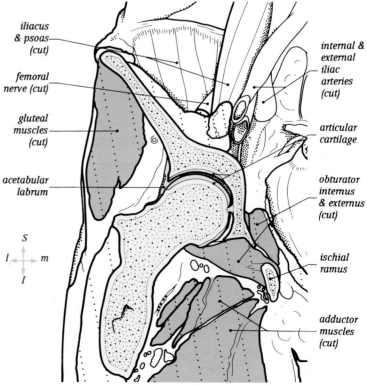

Labels on Fig. 6.64:
- iliacus & psoas (cut)
- femoral nerve (cut)
- gluteal muscles (cut)
- acetabular labrum
- internal & external iliac arteries (cut)
- articular cartilage
- obturator internus & externus (cut)
- ischial ramus
- adductor muscles (cut)

Fig. **6.64** *Coronal section through the hip joint showing its relations.*

KNEE JOINT

The knee joint is a synovial joint between the distal end of the femur, proximal end of the tibia and posterior aspect of the patella (Fig. 6.65). It is a hinge joint with a wide range of flexion and extension and limited lateral and medial rotation. The joint is relatively superficial anteriorly and laterally where some of its bony features are palpable but posteriorly is inaccessible, being deeply placed in the floor of the popliteal fossa (Fig. 6.66).

Anteriorly the ligamentum patellae (Fig. 6.67) passes from the apex of the patella to the tibial tubercle. It is easily palpable and is used clinically for the stretch reflex (knee jerk).

ARTICULAR SURFACES

The medial and lateral condyles of the femur have articular surfaces, covered by hyaline cartilage, which extend over their inferior and posterior aspects and articulate with the respective condyles on the tibia (Fig. 6.65). On the front of the femur lies the patellar (trochlear) articular surface while posteriorly a deep intercondylar notch separates the two condyles. The articular areas on the tibial condyles are separated by the intercondylar eminence, the lateral articular area being flatter and smaller than the medial area (Fig. 6.65).

Fig. 6.65 *Articular surfaces of the patella, femur and tibia.*

Fig. 6.66 *Sagittal section through the knee joint showing the articular surfaces and suprapatellar pouch.*

Fig. 6.67 *Superficial dissection from the anterior aspect showing the ligamentum patellae, capsule, and medial and lateral collateral ligaments.*

CAPSULE

The capsule is thin anteriorly and posteriorly but is reinforced on each side by strong collateral ligaments. On the sides of the femur the capsule attachment extends up to the epicondyles. Posteriorly it attaches along the superior margins of the condyles (Figs. 6.68 & 6.70) and the intercondylar line whilst anteriorly it extends proximally (Fig. 6.67; see Figs. 6.71 & 6.73) to accommodate the synovial membrane which forms the suprapatellar pouch (bursa).

On the sides of the tibia the capsule attaches close to the articular margins. Those parts of the capsule on each side of the joint which loosely anchor the outer borders of the menisci to the femur and tibia are called the coronary ligament. Posteriorly the capsular attachment inclines downwards to include the posterior part of the intercondylar area whilst anteriorly the attachment deviates inferiorly as far as the tibial tubercle. On the patella the capsule is attached close to the articular margins.

Posteriorly part of the insertion of semimembranosus forms the oblique posterior ligament which passes upwards and laterally (Figs. 6.68 & 6.69), reinforcing the capsule. Where the posterior part of the capsule is pierced by popliteus, it thickens to form the arcuate ligament (Fig. 6.68).

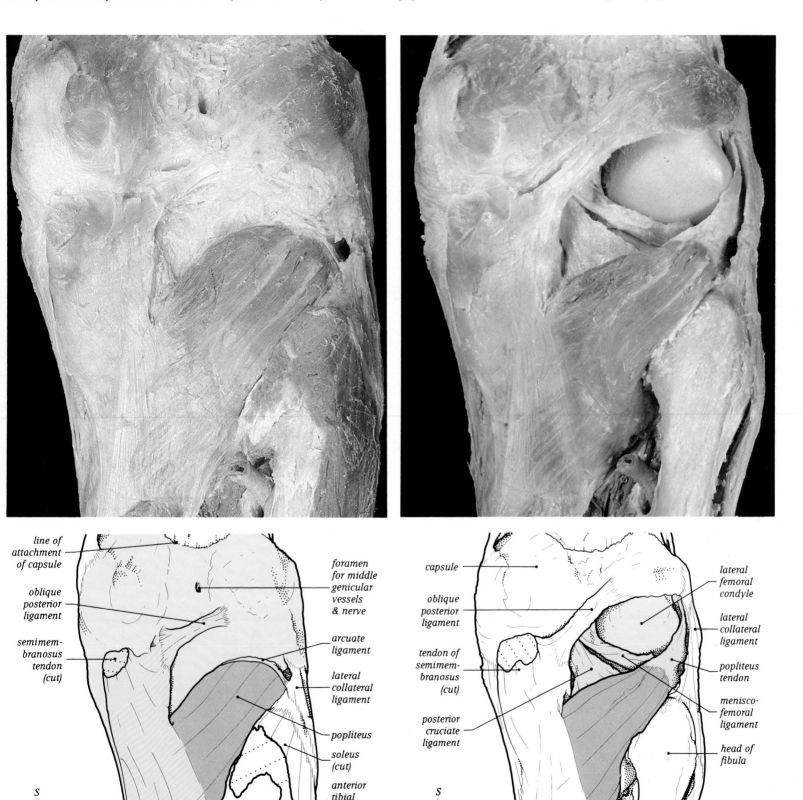

Fig. 6.68 *Superficial dissection from the posterior aspect showing the capsule, semimembranosus insertion and oblique posterior ligament, and popliteus and arcuate ligament.*

Fig. 6.69 *Removal of part of the capsule posteriorly reveals the meniscofemoral and posterior cruciate ligaments and the tendon of popliteus.*

6.37

medial
femoral
condyle

medial
collateral
ligament

posterior
cruciate
ligament

medial
meniscus

lateral
& medial
tibial
condyles

popliteus
(cut)

line of
attachment
of capsule

lateral
femoral
condyle

lateral
collateral
ligament

anterior
cruciate
ligament

popliteus
tendon
(cut)

lateral
meniscus

proximal
tibiofibular
synovial
joint
(capsule
removed)

S
m — l
I

patella

capsule
extending
into supra-
patellar
pouch

ligamentum
patellae

capsule
overlying
meniscus

tibial
tubercle

vastus
medialis

medial
collateral
ligament

gracilis
tendon

sartorius
tendon
(cut)

semi-
tendinosus
tendon

S
A — P
I

Fig. 6.70 *The posterior part of the capsule has been removed to show the anterior and posterior cruciate ligaments and menisci.*

Fig. 6.71 *Superficial dissection from the medial aspect showing the medial collateral ligament, capsule and insertions of sartorius, gracilis and semitendinosus.*

COLLATERAL LIGAMENTS

On the medial side of the joint the thick tibial collateral ligament (Fig. 6.71) broadens as it descends from the medial femoral epicondyle to the upper part of the subcutaneous surface of the tibia. Its deep aspect is attached to the outer margin of the medial meniscus (Fig. 6.70) which diminishes mobility of the meniscus, making it more susceptible to tears. On the lateral side the cord-like fibular collateral ligament (Fig. 6.72) descends from the lateral epicondyle of the femur to the styloid process and head of the fibula, separated from the lateral meniscus by the popliteus tendon (Fig. 6.70).

INTRACAPSULAR LIGAMENTS

The intracapsular ligaments comprise the anterior and posterior cruciate ligaments and the meniscofemoral ligament.

The cruciate ligaments (Fig. 6.70) are named according to their attachment to the intercondylar eminence of the tibia (see Fig. 6.74). The anterior ligament passes upwards, backwards and laterally to attach to the medial surface of the lateral condyle of the femur. The posterior ligament passes upwards, forwards and medially (Fig. 6.70) to attach to the lateral surface of the medial femoral condyle. The meniscofemoral ligament is adjacent to the posterior cruciate ligament (see Fig. 6.69) and attaches the posterior border of the lateral meniscus close to the femoral attachment of the posterior cruciate ligament. It stabilizes the meniscus during rotation of the femur on the tibia. Although within the capsule, the cruciate and meniscofemoral ligaments are covered by reflections of synovial membrane and are therefore not within the synovial cavity.

MENISCI

The medial and lateral menisci are C-shaped (see Fig. 6.74) with their anterior and posterior horns attached to the intercondylar eminence of the tibia and their outer borders to the joint capsule (coronary ligaments). The menisci differ in size and shape, the medial being narrower though slightly larger so that its horns embrace those of the lateral meniscus. Also, the medial is attached to the medial collateral ligament and on cross-section is deeper compared with the lateral meniscus. A transverse ligament (see Fig. 6.74) connects the anterior horn of the medial meniscus with the anterior aspect of the lateral meniscus.

INFRAPATELLAR FAT PAD

Deep to the ligamentum patellae is a quantity of fat (see Fig. 6.66) which bulges the synovial membrane into the interior of the joint. Folds of synovial membrane, the alar folds (Fig. 6.73), extend on either side from the main pad. Another fold, the ligamentum mucosum, lies in the midline between the anterior part of the intercondylar notch and the lower margin of the patella.

SYNOVIAL MEMBRANE AND BURSAE

Synovial membrane lines the interior of the capsule but does not cover the menisci. On the femur it is attached to the margins of the intercondylar notch and covers the front and sides of the cruciate ligaments. Synovial membrane also covers the infrapatellar fat pad and the tendon of popliteus.

The suprapatellar bursa (Fig. 6.73; see also Fig. 6.66) is a large pouch of synovial membrane, passing a hand's breadth proximal to the upper border of the patella, deep to quadriceps. Part of vastus intermedius attaches to it. Since the bursa is continuous with the synovial cavity of the joint, it provides a route for injecting or withdrawing fluid into or from the joint. After injuries to the joint, fluid accumulates (effusion) in the suprapatellar bursa, causing typical fullness around the knee. Several other bursae lie near the knee joint and may enlarge, causing swellings.

Bursae between the capsule and the two heads of gastrocnemius often communicate with the knee joint while that beneath the medial head may also communicate with the overlying semimembranosus bursa. Other bursae, which do not communicate with the joint, are the pre- and infrapatellar bursae beneath the skin covering the patella and ligamentum patellae respectively.

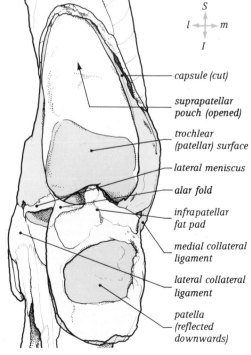

Fig. 6.72 *Lateral aspect showing the lateral collateral ligament and the meniscus, revealed by removal of part of the capsule.*

Fig. 6.73 *Exposure of the interior of the joint and suprapatellar pouch by opening the capsule anteriorly and reflecting the patella downwards.*

6.39

Fig. 6.74 *Attachments of the cruciates and the shape and attachments of the menisci. Cutting of the cruciate and collateral ligaments has allowed separation of femur from tibia.*

POPLITEUS

From its tibial attachment the popliteus passes upwards and laterally (see Fig. 6.68), penetrating the posterior aspect of the capsule of the knee joint deep to the arcuate ligament. Within the joint its tendon, covered by synovial membrane, attaches to the posterior border of the lateral meniscus and to the femur (see Fig. 6.69) immediately below the lateral epicondyle. Popliteus is supplied by the tibial nerve and its actions are considered below.

MOVEMENTS

The principal movements of the knee joint are flexion and extension. Flexion is produced mainly by the hamstrings (semimembranosus, semitendinosus and biceps) assisted by the two heads of gastrocnemius. Extension is produced by quadriceps femoris acting through the ligamentum patellae. Gluteus maximus, acting through the iliotibial tract, maintains stability of the knee in the extended position.

Because of the shape of the articular surfaces, the femur rotates medially during the later stages of extension. The lateral condyle and meniscus (moving in unison because of the meniscofemoral ligament) glide forwards on the lateral tibial condyle whilst the medial condyle completes its movement of extension on the medial meniscus. Full extension is achieved with completion of medial rotation and further movement is prevented by tension in the collateral and oblique posterior ligaments. During the early stages of flexion, lateral rotation of the femur on the tibia is produced by popliteus which also pulls the lateral meniscus posteriorly. During flexion and extension the patella glides over the trochlear surface of the femur.

Slight active rotation of the tibia on the femur can occur when the knee is in a flexed but non-weight-bearing position. Sartorius, gracilis and semitendinosus rotate medially while biceps femoris rotates laterally.

STABILITY

The knee joint is very stable. The most important factors are muscle tone, especially in quadriceps, and the ligaments. The cruciate ligaments stabilize the femur on the tibia, preventing excessive anteroposterior movement. The collateral ligaments assist medial and lateral stability while the iliotibial tract stabilizes the knee during extension. All of these ligaments together with the oblique posterior ligament prevent hyperextension.

Due to angulation of the femur relative to the tibia, contraction of quadriceps femoris tends to displace the patella laterally. This displacement is prevented by, firstly, the lowest fibres of vastus medialis which insert into the medial patellar border and whose active contraction resists lateral movement of the patella, and secondly, by the large size and prominence of the lateral femoral condyle making lateral patellar movement mechanically difficult.

INNERVATION

Branches from the femoral, obturator and sciatic nerves supply the joint, sensory fibres from the femoral nerve travelling with the branches to the vasti and sartorius. Genicular branches from the tibial and common peroneal divisions of the sciatic nerve, together with fibres from the posterior division of the obturator nerve, also supply the joint.

BLOOD SUPPLY

The knee joint receives its blood supply from the extensive genicular anastomosis derived mainly from branches of the popliteal, anterior and posterior tibial arteries.

TIBIOFIBULAR JOINTS

The tibia and fibula articulate at proximal and distal tibiofibular joints and are also connected by an interosseous membrane (Fig. 6.75) which unites the interosseous borders of the bones and separates the flexor and extensor compartments of the leg.

The proximal tibiofibular joint is a plane synovial articulation between the lateral condyle of the tibia and head of the fibula, and is supplied by the common peroneal nerve. The capsule is reinforced by anterior and posterior ligaments, and the synovial cavity does not communicate with the knee joint.

The opposed triangular surfaces at the lower ends of the tibia and fibula are bound together by an interosseous ligament, forming the fibrous distal tibiofibular joint, which is strengthened by anterior and posterior tibiofibular ligaments. The transverse ligament, an inferior extension of the posterior ligament, contributes to the articular socket of the ankle joint (see Fig. 6.77), whose cavity frequently extends for a short distance between the tibia and fibula. The ankle is stabilized by the ligaments of the distal tibiofibular joint which prevent separation of the malleoli. Innervation is by the deep peroneal and tibial nerves.

Very little movement occurs at the tibiofibular joints, but slight rotation of the fibula may accompany flexion and extension of the ankle.

lateral (fibular) collateral ligament

proximal tibiofibular joint (synovial cavity opened)

capsule (cut)

posterior cruciate ligament (cut)

anterior tibial artery

medial (tibial) collateral ligament (cut)

posterior surface of tibia

interosseous membrane

S
m ← → l
I

posterior tibiofibular ligament

Fig. 6.75 *Tibiofibular joints and interosseous membrane. All the muscles of the posterior compartment of the leg have been removed. The lower part of the tibiofibular ligament has been removed.*

ANKLE JOINT

The ankle joint is a synovial hinge joint between the lower ends of the tibia and fibula and the upper part of the talus (Fig. 6.76), and all the articular surfaces are covered by hyaline cartilage. The proximal articular surface comprises the distal end of the tibia and the medial and lateral malleoli, which together form a deep socket (Fig. 6.77), completed posteriorly by the transverse tibiofibular ligament (see below). The socket is wider anteriorly than posteriorly and is completely congruous with the upper part of the talus which is reciprocally wedge shaped (Fig. 6.78). The articular surface on the lateral side of the talus is more extensive than that on the medial side.

CAPSULE AND SYNOVIAL MEMBRANE

The fibrous capsule attaches to the margins of the articular surfaces, but anteriorly extends forwards onto the neck of the talus (Fig. 6.78). The capsule is thin anteriorly and posteriorly, but is reinforced on each side by ligaments. Synovial membrane lines the capsule internally and covers the intracapsular part of the neck of the talus.

Fig. 6.76 *Bones of the ankle joint showing their articulating surfaces.*

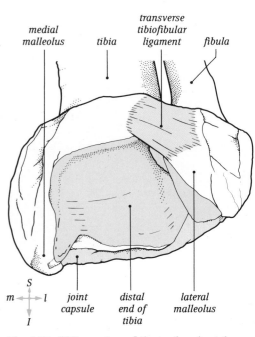

Fig. 6.77 *Oblique view of the wedge-shaped articular socket of the ankle joint.*

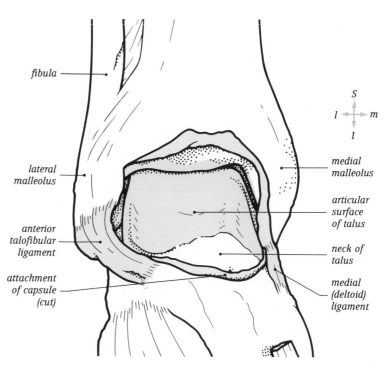

fibula

lateral
malleolus

anterior
talofibular
ligament

attachment
of capsule
(cut)

medial
malleolus

articular
surface
of talus

neck of
talus

medial
(deltoid)
ligament

S
l — m
I

Fig. 6.78 *Anterior view of the ankle joint showing articular surfaces revealed by removal of the capsule.*

S
P — A
I

talus

tendo
calcaneus
(cut)

joint
capsule

lateral
malleolus
of fibula

anterior
talofibular
ligament

calcaneofibular
ligament

calcaneum

attachment
of capsule
(cut)

Fig. 6.79 *Lateral collateral ligament of the ankle joint after removal of the capsule.*

tendon of tibialis anterior (cut)   sus-tentaculum tali   articular surface of talus   medial malleolus of tibia   tendo calcaneus (cut)

long plantar ligament   attachment of tibialis posterior to tuberosity of navicular   'spring' ligament   medial (deltoid) ligament (superficial part)   calcaneum

Fig. 6.80 *Medial collateral ligament of the ankle joint after removal of the capsule.*

LIGAMENTS

The transverse tibiofibular ligament spans the gap between the distal ends of the tibia and fibula, contributing to the articular socket posteriorly (see Fig. 6.77). There are two collateral ligaments. The medial (deltoid) ligament (Fig. 6.80) is attached by its apex to the tip of the medial malleolus. Its deeper fibres descend to the margin of the articular surface on the medial side of the talus and its longer superficial fibres attach to the tuberosity of the navicular, the medial border of the 'spring' ligament and the sustentaculum tali.

The lateral ligament has three components: the anterior and posterior talofibular; and the calcaneofibular ligaments (Figs. 6.79 & 6.81). All attach to the lateral malleolus. The anterior talofibular ligament passes forwards to the lateral side of the neck of the talus, the posterior talofibular ligament medially to the posterior tubercle of the talus, and the calcaneofibular downwards and backwards to the side of the calcaneum.

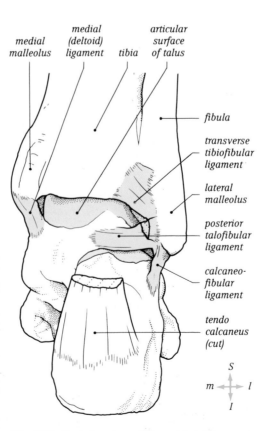

medial malleolus   medial (deltoid) ligament   tibia   articular surface of talus

fibula

transverse tibiofibular ligament

lateral malleolus

posterior talofibular ligament

calcaneo-fibular ligament

tendo calcaneus (cut)

Fig. 6.81 *Posterior view of the ankle joint showing the articular surface of talus after removal of the capsule.*

MOVEMENTS

Only extension (dorsiflexion) and flexion (plantar flexion) occur at the ankle joint, around a transverse axis between the malleoli. Plantar flexion is produced by soleus and gastrocnemius, assisted by tibialis posterior, flexors hallucis longus and digitorum longus, and peroneus longus and brevis. Extension (dorsiflexion) is produced by tibialis anterior, extensors hallucis longus and digitorum longus, and peroneus tertius.

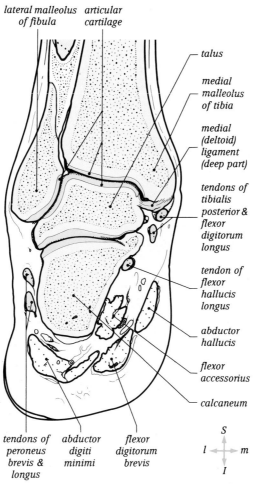

lateral malleolus of fibula — articular cartilage

— talus

— medial malleolus of tibia

— medial (deltoid) ligament (deep part)

— tendons of tibialis posterior & flexor digitorum longus

— tendon of flexor hallucis longus

— abductor hallucis

— flexor accessorius

— calcaneum

tendons of peroneus brevis & longus — abductor digiti minimi — flexor digitorum brevis

S
l ← → m
I

Fig. 6.82 *Coronal section through ankle and talocalcaneal joints showing the articular surfaces.*

STABILITY

The joint is very stable due to the wedge shape of the articulating surfaces and the strong collateral ligaments. During standing and walking, body weight tends to displace the tibiofibular socket forwards so that it becomes closely packed against the wider anterior part of the talus, which further enhances stability during dorsiflexion. Excessive forward displacement of the tibia and fibula on the talus is prevented by the posterior fibres of the medial (deltoid) ligament and by the calcaneofibular and posterior talofibular ligaments. However, in plantar flexion the narrow part of the talus articulates with the wider anterior part of the socket, allowing some side-to-side movement. In this position, forced inversion of the foot may damage the anterior talofibular ligament, one form of 'sprained ankle'.

BLOOD AND NERVE SUPPLY

Branches of the anterior and posterior tibial arteries, including the peroneal, anastomose at the level of the malleoli and supply the joint. Innervation is from the deep peroneal and tibial nerves.

RELATIONS

The sides of the joint, the bony malleoli, are superficial (Fig. 6.82) and easily palpable. Passing subcutaneously in front of the joint are branches of the superficial peroneal nerve and, just anterior to the medial malleolus, the saphenous nerve and long saphenous vein. On a deeper plane are the tendons of tibialis anterior and extensor hallucis longus, the dorsalis pedis artery, the deep peroneal nerve, and the tendons of extensor digitorum longus and peroneus tertius (Fig. 6.83).

Posteriorly the tendo calcaneus (Achillis) lies separated from the joint capsule by a bursa and pad of fat. Behind the medial malleolus are the tendons of tibialis posterior, flexor digitorum longus and flexor hallucis longus (Fig. 6.82), accompanied by the tibial nerve and posterior tibial artery (Fig. 6.83). Passing below the medial malleolus, they enter the foot beneath the flexor retinaculum. Passing superficially behind the lateral malleolus are the short saphenous vein and sural nerve and, more deeply, the tendons of peroneus longus and brevis.

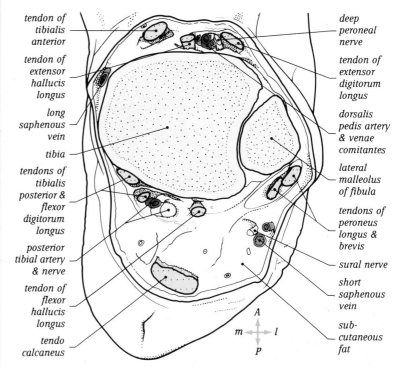

tendon of tibialis anterior —

tendon of extensor hallucis longus —

long saphenous vein —

tibia —

tendons of tibialis posterior & flexor digitorum longus —

posterior tibial artery & nerve —

tendon of flexor hallucis longus —

tendo calcaneus —

— deep peroneal nerve

— tendon of extensor digitorum longus

— dorsalis pedis artery & venae comitantes

— lateral malleolus of fibula

— tendons of peroneus longus & brevis

— sural nerve

— short saphenous vein

— sub-cutaneous fat

A
m ← → l
P

Fig. 6.83 *Transverse section through the ankle immediately above the joint cavity showing its anterior and posterior relations.*

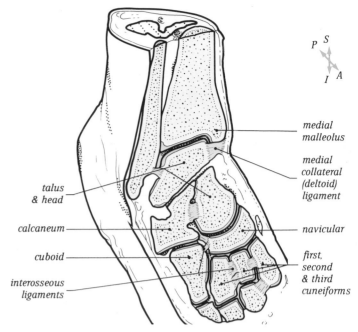

Fig. 6.84 *Vertical and horizontal sectioning of the foot and ankle shows the interrelationships of the tarsal joints.*

These joints include those between the tarsal bones, the metatarsals and the phalanges. They are all synovial and have shapes related to their movements.

TARSAL JOINTS

Whilst the tarsal joints are articulations between individual bones, they are usually classified into groups according to their locations (Fig. 6.84). The posterior tarsal group involves the talus and calcaneum; the midtarsals are between the talus and navicular on the medial side of the foot and between the calcaneum and cuboid on the lateral side; the anterior tarsals include the navicular, three cuneiforms and cuboid. All these joints are extremely stable.

Talocalcaneal joint

There are two articulations between the talus and calcaneum, each with a separate synovial cavity. Posteriorly is a saddle joint between the convex surface on the middle third of the calcaneum and the reciprocally concave surface on the body of the talus (Fig. 6.85). Anteriorly are two small flat facets on the anterior part of the calcaneum, including the sustentaculum tali, which articulate with corresponding facets beneath the head of the talus (Fig. 6.85).

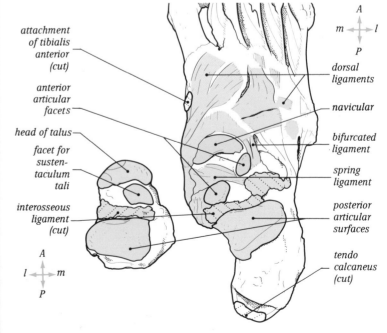

Fig. 6.85 *Talocalcaneal and talonavicular joints. The talus has been disarticulated and turned over.*

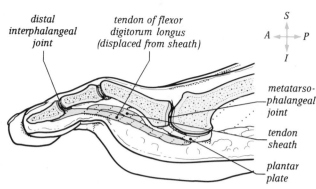

Fig. 6.86 *Sagittal section through the third toe showing the metatarsophalangeal and interphalangeal joints.*

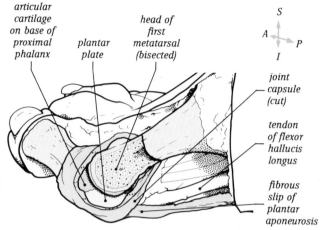

Fig. 6.87 *Internal features of the first metatarsophalangeal joint. Part of the capsule and the distal part of the metatarsal bone have been removed.*

Talonavicular joint

The head of the talus forms a ball-and-socket joint with the posterior surface of the navicular. This joint shares a common synovial cavity with the anterior part of the talocalcaneal articulation. The combined joint, which involves the head of the talus, is termed the talocalcaneonavicular (subtalar) joint.

Calcaneocuboid joint

At this plane joint, the flat anterior surface of the calcaneum articulates with the posterior surface of the cuboid (Fig. 6.84).

Other tarsal joints

Plane joints occur between the opposing surfaces of the navicular, the three cuneiforms and the cuboid (Fig. 6.84) and their synovial cavities freely communicate.

Capsules and ligaments

The fibrous capsules are attached around the margins of the articular surfaces. Short ligaments on the dorsum of the joints (Fig. 6.85) reinforce the capsules and, with the interosseous ligaments (Fig. 6.84), keep the articulating surfaces closely opposed. The strong interosseous talocalcaneal ligament (Fig. 6.85) in the sinus tarsi holds the talus and calcaneum together. The stem of the bifurcated ligament attaches to the anterior part of the calcaneum and its limbs to the navicular and cuboid. Beneath the tarsals, the long and short plantar ligaments (see Fig. 6.49) unite the plantar surfaces of the calcaneum and cuboid. The plantar calcaneonavicular ('spring') ligament (Fig. 6.85) unites the navicular and sustentaculum tali, supporting the head of the talus and completing the socket by which the head articulates with the navicular and calcaneum.

Movements

The most mobile of the tarsal joints is the talocalcaneonavicular joint. Its ball-and-socket shape permits rotation around an oblique axis which passes upwards, forwards and medially through the neck and head of the talus. This rotation, together with gliding movements at the other tarsal joints, enables the anterior part of the foot to twist in respect to the more posterior part. These twisting movements involve raising either the medial or lateral border

of the foot. Raising the medial border is called inversion and is produced by tibialis anterior and posterior, assisted by extensor hallucis longus. Raising the lateral border is called eversion and is brought about by peroneus longus, brevis and tertius.

Because of the oblique axis of the talocalcaneonavicular joint, inversion is always accompanied by plantar flexion and adduction of the foot whilst eversion is accompanied by dorsiflexion and abduction. These additional movements can be compensated by simultaneous movements at other joints. Thus, the plantar flexion accompanying inversion can be offset by slight dorsiflexion at the ankle joint whilst adduction can be offset by lateral rotation of the leg at the knee and hip joints.

Innervation

The tarsal joints are innervated by branches of the medial and lateral plantar nerves and the deep peroneal nerve.

TARSOMETATARSAL AND INTERMETATARSAL JOINTS

These are plane joints in which the bases of the fourth and fifth metatarsals articulate with the cuboid whilst the bases of the first, second and third metatarsals articulate with the respective cuneiforms. Dorsal, plantar and interosseous ligaments reinforce the joint capsules. These joints allow gliding movements during alterations in the height of the arches. Innervation is by plantar and deep peroneal nerves.

METATARSOPHALANGEAL AND INTERPHALANGEAL JOINTS

In each of the ball-and-socket metatarsophalangeal joints the metatarsal head articulates with the base of the proximal phalanx and the associated fibrocartilaginous plantar plate (Figs. 6.86 & 6.87). A capsule enclosing the articular surfaces is reinforced on each side by a collateral ligament and dorsally by the extensor expansion. The principal movements are flexion and extension with only minimal abduction or adduction. The first metatarsophalangeal joint is especially important, bearing body weight during walking. Two sesamoid bones (see Fig. 6.91) are usually present in the plantar plate of this joint, closely associated with the insertions of the intrinsic muscles of the great toe (see page 6.24).

JOINTS OF FOOT

The interphalangeal joints (Figs. 6.86 & 6.88) are hinge joints, allowing flexion and extension. The muscles moving these joints are described on pages 6.23 and 6.24. The joints of the toes are innervated by digital branches of the medial and lateral plantar nerves.

ARCHES OF FOOT

The tarsal and metatarsal bones form two longitudinal arches, medial and lateral. The medial arch is higher, forming the instep of the foot, and consists of the calcaneum, talus, navicular, three cuneiforms, and medial three metatarsals (Figs. 6.89 & 6.90). The lateral arch comprises the calcaneum, cuboid and lateral two metatarsals (Fig. 6.89). Each arch has an anterior and a posterior pillar which together transmit body weight to the ground. The posterior pillar of each arch is the same, namely the tubercles on the inferior surface of the calcaneum. However, the anterior pillars are separate, being formed by the heads of the appropriate metatarsals. The arches are important in relation to human bipedalism as they enhance forward propulsion.

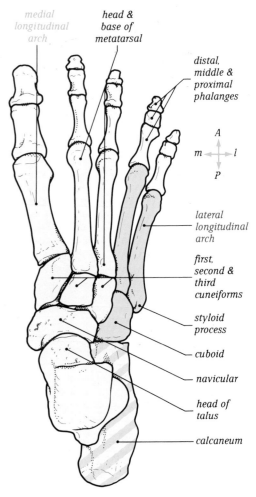

Fig. 6.89 *Dorsal aspect of the bones of the foot showing the medial and lateral longitudinal arches.*

Fig. 6.88 *Longitudinal section through the great toe showing its joints.*

Fig. 6.90 *Medial aspect of the bones of the foot and the medial longitudinal arch (blue).*

STABILITY

Factors in maintaining the arches include skeletal structure, ligaments, the plantar aponeurosis, tendons and muscles. Skeletal structure is important in the medial arch, where at its highest point the head of the talus articulates in a wedge-like manner with the navicular anteriorly and the sustentaculum tali posteriorly (Fig. 6.91). The head of the talus is supported inferiorly by the plantar calcaneonavicular ('spring') ligament (see Fig. 6.85), lying immediately above the tendon of flexor hallucis longus and a slip from the tendon of tibialis posterior which passes backwards to the sustentaculum tali (see Fig. 6.49). Tibialis anterior, through the attachment of its tendon to the first cuneiform and first metatarsal, may also support the medial arch, which it raises during inversion.

The lateral arch is supported by the long and short plantar ligaments and the tendon of peroneus longus. Both longitudinal arches derive support from the long flexor tendons of the toes and from the plantar aponeurosis whose digital slips gain indirect attachment to the proximal phalanges (see Fig. 6.87). When the heel rises from the ground the aponeurosis is passively tightened by extension of the toes at the metatarsophalangeal joints, thereby raising the longitudinal arches.

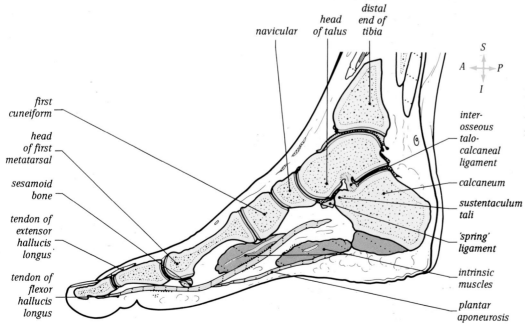

Fig. 6.91 *Sagittal section of foot showing the medial longitudinal arch.*

The cutaneous innervation of the lower limb derives from the lumbar and sacral plexuses as well as other spinal nerves (Fig. 6.92). Each cutaneous nerve supplies an area of skin which is variable from one person to another. There is considerable overlapping of innervation by adjacent nerves; therefore damage to a single nerve usually produces anaesthesia of only the central part of the area of skin it supplies.

L1, L2 & L3

T12 & L1

S1, S2 & S3

femoral branch of genitofemoral nerve

ilioinguinal nerve

obturator nerve

cutaneous nerves of thigh:
lateral
intermediate
medial

lateral cutaneous nerve of calf

saphenous nerve

sural nerve

superficial & deep peroneal nerves

lateral & medial plantar nerves

☐ posterior rami
■ lateral cutaneous branches of spinal nerves
☐ sciatic nerve (sacral plexus)
■ posterior cutaneous nerve of thigh (sacral plexus)
☐ femoral nerve (lumbar plexus)
☐ other branches (lumbar plexus)

Fig. 6.92 *Areas of distribution of cutaneous nerves in the lower limb.*

NECK

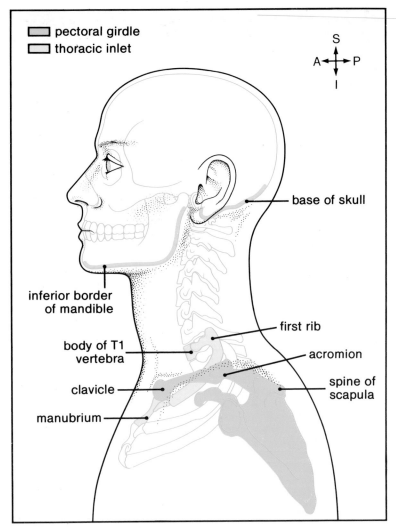

pectoral girdle
thoracic inlet

base of skull

inferior border
of mandible

first rib

body of T1
vertebra

acromion

clavicle

spine of
scapula

manubrium

Fig. 7.1 *Lateral view of the neck and the bones that mark its boundaries.*

The neck is the junctional region between the head and the thorax and upper limbs, bounded above by the base of the skull and mandible and below by the thoracic inlet and pectoral girdle (Fig. 7.1). The neck contains the cervical vertebrae and muscles, the pharynx, larynx, oesophagus, trachea and thyroid gland. Vessels and nerves in the region either supply the various organs, muscles and skin, or are in transit between the head, thorax and upper limbs. All are enclosed by investing and superficial fasciae and skin.

FASCIAL LAYERS

These are complex and are divided into four components: investing fascia, prevertebral fascia, pretracheal fascia and carotid sheaths (Fig. 7.2). The investing fascia is analogous to deep fascia in the limbs. It surrounds the neck, extending from the pectoral girdle below to the base of the skull and mandible above, and splits to enclose trapezius and sternomastoid. Superiorly, the investing fascia is attached to the superior nuchal lines and to the mastoid processes. Between the mastoid process and the angle of the mandible the fascia encloses the parotid gland. Its superficial layer passes superiorly over the surface of the gland to attach to the zygomatic arch; on its deep surface the fascia is thickened to form the stylomandibular ligament. Inferiorly the investing fascia is attached to the superior border of the clavicle, the acromion and the spine of the scapula.

The prevertebral fascia encloses the vertebral column, pre- and paravertebral muscles and origins of the cervical and brachial plexuses. Superiorly it attaches to the base of the skull and inferiorly it extends into the superior mediastinum.

The pretracheal fascia covers the anterior and lateral aspects of the trachea and larynx, limited superiorly by the hyoid bone and by the oblique lines on the thyroid cartilage. It splits to enclose the thyroid gland and inferiorly fuses with the adventitia of the aortic arch in the superior mediastinum. Postero-laterally on each side the pretracheal fascia blends with the carotid sheath.

Each of the two carotid sheaths contains a common, an internal and part of an external carotid artery, a vagus nerve and an internal jugular vein. The sheaths are attached to the base of the skull around the jugular and carotid foramina and pass inferiorly to the aortic arch and brachiocephalic veins to fuse with the adventitia covering these vessels.

For purposes of anatomical description each side of the neck is divided into anterior and posterior triangles separated from one another by sternomastoid.

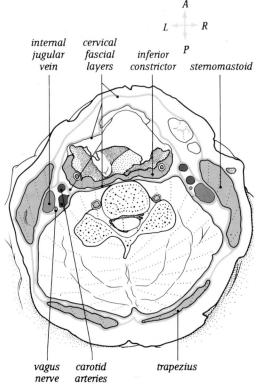

internal jugular vein

cervical fascial layers

inferior constrictor

sternomastoid

vagus nerve

carotid arteries

trapezius

Fig. 7.2 *Transverse section of the neck at the level of C4 showing the layers of cervical fascia. The layers are shown separately in the diagrams on the right.*

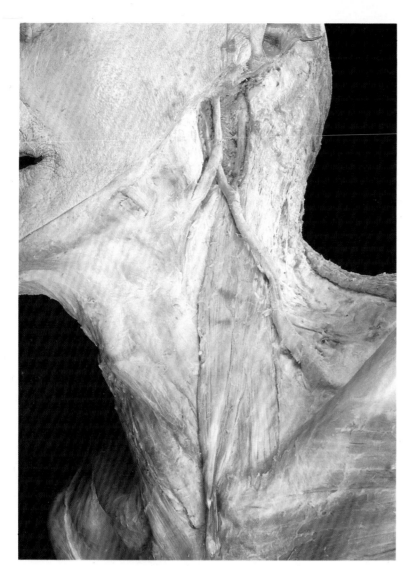

STERNOMASTOID

This muscle passes obliquely upwards and backwards from the manubrium and the medial end of the clavicle to the mastoid process and superior nuchal line of the skull (Fig. 7.3). One sternomastoid acting alone turns the head towards the opposite shoulder, whereas acting together both muscles extend the atlantoccipital joint. Sternomastoid is innervated by the spinal part of the accessory nerve (XI).

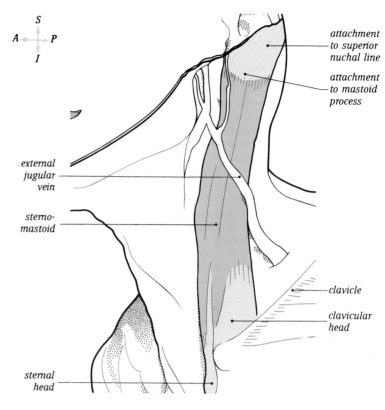

Fig. 7.3 *Oblique view of the neck showing sternomastoid after removal of part of the investing fascia.*

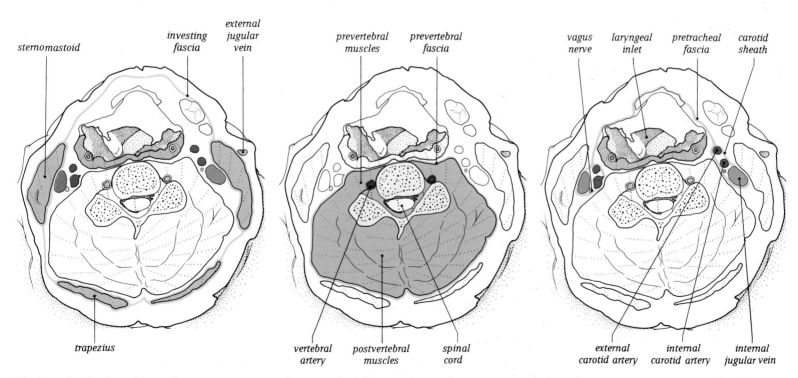

The investing fascia and its enclosures.

The prevertebral fascia and its enclosures.

The pretracheal fascia and carotid sheaths and their enclosures.

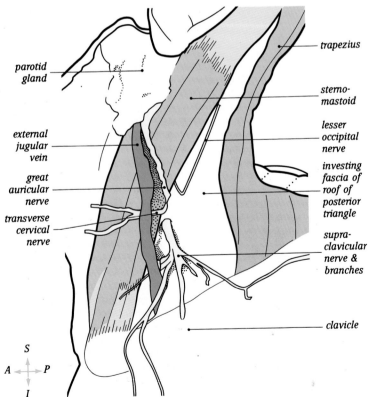

parotid gland

external jugular vein

great auricular nerve

transverse cervical nerve

trapezius

sterno-mastoid

lesser occipital nerve

investing fascia of roof of posterior triangle

supra-clavicular nerve & branches

clavicle

S

A ←→ P

I

Fig. 7.4 *Boundaries and roof of the posterior triangle of the neck. The external jugular vein and cutaneous branches of the cervical plexus, lying superficial to the roof, are also present.*

7.4

POSTERIOR TRIANGLE OF NECK

This triangle is bounded anteriorly by sternomastoid and posteriorly by trapezius. Inferiorly the upper border of the clavicle forms the base whilst superiorly the attachments of sternomastoid and trapezius converge onto the superior nuchal line to form the apex of the triangle. The posterior triangle does not lie in a flat plane but spirals so that the inferior portion is directed anteriorly whilst the apex faces posterolaterally.

Roof

The roof of the triangle is formed by the investing fascia which spans the interval between trapezius and sternomastoid. The external jugular vein initially lies vertically over the sternomastoid just beneath the skin and then passes onto the roof of the lower part of the triangle. The vein pierces the roof just above the clavicle to enter the triangle and drain into the subclavian vein. Cutaneous branches of the cervical plexus (see below) also lie superficial to the roof of the triangle (Fig. 7.4).

Floor

The floor of the posterior triangle is formed by the prevertebral fascia extending laterally to cover the paravertebral muscles which are, from above downwards, splenius capitis, levator scapulae and scalenus posterior, medius and anterior (Fig. 7.5). Deep to the prevertebral fascia are the subclavian artery, the three trunks of the brachial plexus and the cervical plexus. Continuing laterally to reach the axilla, the brachial plexus and the subclavian artery are enclosed in a prolongation of the prevertebral fascia, the axillary sheath. Below the scalene muscles, subclavian vessels and brachial plexus are the pleura and apex of the lung.

Contents

Between the floor and the roof of the triangle lie the contents (Fig. 7.6) which include a number of vascular structures, the spinal part of the accessory (XI) nerve, components of the cervical plexus and supraclavicular and occipital lymph nodes. The spinal part of the accessory nerve passes obliquely across the triangle from beneath the posterior border of sternomastoid to leave deep to the anterior border of trapezius. It supplies both of these muscles. In the lower part of the triangle the inferior belly of omohyoid passes towards its scapular attachment. Two branches of the thyrocervical trunk, namely the transverse cervical and suprascapular arteries, also pass laterally across the triangle to the scapula. At the apex of the triangle the occipital artery emerges to supply part of the scalp. The subclavian vein is sometimes visible just above the clavicle.

CERVICAL PLEXUS

The cervical plexus is formed from the anterior rami of the first four cervical spinal nerves and supplies the paravertebral muscles with segmental branches. It provides a branch from C1 to the hypoglossal nerve and branches from C2 and C3 which all contribute to the ansa cervicalis (see below). The phrenic nerve, the principal innervation of the diaphragm, is formed from C3, C4 and C5 and runs vertically downwards on the anterior surface of scalenus anterior, behind the prevertebral fascia.

Sensory branches from the cervical plexus (Fig. 7.4) pass through the triangle and emerge by piercing the roof near the midpoint of the posterior border of sternomastoid. These convey sensation from the neck, the lower part of the face and pinna, the side of the scalp and the upper part of the thoracic wall. The lesser occipital nerve (C2) ascends along the posterior border of sternomastoid and supplies the side of the occipital region of the scalp. The great auricular nerve (C2 & C3) runs vertically upwards across sternomastoid and conveys sensation from the lower part of the pinna and the skin over the parotid gland. The transverse cervical nerve (C2 & C3) passes horizontally, supplying the skin over sternomastoid and the anterior triangle. Finally, the supraclavicular nerves (C3 & C4) radiate downwards to convey sensation from skin over the upper part of the anterior thoracic wall and the shoulder region.

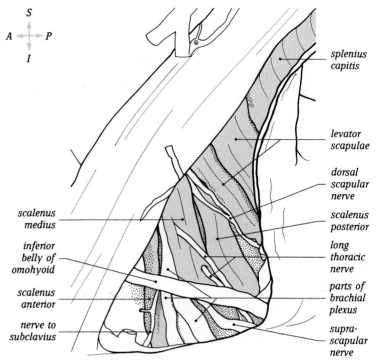

Fig. 7.5 *Floor of the posterior triangle of the neck. The inferior belly of the omohyoid muscle, one of the contents of the triangle, is still present.*

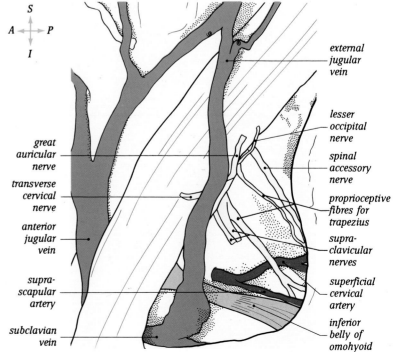

Fig. 7.6 *Roof of the posterior triangle has been removed to reveal the contents. The external jugular vein is in continuity with the anterior jugular system.*

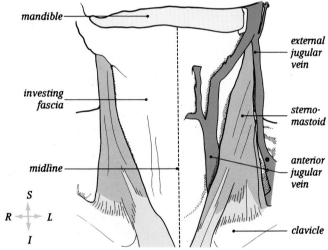

Fig. 7.7 *Boundaries and roof of both anterior triangles of the neck. The midline is the division between the two anterior triangles.*

Fig. 7.8 *The right omohyoid and sternohyoid muscles have been removed to show the deeper thryohyoid and sternothyroid muscles.*

ANTERIOR TRIANGLE OF NECK

By convention, the two anterior triangles of the neck extend medially as far as the median plane. Posterolaterally each triangle is bounded by the anterior border of sternomastoid and superiorly by the inferior border of the mandible. For convenience, that part of the triangle lying above the hyoid bone will be described in the section concerning mylohyoid and related structures.

Roof

The roof of the anterior triangle (Fig. 7.7) is formed by the investing fascia of the neck in a manner similar to that of the posterior triangle. Superficial to the fascia are platysma (see page 7.11) and the anterior jugular vein. This vessel pierces the roof and passes deep to sternomastoid to drain into the external jugular vein just before its termination in the subclavian vein. The cutaneous innervation of the skin over the triangle has already been described (see page 7.4).

Floor

The floor of the anterior triangle is composed of the pretracheal fascia and posterolaterally the carotid sheath. The pretracheal fascia encloses the thyroid gland (Fig. 7.10) whilst the larynx and trachea lie deep to the

gland. Laterally the carotid arteries, internal jugular vein and vagus (X) nerve all lie within the carotid sheath.

Contents

The contents of the anterior triangle (Fig. 7.8) comprise infrahyoid or strap muscles (sternohyoid, sternothyroid, thyrohyoid and omohyoid) and their immediate nerve supply. The sternohyoid is the most superficial strap muscle and is attached inferiorly to the deep surface of the manubrium. Superiorly it is attached to the lower border of the body of the hyoid bone. Deep to sternohyoid are both sternothyroid and thyrohyoid. Sternothyroid extends from the manubrium to the oblique line on the lamina of the thyroid cartilage. In the same plane the thyrohyoid runs from the thyroid cartilage to the inferior edge of the body of the hyoid bone. Omohyoid consists of two bellies linked by an intermediate tendon. The inferior belly is attached to the suprascapular ligament and the adjacent part of the scapula. It is this belly which crosses the posterior triangle and ends deep to sternomastoid in the intermediate tendon. The tendon is anchored to the clavicle by a loop of investing fascia. The superior belly continues almost vertically to its attachment on the lower border of the hyoid bone lateral to the other muscles.

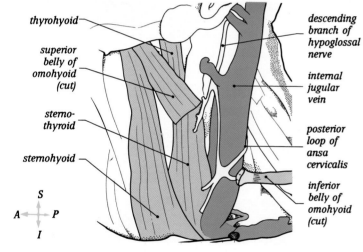

Fig. 7.9 *Ansa cervicalis, lying on the internal jugular vein, has branches passing to the strap muscles.*

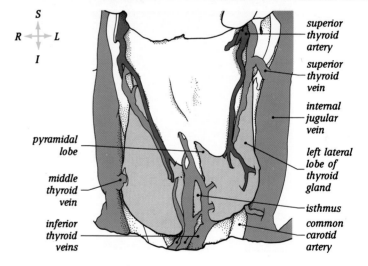

Fig. 7.10 *Thyroid gland and its immediate blood supply is revealed after removal of the pretracheal fascia.*

All four muscles are supplied segmentally by branches from the first three cervical spinal nerves. Thyrohyoid is supplied by fibres from C1 which have travelled with the hypoglossal (XII) nerve; the remaining muscles are supplied via the ansa cervicalis. Functionally the infrahyoid muscles serve to depress the hyoid bone and the larynx.

ANSA CERVICALIS

Under cover of sternomastoid two nerves unite to form a loop, the ansa cervicalis (Fig. 7.9), which provides the motor supply to the strap muscles. The anterior part of the loop is formed by the descending branch of the hypoglossal nerve which consists solely of C1 fibres. C2 and C3 fibres from the cervical plexus form the posterior loop of the ansa.

THYROID GLAND

The thyroid gland (Fig. 7.10) is a vascular endocrine gland enclosed by the pretracheal fascia and closely applied to the anterior and lateral surfaces of the trachea. The fascia links the gland to the larynx so that during swallowing both structures are elevated simultaneously. The two lateral lobes of the gland are joined across the midline by a narrow isthmus at the level of the third tracheal ring. A single pyramidal lobe is often present and projects

upwards from the isthmus. Each lateral lobe is pear-shaped with its superior extremity reaching the oblique line on the thyroid cartilage whilst its lower pole lies at the level of the fifth tracheal ring.

Lying anterior to the isthmus of the gland are the sternothyroid muscles and the anterior jugular veins. The lateral lobes are covered anterolaterally by the other infrahyoid muscles and the anterior borders of the sternomastoid muscles. Posterolaterally lie the carotid sheaths whilst posteromedially are the trachea, larynx and oesophagus. In the interval between the oesophagus and trachea the recurrent laryngeal nerves course upwards towards the larynx. A superior and an inferior parathyroid gland are embedded in the posterior surface of each lateral lobe.

The thyroid gland is a highly vascular organ and is supplied on each side by a superior and an inferior thyroid artery. The superior thyroid artery, a branch of the external carotid artery, descends to the upper pole of the gland. The inferior thyroid artery, from the thyrocervical trunk of the subclavian artery, ascends to enter the posterolateral aspect of the gland from behind the carotid sheath. A venous plexus on the surface of the gland drains via superior and middle thyroid veins into the internal jugular veins and via inferior thyroid veins that descend to the left brachiocephalic vein. Lymph drains from the gland into the jugular chain of nodes.

ROOT OF NECK

The root of the neck is the region immediately above the thoracic inlet (see page 7.2). In the midline are the trachea and oesophagus descending into the superior mediastinum (Fig. 7.11) between the apices of the lungs covered with pleura and suprapleural membrane (Fig. 7.12). The other major structures in the root of the neck are vessels and nerves which will be described in relation to scalenus anterior and its attachment to the scalene tubercle of the first rib (see page 2.3).

Veins

Each subclavian vein (Fig. 7.11) begins at the outer border of the first rib as the continuation of the axillary vein (see page 3.8). The vessel passes over the rib in front of the attachment of scalenus anterior and receives the external jugular vein from above. The subclavian and internal jugular veins unite at the medial border of the scalenus anterior to form the brachiocephalic vein which enters the thorax anteriorly alongside the trachea. On each side of the neck a major lymphatic trunk terminates by drainage into the angle where the subclavian and internal jugular veins unite. On the left, this lymphatic vessel is the thoracic duct which arches laterally over the apex of the lung from its position alongside the oesophagus. The duct passes between the carotid sheath and the vertebral vessels, crossing in front of the phrenic nerve and the subclavian artery. The thoracic duct is the ultimate drainage channel for lymph from the lower limbs, pelvis, abdomen, left upper limb and the left side of the thorax, head and neck. On the right side of the neck the smaller right lymphatic trunk terminates in the veins in a manner similar to the thoracic duct. However, it drains lymph only from the right upper limb and the right side of the thorax, head and neck.

Arteries

The left common carotid and left subclavian arteries emerge from the thorax on the left of the trachea and oesophagus (Fig. 7.11). On the right, the brachiocephalic artery divides at the level of the thoracic inlet to form the right common carotid and right subclavian arteries (Fig. 7.11). Each common carotid artery ascends into the neck within its sheath and gives no branches before its termination. Each subclavian artery passes laterally over the upper surface of the first rib posterior to scalenus anterior and continues into the axilla as the axillary artery (see page 3.7).

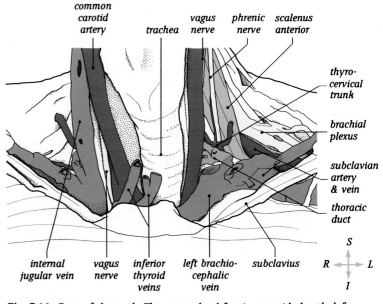

Fig. 7.11 *Root of the neck. The pretracheal fascia, carotid sheath, left internal jugular vein and clavicles have been removed.*

Three branches of the subclavian artery, namely internal thoracic, thyrocervical and vertebral arteries (Figs. 7.11 & 7.12), arise medial to scalenus anterior. The internal thoracic artery (see page 2.11) descends into the thorax to supply the anterior thoracic and abdominal walls. The thyrocervical trunk is short and divides into three branches, the inferior thyroid (page 7.7), suprascapular and superficial cervical arteries. The latter two vessels cross the posterior triangle of the neck. The suprascapular artery supplies the scapula and related structures and the superficial cervical artery supplies superficial structures in the posterior part of the neck. The vertebral artery (Fig. 7.12) inclines upwards and backwards medial to scalenus anterior and crosses in front of the transverse process of the seventh cervical vertebra. Continuing superiorly through the foramina transversaria of the upper six cervical vertebrae, it eventually enters the skull through the foramen magnum (see page 7.44).

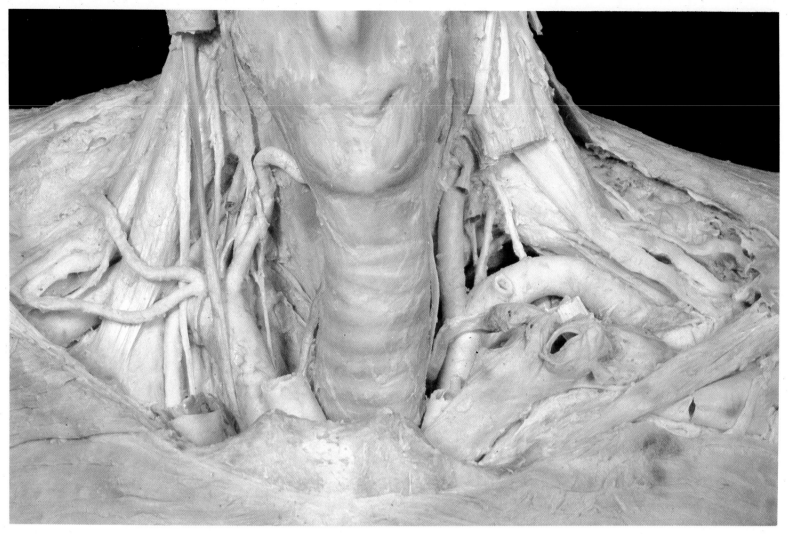

The costocervical trunk (Fig. 7.12) arises from the subclavian artery behind scalenus anterior and arches backwards over the suprapleural membrane as far as the neck of the first rib, where it divides to form the superior intercostal artery supplying the upper two intercostal spaces (see page 2.9) and the deep cervical artery which supplies the muscles of the back of the neck.

Nerves

The vagus (X) and phrenic nerves, both sympathetic chains and parts of both brachial plexuses all traverse the root of the neck. Each vagus nerve (Fig. 7.11) descends within the carotid sheath and enters the superior mediastinum between the main arterial and venous structures medial to the phrenic nerve. On the right side of the neck the recurrent laryngeal nerve arises from the vagus, hooking under the subclavian artery to ascend in the groove formed by the lateral surfaces of the trachea and oesophagus. On the left, the recurrent laryngeal nerve follows a similar course but arises from the vagus in the thorax (see page 2.34).

The phrenic nerve (Fig. 7.12), formed from the anterior rami of the third, fourth and fifth cervical spinal nerves, passes inferiorly on the anterior surface of scalenus anterior beneath the prevertebral fascia and leaves the medial side of the muscle near its lower end. It then enters the thorax between the main arterial and venous structures lateral to the vagus nerve.

The sympathetic trunks (Fig. 7.12), covered by the prevertebral fascia, lie alongside the bodies of the cervical vertebrae. In the neck each trunk bears only three sympathetic ganglia, the superior, middle and inferior. The lowest ganglion fuses frequently with the first thoracic ganglion to form the stellate ganglion. The trunk continues into the thorax in front of the neck of the first rib. The middle and inferior cervical sympathetic ganglia are often linked by a nerve, the ansa subclavia, which curves around the subclavian artery.

The brachial plexus (Fig. 7.11) originates from the anterior rami of the lowest four cervical and first thoracic spinal nerves. These nerves, partly covered by scalenus anterior, constitute the roots of the plexus. They combine to form the trunks of the plexus which emerge from behind the lateral border of the muscle. The plexus continues into the upper limb enclosed with the axillary artery in a prolongation of the prevertebral fascia called the axillary sheath. (A detailed account is given on page 3.8).

Fig. 7.12 labels (top): *superficial cervical & inferior thyroid arteries* — *vagus nerve* — *phrenic nerve* — *sympathetic trunk* — *scalenus medius* — *deep cervical arteries*

Right-side labels: *superior intercostal artery*; *pleural cavity*; *costo-cervical trunk*

Bottom labels: *suprascapular & internal thoracic arteries* — *supra-pleural membrane* — *ansa subclavia* — *cardiac nerve* — *recurrent laryngeal nerves* — *vertebral artery*

Orientation: S / R — L / I

Fig. 7.12 *Deeper structures of the root of neck revealed by removal of left vagus and phrenic nerves, the left scalenus anterior, both common carotid arteries and most of the veins.*

Scalene muscles

Scalenus anterior (Fig. 7.12) is the most anterior of the prevertebral group of muscles. Superiorly it is attached to the transverse processes of the third, fourth, fifth and sixth cervical vertebrae. Inferiorly it gains attachment to the scalene tubercle on the first rib (see page 2.3). Behind it lie scalenus medius (Fig. 7.12) and scalenus posterior, which arise from the transverse processes of the lower six cervical vertebrae and attach inferiorly to the upper surfaces of the first and second ribs respectively. These prevertebral muscles are supplied segmentally by cervical spinal nerves. They elevate the first and second ribs and laterally flex the neck.

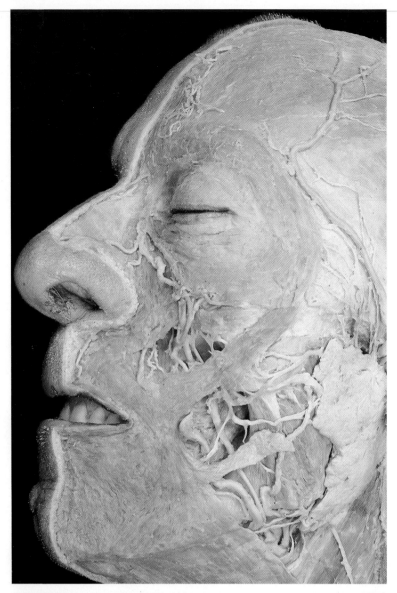

The superficial fascia of the face and scalp is highly vascular and is traversed by several nerves. Most of the nerves are sensory to the skin of the region and include branches of the trigeminal (V) and upper cervical spinal nerves. In addition, there are branches which are motor from the facial (VII) nerve to a group of muscles in the subcutaneous tissues of the face, scalp and front of the neck, known collectively as the muscles of facial expression.

MUSCLES OF FACIAL EXPRESSION

In general, these muscles are arranged as sphincters or dilators around the orifices of the face (Fig. 7.13). Most are anchored to bone at one end and attached to skin at the other.

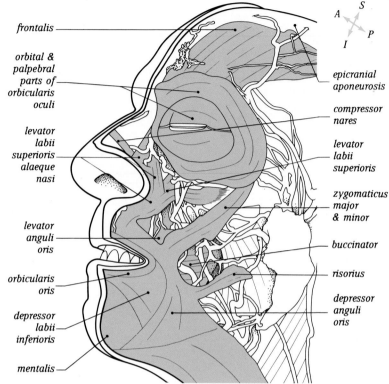

Fig. 7.13 *Muscles of facial expression. The skin and subcutaneous fat have been removed.*

Palpebral fissure

The sphincter of the orbit is orbicularis oculi which is divided into inner palpebral and outer orbital parts. The palpebral part lies within the eyelids and is attached to the medial and lateral palpebral ligaments. The orbital portion is attached only to the medial palpebral ligament and its fibres lie around the orbital margin. Both parts close the palpebral fissure, the palpebral part gently and the orbital part forcefully as when 'screwing up the eyes'. The dilator components are provided by levator palpebrae superioris within the orbit (see page 7.49), and by occipitofrontalis in the scalp. The latter muscle has two bellies, occipital and frontal, linked by an extensive intermediate tendon, the epicranial aponeurosis. This aponeurosis forms a mobile layer over the vault of the skull. From its posterior extremity the occipital belly (occipitalis) descends to its attachment on the highest nuchal line of the occipital bone (Fig. 7.14); from its anterior end the frontal belly (frontalis) descends in the forehead and its fibres interdigitate with those of orbicularis oculi and attach to skin near the eyebrow. Occipitalis fixes the epicranial aponeurosis allowing frontalis to raise the eyebrows.

Nose

Around each nostril are two feeble muscles, the dilator and compressor nares.

Mouth

Orbicularis oris, the sphincter of the mouth, is embedded in the lips and attaches near the midline to the mandible and maxilla. In addition there are dilators around the mouth whose fibres continue into orbicularis oris. The most medial dilator of the upper lip is levator labii superioris alaeque nasi. This muscle attaches near the medial margin of the orbit and runs to the alar cartilage of the nose and to the upper lip. Levator labii superioris is attached to bone beneath the orbital margin, whereas levator anguli oris lies slightly deeper and its fibres incline towards the angle of the mouth. Two of the dilator muscles take attachment from the zygoma, namely zygomaticus major and minor. Attached to the mandible are three muscles called, from lateral to medial, depressor anguli oris, depressor labii inferioris and mentalis.

Fig. 7.14 *Posterior view to show occipitalis attached to the highest nuchal line.*

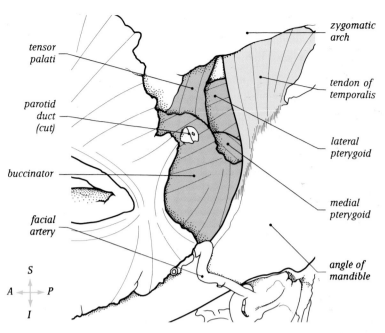

Fig. 7.15 *Buccinator seen after removal of most of the superficial facial muscles, the parotid gland and most of its duct, and masseter.*

The buccinator muscle (Figs. 7.13 & 7.15) lies deep to the other dilator muscles in the wall of the cheek. Anteriorly it blends with the deep surface of orbicularis oris. Posteriorly it gains attachment to the outer surface of the mandible from the level of the first to the third molar teeth. Passing behind the third molar tooth, buccinator is attached to the pterygomandibular raphe and the pterygoid hamulus. The muscle attachment continues forwards along the outer surface of the maxilla as far as the first upper molar tooth. Buccinator controls the size of the vestibule of the mouth (that part of the buccal cavity lying between the cheek and the teeth).

Neck
The platysma (Fig. 7.16), the most extensive muscle of facial expression, descends in the superficial fascia of the neck from the inferior border of the mandible and fades out on the anterior surface of the thorax. A few fibres may run horizontally from the angle of the mouth as risorius. Platysma is most easily seen in action during respiratory distress when the skin of the neck is pulled taut.

Ear
In the human the auricular muscles are vestigial.

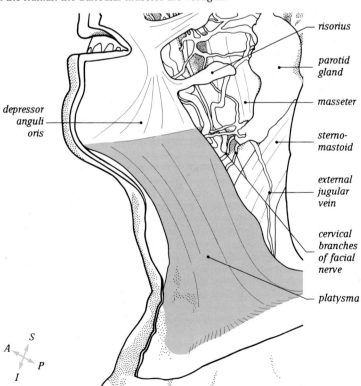

Fig. 7.16 *Platysma, the largest muscle of facial expression, extends down onto the surface of the thorax.*

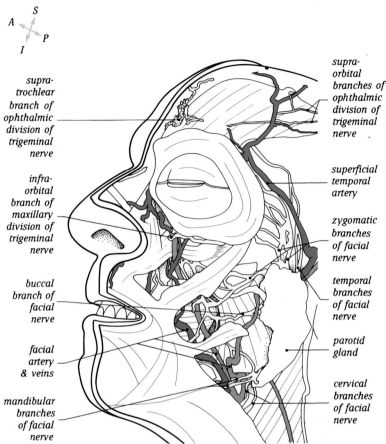

Fig. 7.17 *Neurovascular structures of the face. In this specimen the facial vein is duplicated, a common variation.*

FACIAL NERVE

All the muscles of facial expression derive their motor nerve supply from the facial (VII) nerve. Occipitalis is innervated by the posterior auricular branch of the nerve (see page 7.15) while the remaining muscles are supplied by the five sets of branches (Fig. 7.17) that emerge from the anterior border of the parotid gland (see page 7.15). The temporal branch of the facial nerve ascends to supply the auricular muscles and frontalis. The zygomatic branch is directed towards the eye and supplies muscles above and below the palpebral fissure. The third branch, the buccal, runs horizontally forwards to innervate buccinator and the muscles of the upper lip. The mandibular branch supplies the muscles of the lower lip, dipping below the mandible in its course. The cervical branch descends to supply platysma.

BLOOD SUPPLY OF FACE

Most of the superficial structures of the face obtain their blood supply from the facial artery (Fig. 7.17), a branch of the external carotid artery. The facial artery enters the face by hooking under the inferior border of the mandible where it is easily palpated. The vessel then pursues a tortuous course across the face towards the inner angle of the orbit. The area of the face in front of the ear is supplied by the transverse facial artery, an anterior branch of the superficial temporal artery. Emerging from the orbit to supply the forehead are the supraorbital and supratrochlear branches of the ophthalmic artery.

Blood from the face drains into the facial vein (Fig. 7.17) which accompanies the facial artery. The vein also receives the supratrochlear and supraorbital veins and thus communicates with ophthalmic veins in the orbit. Blood from the lateral part of the face drains into the superficial temporal vein (see page 7.13).

ophthalmic ⎤
maxillary ⎥ — divisions
mandibular ⎦
cervical nerves

Fig. 7.18 *Dermatomes of face and neck. Areas of the face are supplied with sensory fibres from the different divisions of the trigeminal nerve.*

SENSORY SUPPLY

The sensory nerve supply of the face is conveyed in branches of the three divisions of the trigeminal (V) nerve (Fig. 7.18).

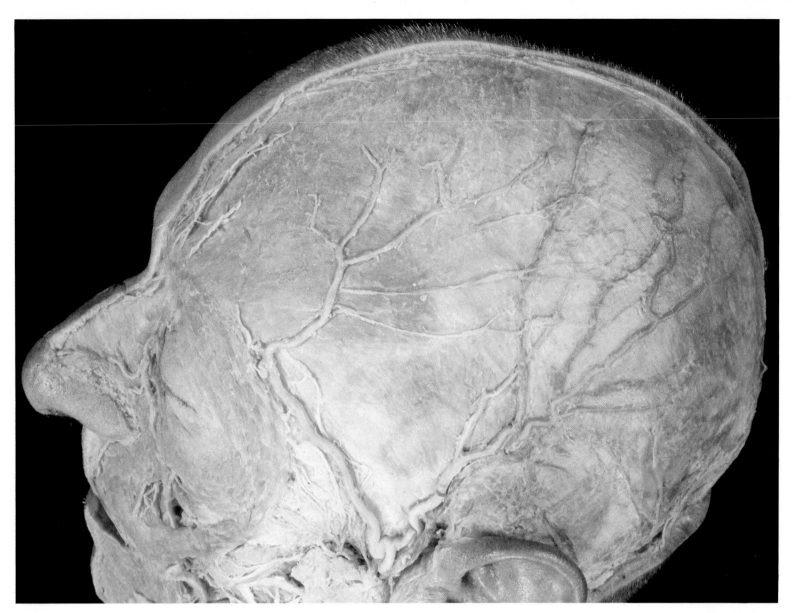

SCALP

The scalp (Fig. 7.19) extends from the superior nuchal line posteriorly to the superior orbital margin anteriorly, and to the external acoustic meatus and zygomatic arch laterally. It comprises two functional layers applied to the outer surface of the vault of the skull. Close to the bones lies the pericranium which forms the periosteum of the skull. This is loosely attached over each constituent bone but is firmly bound to the sutures so that subperiosteal bleeding is limited to the area of the bones involved. Superficial to the pericranium, but separated from it by a layer of loose connective tissue, lie the epicranial aponeurosis (intermediate tendon of occipitofrontalis) and the skin of the scalp firmly bound to each other so that they move as one over the underlying pericranium and skull.

The arteries and nerves that supply the scalp enter at its circumference and because they accompany each other they will be described together starting anteriorly. Near the midline are the supratrochlear and supraorbital nerves, arteries and veins. The nerves are derived from the ophthalmic division of the trigeminal (V) nerve. The vessels communicate with their ophthalmic counterparts within the orbit.

Lateral to the orbit the zygomaticotemporal nerve from the maxillary division of the trigeminal nerve, accompanied by its vessels, ascends a short distance into the scalp. Just in front of the ear the auriculotemporal nerve from the mandibular

Fig. 7.19 *Vessels and nerves of the scalp lying on the epicranial aponeurosis. Not all branches are present in this specimen.*

division of the fifth cranial nerve, passes into the scalp. The superficial temporal artery and vein follow a similar course.

The area of the scalp behind the ear is supplied by the lesser occipital nerve (C2 anterior ramus) accompanied by the posterior auricular artery and

vein. Posteriorly near the midline the scalp receives the greater occipital nerve (C2 posterior ramus) and the occipital artery and vein.

In addition, venous blood may drain via the diploic veins of the skull into the intracranial venous sinuses.

7.13

PAROTID GLAND

The parotid is the largest of the salivary glands and is pyramidal in shape (Fig. 7.20). Its base faces laterally between the anterior border of sternomastoid and the ramus of the mandible, while its apex lies deeply against the styloid process. The gland extends upwards between the external auditory meatus and the temporomandibular joint, movements of which may be painful when the parotid is inflamed.

The investing fascia of the neck splits into two layers to enclose the gland (see page 7.2). The superficial layer attaches above to the zygomatic arch whilst anteriorly it merges with the tissues of the cheek. The deep layer is attached to the tympanic part of the temporal bone and is thickened between the styloid process and the angle of the mandible to form the stylomandibular ligament.

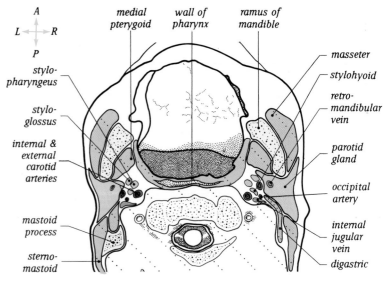

Fig. 7.20 *Transverse section of the head through the parotid glands. They extend deeply as far as the styloid processes.*

The parotid gland is deeply indented in front by the mandible, masseter and medial pterygoid. Deep to the gland are the infratemporal fossa and the styloid apparatus, the latter separating it from the carotid sheath and the pharyngeal wall.

The parotid duct (Fig. 7.21) passes forwards across the surface of masseter, turns medially and pierces buccinator to open obliquely into the vestibule of the mouth opposite the upper second molar tooth. When masseter contracts, the duct may be palpated over the anterior edge of the muscle. An accessory part of the gland may lie alongside the duct.

Fig. 7.21 *Parotid gland and branches of the facial nerve exposed by the removal of the superficial layer of parotid fascia.*

Fig. 7.22 labels: superficial temporal vein, maxillary vein, retro-mandibular vein, masseter, facial vein, external jugular vein, external auditory meatus, deep part of parotid gland, posterior auricular vein, posterior & anterior divisions of retro-mandibular vein, sterno-mastoid

Fig. 7.22 *The superficial portion of the parotid gland has been removed to expose the retromandibular vein and its tributaries.*

Fig. 7.23 labels: transverse facial artery, ramus of mandible, external carotid artery, masseter, superficial temporal artery, maxillary artery, facial nerve, posterior belly of digastric, accessory nerve, internal jugular vein

Fig. 7.23 *The parotid gland has been completely removed to reveal the external carotid artery and its terminal branches.*

STRUCTURES TRAVERSING PAROTID GLAND

Of these, the most superficial are branches of the facial (VII) nerve which run forwards to reach the face and pass superficial to the retromandibular vein and its tributaries. Deepest of all is the termination of the external carotid artery.

Facial (VII) nerve

The facial nerve emerges from the skull through the stylomastoid foramen and turns forwards to enter the posterior surface of the parotid gland. Before penetrating the gland it gives two branches. The posterior auricular branch passes behind the external auditory meatus to supply occipitalis and the auricular muscles. The other supplies the posterior belly of digastric and stylohyoid. Within the gland the facial nerve forms a plexus from which five groups of branches (Fig. 7.21) emerge at the periphery of the gland to supply the muscles of facial expression (see page 7.12).

Retromandibular vein

Within the parotid gland the superficial temporal and maxillary veins unite to form the retromandibular vein (Fig. 7.22). Inferiorly this short vein terminates as anterior and posterior divisions which escape from the gland. The anterior division joins the facial vein to form the common facial vein which drains into the internal jugular vein. The posterior division unites with the posterior auricular vein to form the external jugular vein (see page 7.4).

Termination of external carotid artery

Entering the parotid from below, the external carotid artery ascends through the gland and at the level of the neck of the mandible divides into the maxillary and superficial temporal arteries (Fig. 7.23). The former runs anterosuperiorly to leave the gland and enter the infratemporal fossa. The superficial temporal artery continues between the external auditory meatus and the temporomandibular joint to supply the temple. Its pulsation can be felt just above the joint.

Several lymph nodes lie just under the fascia covering the parotid gland or within the gland itself.

NEUROVASCULAR SUPPLY

The gland receives its vascular supply from the vessels traversing it. Parasympathetic secretomotor fibres follow a tortuous route to the gland. The preganglionic fibres arise from the inferior salivatory nucleus in the brain stem and pass in the tympanic branch of the glossopharyngeal (IX) nerve to the tympanic plexus in the middle ear, leaving the skull in the lesser petrosal nerve to synapse in the otic ganglion (see page 7.18). Postganglionic parasympathetic fibres travel to the gland in the auriculotemporal branch of the mandibular (Vc) division. By contrast, postganglionic sympathetic nerves are conveyed to the gland in the plexus accompanying the external carotid artery.

zygomatic arch

superficial temporal artery

external auditory meatus

masseter

ramus of mandible

parotid duct

facial artery

S

A ← → P

I

Fig. 7.24 *Lateral view of masseter showing its attachment to the zygomatic arch and the angle of the mandible, after removal of the parotid gland.*

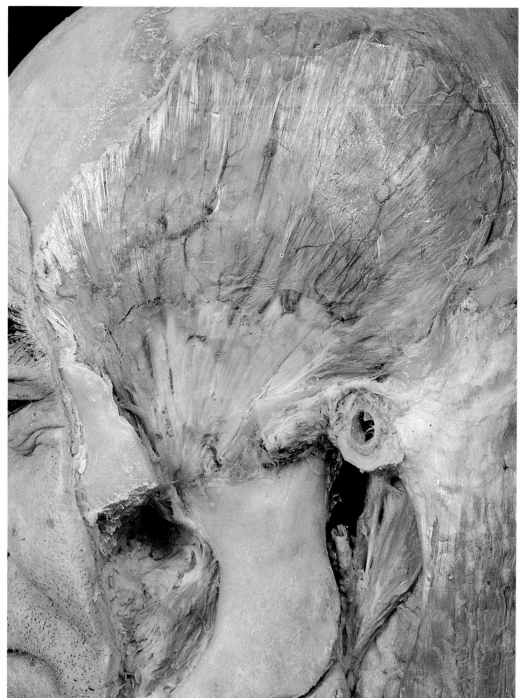

MASSETER

Masseter (Fig. 7.24) attaches along the length of the zygomatic arch and its fibres slope downwards and backwards to the lateral surface of the ramus of the mandible adjacent to the angle. This muscle is a powerful elevator of the mandible and is easily palpated when the teeth are clenched. It is supplied by the masseteric branch of the mandibular (Vc) division of the trigeminal nerve.

TEMPORALIS

Temporalis (Fig. 7.25) is a large fan-shaped muscle occupying the temporal fossa and taking attachment from the area of bone bounded by the inferior temporal line. The more superficial fibres arise from the temporal fascia which covers the muscle and is attached to the superior temporal line. All the fibres descend deep to the zygomatic arch to attach to the coronoid process and anteromedial aspect of the ramus of the mandible. Temporalis elevates the mandible, as in closing the mouth, and its posterior fibres retract the mandible. The deep temporal branches of the mandibular (Vc) division of the trigeminal nerve supply the muscle from its deep surface.

INFRATEMPORAL FOSSA

This fossa lies deep to the ramus of the mandible and is limited on its medial aspect by the lateral wall of the pharynx and the medial pterygoid plate of the sphenoid bone. The fossa is bounded by the posterior surface of the maxilla in front and by the styloid process and its attached muscles behind. The roof is provided by the temporal and sphenoid bones in the base of the skull whilst inferiorly the fossa is continuous with the neck.

Within the fossa are the two pterygoid muscles, the mandibular (Vc) division of the trigeminal nerve and its branches, and the maxillary vessels and their branches. Adjacent to the fossa is the temporomandibular joint.

Fig. 7.25 *Temporalis seen after removal of masseter, part of the zygomatic arch and the temporal fascia.*

Pterygoid muscles

The lateral and medial pterygoid muscles (Figs. 7.26 & 7.27) each have two attachments to the skull. The upper head of the lateral pterygoid attaches to the inferior surface of the greater wing of the sphenoid. The lower head attaches to the lateral surface of the lateral pterygoid plate. Both heads converge on the neck of the mandible and the capsule of the temporomandibular joint. The lateral pterygoid pulls forward both the neck of the mandible and the articular disc, thus depressing the mandible and opening the mouth.

The lower head of the lateral pterygoid is clasped by the two heads of the medial pterygoid. The deep head of the latter is larger and attaches to the medial surface of the lateral pterygoid plate. The superficial head is attached to the tuberosity of the maxilla. The fibres of both heads incline obliquely downwards and backwards to attach to the medial surface of the angle of the mandible. The muscle is a powerful elevator of the mandible.

Temporomandibular joint

The temporomandibular joint (Fig. 7.26) is a synovial joint. The head of the mandible articulates with the glenoid fossa and articular eminence of the temporal bone. Fibrocartilage covers the articular surfaces and also forms an articular disc which divides the joint into two separate cavities. Within these cavities the non-cartilaginous surfaces are lined with synovial membrane.

The fibrous capsule surrounding the joint is attached to the margin of the articular cartilage and to the neck of the mandible. Anteriorly it receives the attachment of the lateral pterygoid while its deep surface is firmly adherent to the periphery of the articular disc.

Laterally the capsule (see Fig. 7.25) is thickened to form the temporomandibular ligament, which inclines posteroinferiorly from the root of the zygomatic arch to the neck of the mandible. Two accessory ligaments lie medial to the joint, although not in contact with the capsule. The sphenomandibular ligament extends from the spine of the sphenoid to the lingula adjacent to the mandibular foramen. The stylomandibular ligament, a thickening of the parotid fascia, passes from the styloid process to the angle of the mandible.

The joint receives its nerve supply from the auriculotemporal and masseteric branches of the mandibular (Vc) division of the trigeminal nerve.

Movements at the joint include elevation, depression, protraction and retraction of the mandible. The head of the mandible does not merely rotate in the glenoid fossa but also moves forwards onto the articular eminence of the temporal bone, taking the articular disc with it. The alternate protraction and retraction of right and left sides produces the grinding movements used in chewing. The muscles responsible for these movements are known collectively as the muscles of mastication. The mouth is closed by contraction of masseter, temporalis and medial pterygoid. The lateral pterygoid protracts the mandible and, assisted by digastric and mylohyoid (see page 7.21), also opens the mouth. Retraction is produced by the posterior fibres of temporalis. When the mandible is fully depressed the joint is relatively unstable and dislocation may occur, the head of the mandible moving in front of the articular eminence and resulting in an inability to close the mouth.

Mandibular (Vc) division of trigeminal nerve

The mandibular division of the trigeminal nerve (Figs. 7.27 & 7.28) contains sensory and motor fibres and enters the infratemporal fossa through the foramen ovale in the sphenoid. Two small branches arise from the short main trunk of the nerve. The first branch ascends through the foramen ovale to receive sensation from the meninges of the middle cranial fossa. The other branch is motor, supplying the medial pterygoid and also giving a small branch which passes through the otic ganglion (lying just medial to the main trunk of the mandibular division) to supply tensor tympani and tensor palati.

The main trunk descends between the lateral pterygoid and tensor palati muscles, dividing into anterior and posterior divisions. The anterior division is mainly motor and gives masseteric, deep temporal, lateral pterygoid and buccal branches. The masseteric nerve (Fig. 7.26) curves laterally above the lateral pterygoid to enter the deep surface of masseter. Two or three deep temporal nerves (Fig. 7.28) ascend deep to temporalis which they supply and further branches enter the deep surface of the lateral pterygoid. The buccal nerve (Figs. 7.27 & 7.28) is a sensory branch which passes forwards between the two heads of the lateral pterygoid to supply the skin over the cheek and the mucosa lining the cheek which it reaches by piercing, but not supplying, buccinator.

The posterior division of the main trunk is mainly sensory and has three branches, the auriculotemporal, lingual and inferior alveolar nerves. The

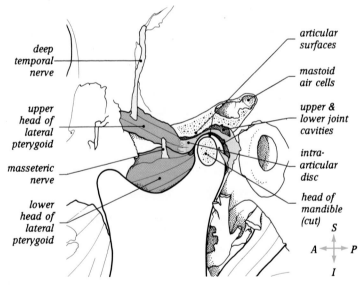

Fig. 7.26 *Temporomandibular joint opened by the excision of the lateral part of its capsule.*

auriculotemporal nerve (Fig. 7.28) arises by two roots which clasp the origin of the middle meningeal artery. The nerve passes backwards before turning superiorly behind the temporomandibular joint to ascend in company with the superficial temporal vessels. It gives secretomotor branches to the parotid gland (see page 7.15) and conveys sensation from the temporal region, the upper half of the pinna and most of the external auditory meatus.

The lingual nerve (Figs. 7.27 & 7.28) inclines downwards and forwards between the pterygoids, deviating medially to pass below the superior constrictor of the pharynx. In the floor of the mouth it runs forwards lateral to the hyoglossus muscle, at whose anterior border it again turns medially to pass inferior to the submandibular duct and enter the base of the tongue. It conveys general sensation from the anterior two-thirds of the tongue. Near the lower border of the lateral pterygoid the lingual nerve is joined by the chorda tympani (a branch of the facial nerve). Arising within the temporal bone, the chorda tympani emerges from the petrotympanic fissure. It carries taste fibres which have travelled in the lingual nerve from the

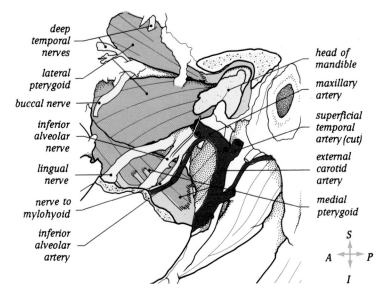

deep temporal nerves

lateral pterygoid

buccal nerve

inferior alveolar nerve

lingual nerve

nerve to mylohyoid

inferior alveolar artery

head of mandible

maxillary artery

superficial temporal artery (cut)

external carotid artery

medial pterygoid

S
A ← → P
I

Fig. 7.27 *Contents of the infratemporal fossa seen after excision of part of the ramus of the mandible.*

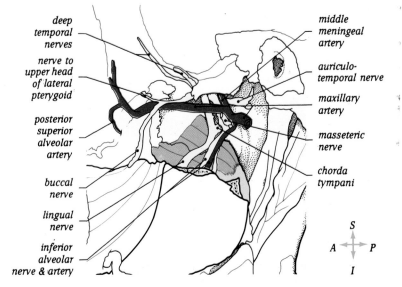

deep temporal nerves

nerve to upper head of lateral pterygoid

posterior superior alveolar artery

buccal nerve

lingual nerve

inferior alveolar nerve & artery

middle meningeal artery

auriculo-temporal nerve

maxillary artery

masseteric nerve

chorda tympani

S
A ← → P
I

Fig. 7.28 *Branches of the mandibular division of the trigeminal nerve and the maxillary artery revealed by removal of the mandibular head, lateral pterygoid and lateral root of the auriculotemporal nerve.*

anterior two-thirds of the tongue and preganglionic parasympathetic fibres destined for the submandibular ganglion (see page 7.25).

The inferior alveolar nerve (Figs. 7.27 & 7.28) descends medial to the lateral pterygoid and gives rise to a motor branch which curves downwards to supply mylohyoid and the anterior belly of digastric. The inferior alveolar nerve then enters the mandibular foramen in the ramus of the mandible and runs forwards in the mandibular canal, supplying the lower teeth. Its mental branch emerges from the mental foramen to supply skin overlying the chin.

Maxillary artery

This artery (Figs. 7.27 & 7.28) arises in the parotid gland (see page 7.15) as a terminal branch of the external carotid artery, passes anterosuperiorly across the infratemporal fossa, usually lateral to the lateral pterygoid, and enters the pterygopalatine fossa where terminal branches arise. These correspond to branches of the maxillary nerve (see page 7.27).

In the infratemporal fossa the maxillary artery gives branches to supply the pterygoid muscles, masseter and temporalis. In addition, the middle meningeal artery arises deep to the lateral pterygoid embraced by the two roots of the auriculotemporal nerve. It traverses the foramen spinosum and within the cranium supplies the meninges of the middle cranial fossa and the cranial vault.

The maxillary artery also gives rise to the inferior alveolar artery which accompanies the nerve into the mandibular canal. Further small branches supply the middle ear and the lining of the external auditory meatus.

Pterygoid venous plexus

Veins within the pterygopalatine fossa form a plexus which extends into the infratemporal fossa where it is related to the pterygoid muscles. This pterygoid plexus has important connections to the cavernous sinus in the skull and infraorbital and ophthalmic veins. The plexus drains by the maxillary vein into the retromandibular vein (see page 7.15).

7.19

inferior
alveolar
nerve

lingual
nerve

nerve to
mylohyoid

styloglossus

stylohyoid

anterior
belly of
digastric

nerve to
thyrohyoid

styloid
process

posterior
belly of
digastric

external carotid
artery (cut)

facial artery

hypoglossal nerve

lingual artery

Fig. 7.29 *Digastric and stylohyoid seen after
removal of part of the mandible. The superficial
part of the submandibular gland has also been
excised.*

DIGASTRIC

The digastric muscle (Fig. 7.29) consists of anterior and posterior bellies united by an intermediate tendon. The posterior belly attaches to the medial surface of the mastoid process and inclines forwards and downwards, becoming continuous with the intermediate tendon close to the hyoid bone. This tendon pierces stylohyoid and is anchored by a fascial sling to the hyoid bone. The anterior belly continues forwards from the intermediate tendon to attach to the inferior border of the mandible near the midline. Digastric elevates the hyoid bone during swallowing and assists mylohyoid and the lateral pterygoid in depressing the mandible when opening the mouth. The posterior belly is innervated by the facial (VII) nerve (see page 7.15). The anterior belly receives its motor supply from the mandibular (Vc) division of the trigeminal nerve via the mylohyoid branch of the inferior alveolar nerve (see page 7.19).

MUSCLES OF STYLOID PROCESS

Three muscles, stylohyoid, stylopharyngeus and styloglossus, attach to the styloid process but diverge to reach the hyoid bone, the pharynx and the tongue respectively.

Stylohyoid (Fig. 7.29) inclines downwards and forwards from the posterior surface of the styloid process to attach to the body of the hyoid bone alongside the lesser horn. The muscle or its tendon is pierced by the intermediate tendon of digastric near the hyoid bone. Stylohyoid elevates the hyoid and is innervated by the facial (VII) nerve.

Stylopharyngeus (Fig. 7.30) is attached to the medial side of the root of the styloid process and passes inferomedially on the lateral surface of the superior pharyngeal constrictor. It enters the wall of the pharynx between the superior and middle constrictors and blends with the other longitudinal muscles of the pharynx. The muscle elevates the pharynx and larynx during swallowing and is the only muscle innervated by the glossopharyngeal (IX) nerve.

Styloglossus (Fig. 7.30) inclines anteromedially from the tip of the styloid process and upper end of the stylohyoid ligament and passes between the superior and middle constrictors of the pharynx to enter the tongue. It elevates and retracts the tongue and, in common with other muscles of the tongue, is supplied by the hypoglossal (XII) nerve.

styloid
process

occipital
artery

stylo-
pharyngeus

glosso-
pharyngeal
nerve

ascending
palatine
artery

sterno-
mastoid

stylohyoid
ligament
(cut ends)

styloglossus

mylohyoid

Fig. 7.30 *Stylopharyngeus and styloglossus seen after excision of digastric, stylohyoid and the middle portion of the stylohyoid ligament.*

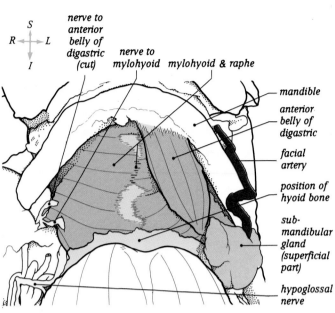

Fig. 7.31 *Mylohyoid revealed by removal of the right anterior belly of digastric and superficial part of the submandibular gland.*

Fig. 7.32 *The hypoglossal nerve, lingual nerve and submandibular duct pass above mylohyoid.*

Suspended from the body of the mandible is a thin sheet of muscle formed by the two mylohyoid muscles. The fibres of each muscle incline downwards and medially, meeting each other in the midline to form a shallow gutter. This gutter slopes downwards and backwards and ends at the free posterior borders of the two muscles on either side of the hyoid bone.

Each mylohyoid separates the superficial tissues in the upper part of the neck from the tongue and related structures within the mouth. Below the muscle lie the anterior belly of digastric (see page 7.21), part of the platysma (see page 7.11), the facial artery and vein, and the superficial part (the bulk) of the submandibular salivary gland (Fig. 7.31). This gland curves around the posterior border of mylohyoid so that its deep part and the submandibular duct lie above the muscle. Also located on the superior aspect of mylohyoid are the sublingual glands, the tongue with its vessels and nerves, and the geniohyoid muscles.

MYLOHYOID

This muscle (Figs. 7.31 & 7.32) takes attachment from the mylohyoid line on the inner aspect of the body of the mandible. Most of its fibres reach a midline raphe where they interdigitate with those from the opposite side. However, the fibres close to the posterior edge of the muscle descend to the body of the hyoid bone. The mylohyoid muscles raise the hyoid bone and the tongue during swallowing; they also help to depress the mandible when the hyoid bone is fixed from below. The muscle is innervated by the mylohyoid nerve, a branch of the inferior alveolar nerve from the mandibular division of the trigeminal nerve.

GENIOHYOID

Above mylohyoid a small muscle, geniohyoid (Fig. 7.33), lies close to the midline, passing from the inferior genial tubercle on the mandible to the body of the hyoid bone. Innervated by C1 spinal nerve fibres that are conveyed in the hypoglossal nerve, geniohyoid either elevates the hyoid or depresses the mandible.

Fig. 7.33 *Removal of part of the mandible and mylohyoid reveals structures deep to mylohyoid. The submandibular ganglion is thin and elongated in this specimen.*

7.23

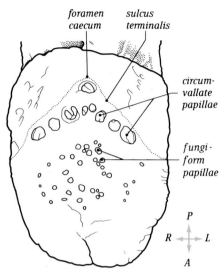

Fig. 7.34 *Surface features of the tongue.*

TONGUE

The tongue is a muscular organ and lies mostly within the oral cavity although its posterior part projects into the oropharynx.

Surface features

The tongue is covered by mucosa which is reflected anteriorly and laterally onto the inferior surface of the organ. Under the tip of the tongue the mucous membrane forms a midline fold, the frenulum. The upper surface of the tongue (Fig. 7.34) is divided into anterior two-thirds and posterior one-third by a V-shaped groove, the sulcus terminalis. A midline depression, the foramen caecum, lies at the apex of the sulcus terminalis. A row of round elevations, the circumvallate papillae, lie just in front of the sulcus. From the mucosa of the tongue, somatic sensory and taste fibres pass centrally to reach the brain. From the anterior two-thirds of the tongue (and adjacent oral mucosa) these fibres travel in the lingual nerve (see page 7.18). Somatic sensory fibres continue in the mandibular division of the trigeminal nerve to the brain. However, taste fibres leave the lingual nerve and are conveyed via the chorda tympani nerve to the facial nerve (see pages 7.18 & 7.19). Both taste and somatic sensory nerve fibres from the posterior third of the tongue (including the circumvallate papillae) are conveyed in the glossopharyngeal (IX) nerve.

Muscles

The musculature of the tongue, divided into two functional halves by a fibrous septum, consists of both extrinsic and intrinsic muscles. In general, the extrinsic muscles alter the position of the tongue and the intrinsic muscles alter its shape.

The extrinsic muscles comprise styloglossus (see page 7.21), hyoglossus and genioglossus. Hyoglossus (see Fig. 7.33) is attached to the body and greater horn of the hyoid bone and its fibres pass upwards and forwards to reach the side of the tongue. Hyoglossus depresses the tongue, particularly at the sides. Genioglossus (Figs. 7.35 & 7.36) forms much of the bulk of the tongue, its fibres radiating from the superior genial tubercle close to the midline to most parts of the tongue. The superior fibres reach the tip whilst the inferior fibres pass into the postero-inferior part of the organ. Genioglossus draws the tongue forwards and downwards and its anterior fibres retract the tip.

Palatoglossus descends from the soft palate and enters the side of the tongue posteriorly. Although it helps to elevate the tongue it is usually considered to be a muscle of the palate (see page 7.30).

Fig. 7.35 *Deeper structures in the base of the tongue revealed by removal of the sublingual gland and part of hyoglossus.*

The intrinsic muscles comprise interlacing longitudinal, transverse and vertical groups of fibres on either side of the midline fibrous septum. The shape of the tongue is changed by integrated contractions of the various groups.

The hypoglossal (XII) nerve (see Fig. 7.33) supplies all the muscles of the tongue, both intrinsic and extrinsic. (The nerve supply to palatoglossus is described with the other muscles of the palate; see page 7.30.)

Blood supply

Arising from the front of the external carotid artery, the lingual artery (Fig. 7.35) loops upwards above the greater horn of the hyoid bone and continues forwards into the base of the tongue deep to hyoglossus. Having supplied structures in the tongue, the lingual artery terminates in the tip. Venous drainage follows a reciprocal course into the internal jugular vein.

SUBMANDIBULAR AND SUBLINGUAL GLANDS

The superficial part of the submandibular salivary gland (see Fig. 7.31) lies inferior to mylohyoid and extends below the medial surface of the mandible. It is continuous around the posterior border of mylohyoid with the smaller deep part (see Fig. 7.32) of the gland which lies above the muscle. The lateral surface of the superficial part of the gland is indented by the facial artery as the vessel arches forwards to reach the inferior border of the mandible (see page 7.12). From the deep part of the gland the submandibular duct passes forwards and medially to open close to the midline at the base of the frenulum of the tongue. A number of small sublingual glands (see Fig. 7.33) lie beneath the mucosa adjacent to the submandibular duct. These glands are drained by ducts which open either into the submandibular duct or directly into the mouth. Both the sublingual and submandibular glands receive postganglionic parasympathetic secretomotor fibres from the submandibular ganglion (see Fig. 7.33). Preganglionic fibres reach the submandibular ganglion from the facial nerve by way of the chorda tympani and lingual nerves.

Fig. 7.36 *Sagittal section through the tongue and its surrounding structures.*

HYPOGLOSSAL (XII) NERVE

The twelfth cranial nerve (see Fig. 7.32) leaves the skull through the hypoglossal canal and descends between the internal jugular vein and internal carotid artery to turn forwards close to the origin of the occipital artery from the external carotid artery, where the descending limb of the ansa cervicalis (see page 7.7) arises. The hypoglossal nerve then continues forwards across the loop of the lingual artery and passes between mylohyoid and hyoglossus to enter the tongue whose muscles it supplies. The branches given to thyrohyoid and geniohyoid are composed of C1 fibres which are distributed via the hypoglossal nerve.

GLOSSOPHARYNGEAL (IX) NERVE

The glossopharyngeal nerve (Fig. 7.35) emerges from the skull through the jugular foramen. Initially contained within the carotid sheath, the nerve curves forwards around the stylopharyngeus muscle (which it also supplies) and passes between the superior and middle constrictors of the pharynx to enter the posterior part of the tongue. The glossopharyngeal nerve conveys both somatic and taste sensation from the posterior third of the tongue, oropharynx and lateral parts of the soft palate. The nerve has an autonomic sensory branch, the carotid sinus nerve, which ascends from the carotid sinus and carotid body. In addition, a tympanic branch passes to the tympanic plexus in the middle ear. The lesser petrosal nerve arises from this plexus.

PTERYGOPALATINE FOSSA

The pterygopalatine fossa lies between the pterygoid process of the sphenoid bone posteriorly, the palatine bone medially and the maxilla anteriorly (Fig. 7.37). It is slitlike and opens laterally into the infratemporal fossa. It contains part of the maxillary (Vb) division of the trigeminal nerve, the pterygopalatine ganglion and its branches and the termination of the maxillary artery, together with accompanying veins and lymphatics. The pterygopalatine fossa communicates with the middle cranial fossa through the foramen rotundum and the pterygoid canal, with the orbit through the inferior orbital fissure, with the walls of the nasal cavity through the sphenopalatine foramen and with the palate via the greater and lesser palatine canals.

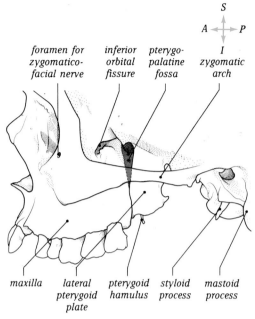

Fig. 7.37 *The pterygopalatine fossa is bounded by the maxilla and lateral pterygoid plate.*

Maxillary (Vb) division of the trigeminal nerve
The maxillary division (Fig. 7.38) leaves the cranial cavity through the foramen rotundum, crosses the pterygopalatine fossa and continues forwards through the inferior orbital fissure into the orbit. It terminates as the infraorbital nerve which traverses the infraorbital canal to reach the face. The maxillary division has several branches arising in the pterygopalatine fossa, the floor of the orbit and on the face. In the pterygopalatine fossa (Fig. 7.39), two branches suspend the pterygo-palatine ganglion from the parent nerve. Also arising in the fossa are the posterior superior alveolar nerves (Figs. 7.38 & 7.39) which descend in the posterior wall of the maxillary air sinus to reach the upper molar teeth. In the floor of the orbit the middle and anterior superior alveolar nerves (Fig. 7.38) arise and descend in the lateral and anterior walls of the maxilla. Collectively the superior alveolar nerves supply the maxilla and its air sinus, the alveolar ridge and all the upper teeth. The zygomatic nerve (Fig. 7.38) also arises in the floor of the orbit and ascends on the lateral wall, dividing into zygomaticotemporal and zygomatico-facial nerves. These branches pierce the zygomatic bone to supply the overyling facial skin. A branch from the zygomaticotemporal nerve conveys postganglionic parasympathetic fibres from the pterygopalatine ganglion to the lacrimal gland. The infraorbital nerve (Fig. 7.38) emerges onto the face through the infraorbital foramen and supplies the skin of the cheek, lower eyelid, upper lip and lateral surface of the external nose.

Fig. 7.38 *The maxillary nerve and artery seen after excision of part of the lateral walls of the orbit and maxillary air sinus.*

Pterygopalatine ganglion

The pterygopalatine ganglion (Fig. 7.39) is suspended from the maxillary division in the pterygopalatine fossa and transmits sensory, parasympathetic, and sympathetic nerve fibres. Sensory fibres originating in the palate, nose and nasopharynx pass through the ganglion without synapsing to enter the maxillary division. Preganglionic parasympathetic fibres destined for the ganglion leave the brain in the facial (VII) nerve and travel via the greater petrosal nerve. These fibres emerge from the petrous temporal bone and pass along the floor of the middle cranial fossa to enter the foramen lacerum, where they accompany postganglionic vasomotor sympathetic fibres from the carotid plexus as the nerve of the pterygoid canal. This nerve traverses the pterygoid canal to reach the pterygopalatine ganglion. In the ganglion the parasympathetic fibres synapse, and postganglionic fibres are distributed through the appropriate branches of the ganglion to the mucous glands in the nose and palate. Secretomotor parasympathetic fibres destined for the lacrimal gland enter the maxillary division and travel in its zygomatic branch. The ganglion earns its nickname, the hay fever ganglion, by virtue of its parasympathetic component. Sympathetic fibres are also distributed in the branches of the ganglion.

maxillary
(Vb) division

nerve of
pterygoid canal

pterygopalatine
ganglion

pharyngeal
branch

lesser & greater
palatine nerves

lateral
nasal nerve

posterior superior
alveolar nerve

maxillary
artery (cut)

Fig. 7.39 *Contents of the pterygopalatine fossa revealed by removal of much of the bone of the lateral wall of the nasal cavity.*

There are five groups of branches from the pterygopalatine ganglion (Fig. 7.39), namely lateral nasal, pharyngeal, nasopalatine, and greater and lesser palatine. Lateral nasal nerves, entering via the sphenopalatine foramen, supply the lateral wall of the nasal cavity. The pharyngeal branch innervates the nasopharynx. The nasopalatine nerve (Fig. 7.40) crosses the anterior surface of the body of the sphenoid bone to enter the nasal septum, then angles anteroinferiorly in a groove on the upper edge of the vomer, eventually passing through the incisive canal onto the lower surface of the anterior part of the hard palate. The nerve conveys sensation from the front of the palate and the inferior part of the nasal septum. The greater and lesser palatine nerves traverse the palatine canal to emerge from the appropriate palatine foramina on the lower surface of the hard palate. The greater palatine nerve supplies the hard palate whilst the lesser innervates the soft palate.

Vessels

The maxillary artery (Figs. 7.38 & 7.39) enters the pterygopalatine fossa from the infratemporal fossa and divides into its terminal branches. These accompany the branches of the ganglion and, having similar distributions, bear corresponding names. Venous blood drains into the pterygoid plexus which continues into the infratemporal fossa and communicates with the cavernous sinus via the inferior and superior orbital fissures.

sphenoidal
air sinus

nasopalatine
nerve

hard palate

incisive
foramen

soft palate

upper lip

Fig. 7.40 *Sagittal section showing the left nasopalatine nerve in situ after removal of the nasal septum.*

NASAL CAVITIES AND PARANASAL AIR SINUSES

NASAL CAVITIES

The paired nasal cavities lie centrally within the facial skeleton, medial to the orbits and the maxillary air sinuses (Fig. 7.41). They are separated from the oral cavity by the palate, from the anterior cranial fossa by the cribriform plates and from each other by the midline nasal septum. Anteriorly the cavities lead into the vestibules, which are surrounded by the cartilaginous external nose and open onto the face at the nostrils. Posteriorly the nasal cavities are limited by the free edge of the nasal septum at the posterior nares which open into the nasopharynx. Each cavity is partially subdivided by three shelf-like projections from the lateral wall, the superior, middle and inferior conchae. The parts of the nasal cavity beneath each of these are called correspondingly the superior, middle and inferior meatuses, whilst above the superior concha is the sphenoethmoidal recess. Into this recess and the meatuses drain the paranasal air sinuses and the nasolacrimal duct. Respiratory epithelium lines the cavity and paranasal air sinuses whilst the vestibule has a stratified squamous epithelium bearing nasal vibrissae (hairs).

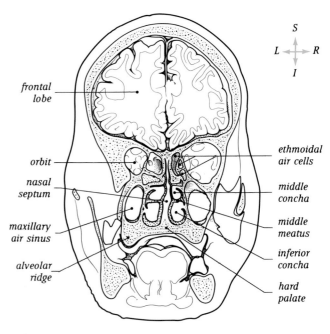

Fig. 7.41 *Near coronal section of the head through the orbits and nasal cavities. (Dentures remain in this specimen.)*

Bony walls

The medial wall is the nasal septum (Fig. 7.42), common to both cavities and formed superiorly by the perpendicular plate of the ethmoid. This plate continues upwards as the crista galli which projects into the anterior cranial fossa. The bony septum is completed posteroinferiorly by the vomer. Anteriorly the septum is composed of hyaline cartilage which extends into the external nose.

The roof of each cavity comprises, from in front backwards, the nasal and frontal bones, the cribriform plate of the ethmoid and, finally, the body of the sphenoid bone containing the sphenoidal air sinuses. Olfactory (I) nerves from the olfactory mucosa traverse the many small foramina in the cribriform plate to reach the olfactory bulbs in the anterior cranial fossa (Fig. 7.43).

The floor of each nasal cavity is formed by the hard palate, consisting of the palatine process of the maxilla and the horizontal process of the palatine bone.

Numerous bones contribute to the lateral wall (Figs. 7.43 & 7.44) including, from in front backwards, the maxilla, lacrimal, ethmoid, palatine and sphenoid bones. The maxilla forms the anteroinferior portion of the lateral wall and contains the maxillary air sinus. Between the maxilla and the ethmoid, part of the lacrimal bone covers the nasolacrimal canal which opens into the inferior meatus. Each lateral mass of the ethmoid is attached to the lateral part of the cribriform plate and contains numerous air cells. From the medial surface of the lateral mass project the small superior and the larger middle conchae. The ethmoidal air cells bulge into the middle meatus forming the bulla beneath which a curved groove, the hiatus semilunaris, separates the ethmoid from the maxilla. Forming the posterior limit of the hiatus semilunaris is the vertical plate of the palatine bone. The most posterior component of the lateral wall is the medial pterygoid plate of the sphenoid. Overlying the maxilla and palatine bones is a separate bone, the inferior concha.

Fig. 7.42 *Sagittal section just to right of midline with intact nasal septum.*

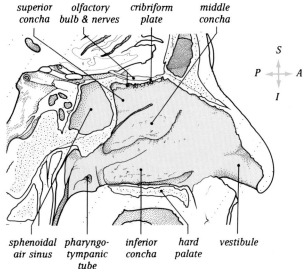

superior concha | olfactory bulb & nerves | cribriform plate | middle concha

sphenoidal air sinus | pharyngo-tympanic tube | inferior concha | hard palate | vestibule

Fig. 7.43 *Sagittal section with the nasal septum removed to show the lateral wall of the nasal cavity.*

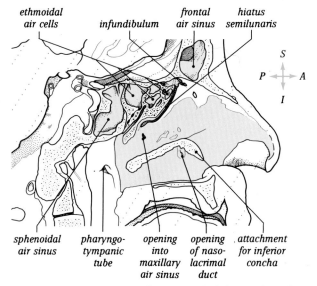

ethmoidal air cells | infundibulum | frontal air sinus | hiatus semilunaris

sphenoidal air sinus | pharyngo-tympanic tube | opening into maxillary air sinus | opening of naso-lacrimal duct | attachment for inferior concha

Fig. 7.44 *Sagittal section after removal of the conchae, the ethmoid bulla and the upper part of the lateral nasal wall.*

Sensory nerve supply

The somatic sensory nerve supply to the walls of the nasal cavity is derived mainly from the maxillary (Vb) division of the trigeminal nerve. The lateral nasal nerves from the pterygopalatine ganglion (see page 7.27) supply most of the lateral wall, while the nasopalatine nerve supplies the septum. Lesser and greater palatine nerves supply the posterior part of the lateral wall and the floor. In addition, fibres from the ophthalmic (Va) division reach the nasal cavity via the anterior ethmoidal nerve. This nerve supplies the anterosuperior parts of the septum and the lateral wall and continues as the external nasal nerve to supply most of the external nose.

Blood supply

Most of the blood supply to the walls of the nasal cavity is provided by branches of the maxillary artery. These vessels arise in the pterygopalatine fossa and are named according to the branches of the pterygopalatine ganglion they accompany. The anteroinferior part of the nasal septum is highly vascular (Little's area) and commonly gives rise to nasal haemorrhage (epistaxis).

Venous blood passes to the pterygoid plexus, the facial vein and the ophthalmic veins.

PARANASAL AIR SINUSES

There are four paired groups of paranasal air sinuses (Figs. 7.41 & 7.44) contained within the frontal, maxillary, ethmoid and sphenoid bones. Each

sinus communicates with the nasal cavity, is lined with mucous membrane and normally contains air. The frontal air sinuses are situated in the vertical and horizontal parts of the frontal bone, closely related to the frontal lobes of the brain. They are variable in size and open into the middle meatus at the infundibulum, the most anterior part of the hiatus semilunaris. The frontal air sinus is supplied by the supraorbital branch of the ophthalmic (Va) division of the trigeminal nerve.

The maxillary air sinus (antrum) occupies the body of the maxilla, lying above the oral cavity and alveolar ridge and below the orbit. Its opening at the posterior end of the hiatus semilunaris lies high on the medial wall of the antrum, permitting limited drainage for contents such as mucus or pus. Sensory innervation is from the superior alveolar nerves. The ethmoidal air sinuses are subdivided into three groups of air cells which communicate with the nose through many tiny foramina. The anterior cells open into the floor of the hiatus whilst the middle cells open onto the bulla, both groups being supplied by the anterior ethmoidal nerve. The posterior group, innervated by the posterior ethmoidal nerve, drains into the superior meatus under the superior concha.

The sphenoidal air sinus lies just below the sella turcica in the body of the sphenoid, through the anterior wall of which it opens into the spheno-ethmoidal recess. Its sensory supply is from the pharyngeal branch of the pterygopalatine ganglion.

Infection of the paranasal air sinuses (sinusitis) causes thickening of the mucosal lining which may block the openings into the nasal cavities.

PALATE

The palate consists of hard and soft parts covered by mucous membrane (Fig. 7.45). The hard palate separates the oral and nasal cavities whilst posteriorly the soft palate separates the nasopharynx from the oropharynx.

HARD PALATE

The bones which comprise the hard palate are the palatine processes of the maxillae anteriorly and the horizontal plates of the palatine bones posteriorly (see Fig. 7.72). The hard palate is bounded in front and laterally by the superior alveolar ridge. The soft palate is attached to the free posterior border of the hard palate. Sensory fibres reach the palate in branches of the maxillary (Vb) division of the trigeminal nerve. The nasopalatine nerve emerges from the incisive foramen and supplies the anterior part of the hard palate. The greater palatine nerve gains the hard palate via the greater palatine foramen and innervates its posterior portion.

SOFT PALATE

The soft palate projects into the cavity of the pharynx from its attachment to the posterior edge of the hard palate. When elevated it separates the oropharynx from the nasopharynx. Five paired muscles attach to the soft palate and contribute to its structure. In the midline the uvula projects downwards from its posterior free border.

Muscles

Tensor palati (Fig. 7.47) attaches to the scaphoid fossa and spine of the sphenoid and to the lateral surface of the cartilaginous portion of the pharyngotympanic (Eustachian) tube. Its fibres descend between the lateral and medial pterygoid plates on the lateral aspect of the pharyngeal wall and give way to a tendon just above the pterygoid hamulus. The tendon hooks under the hamulus and turns medially to enter the soft palate where it forms the palatine aponeurosis by fanning out and attaching to the posterior border of the hard palate. The palatine aponeurosis forms the basic structure of the soft palate to which other muscles gain attachment. Tensor palati is supplied by the mandibular (Vc) division of the trigeminal nerve and tenses the soft palate.

Levator palati (Figs. 7.46 & 7.47) attaches to the inferior surface of the petrous temporal bone just medial to the opening of the pharyngotympanic tube and to the adjacent part of the tube. Its fibres descend medial to the medial pterygoid plate within the pharynx and attach to the upper surface of the palatine aponeurosis. The muscle is innervated by the pharyngeal plexus (see page 7.32). Levator palati elevates the soft palate during swallowing, preventing regurgitation of food into the nasal cavities.

Palatoglossus (Fig. 7.46) descends from the inferior surface of the palatine aponeurosis and inclines slightly forwards to enter the posterolateral part of the tongue. The position of palatoglossus is evident on the inner surface of the oral cavity as a mucosal elevation, the palatoglossal ridge (anterior pillar of the fauces; Fig. 7.45). The two palatoglossal ridges form the oropharyngeal isthmus, which marks the posterior boundary of the mouth. Innervated by fibres from the pharyngeal plexus, palatoglossus lowers the soft palate, raises the posterior part of the tongue and moves the palatoglossal ridge towards the midline, thus narrowing the isthmus.

Palatopharyngeus (Figs. 7.46 & 7.47) attaches to the undersurface of the soft palate. Most of its fibres run posteroinferiorly as part of the longitudinal layer of muscle inside the pharynx and form the palatopharyngeal ridge (posterior pillar of the fauces). On contraction these fibres depress the soft palate. Other fibres pass horizontally backwards, raising the mucosa into a ridge against which the soft palate is elevated. The palatopharyngeus receives its motor supply from the pharyngeal plexus.

The uvular muscle (Figs. 7.46 & 7.47), also supplied by the pharyngeal plexus, lies entirely within the soft palate and elevates the uvula. In cases of unilateral paralysis of the soft palate the uvula rises asymmetrically, being pulled away from the paralysed side.

Sensory and secretomotor innervation to the soft palate is from the lesser palatine nerves of the maxillary (Vb) division of the trigeminal nerve, supplemented laterally on the undersurface of the palate by the glossopharyngeal (IX) nerve.

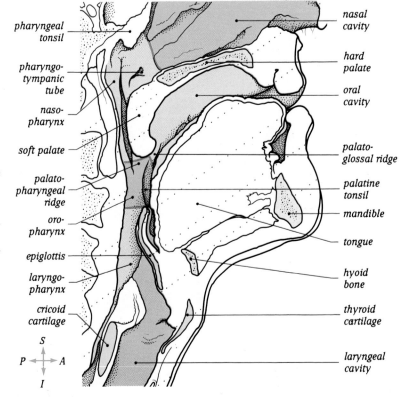

Fig. 7.45 *Sagittal section of palate and pharynx showing communications with the nasal, oral and laryngeal cavities.*

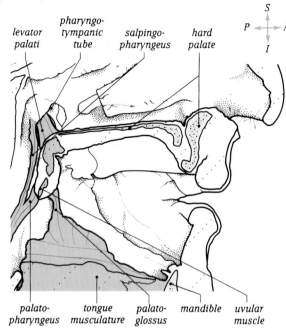

Fig. 7.46 *Further dissection of Fig. 7.45 to show some of the muscles of the soft palate.*

Fig. 7.47 *Posterior view of soft palate after removal of cervical vertebral column and posterior wall of pharynx. On one side, the medial pterygoid and the mucosa of the soft palate has been removed to reveal the muscles.*

7.31

PHARYNX

The pharynx is a muscular tube which is continuous inferiorly with the oesophagus and into which the nasal, oral and laryngeal cavities open (see Fig. 7.45). For descriptive purposes the pharynx is divided into nasopharynx, oropharynx and laryngopharynx. The nasopharynx is attached to the base of the skull and is bounded anteriorly by the posterior nares. Inferiorly it is continuous with the oropharynx at the level of the soft palate. The oropharynx begins anteriorly at the palatoglossal ridge and extends inferiorly to the level of the upper border of the epiglottis where it is in continuity with the laryngopharynx. The laryngopharynx lies behind the laryngeal inlet, the arytenoids and the cricoid lamina, and on either side of the inlet forms recesses, the piriform fossae. At the inferior border of the cricoid cartilage, it is continuous with the oesophagus. The musculature of the pharynx consists of incomplete outer circular and inner longitudinal layers. The pharyngobasilar fascia lies internal to the muscle coat and is lined by mucous membrane.

MUSCLES
The circular layer of muscles comprises three overlapping constrictors, attaching posteriorly to the midline raphe (Figs. 7.48 & 7.49) and suspended from the pharyngeal tubercle of the sphenoid bone.

The superior constrictor attaches anteriorly to the lower part of the medial pterygoid plate, the pterygomandibular raphe (in company with buccinator, see page 7.11) and the posterior end of the mylohyoid line on the mandible. Posteriorly its fibres attach to the pharyngeal tubercle and the pharyngeal raphe.

The middle constrictor attaches to the lower part of the stylohyoid ligament and to the angle between the greater and lesser horns of the hyoid bone. Posteriorly it attaches to the raphe, the upper fibres overlapping those of the superior constrictor.

The inferior constrictor has an anterior attachment to the oblique line on the thyroid cartilage, the lateral surface of the cricoid cartilage and the intervening fascia covering the cricothyroid muscle. Its superior fibres curve upwards to the pharyngeal raphe, overlapping those of the middle constrictor. The lower fibres, sometimes called cricopharyngeus, pass horizontally around the lumen of the pharynx, bypassing the raphe.

The inner longitudinal layer consists of the stylopharyngeus, palatopharyngeus and salpingopharyngeus muscles. Stylopharyngeus (see page 7.21) attaches to the styloid process and lies lateral to the superior constrictor. Its fibres descend between the superior and middle constrictors (Fig. 7.49) to blend with the other longitudinal muscles on the medial surface of the two lower constrictors. Palatopharyngeus inclines posteroinferiorly from the soft palate whilst salpingopharyngeus descends from the pharyngotympanic tube, both muscles lying on the inner surface of the constrictors (see Fig. 7.46). The longitudinal muscles attach inferiorly to the posterior border of the lamina of the thyroid cartilage.

During swallowing, the pharyngeal constrictors contract sequentially from above downwards to propel the bolus of food into the oesophagus. Simultaneously the longitudinal muscles shorten the pharynx and elevate the larynx, thus closing its inlet against the base of the tongue. Due to the shape of the epiglottis, the bolus tends to traverse the piriform fossae. At the same time, the soft palate is raised to prevent food entering the nasopharynx and the cricopharyngeus relaxes to allow the bolus to enter the oesophagus.

NERVE SUPPLY
The pharyngeal plexus (Fig. 7.48) consists of nerve fibres lying on the outer surface of the pharynx and receives the pharyngeal branches of the glossopharyngeal (IX) and vagus (X) nerves. The motor component of the plexus is derived from the cranial part of the accessory (XI) nerve via the vagus nerve. It supplies the muscles of the pharynx except for stylopharyngeus (glossopharyngeal nerve, see page 7.25).

Sensory fibres from the glossopharyngeal nerve traverse the plexus to supply the oropharynx whilst the vagal fibres of the plexus, assisted by those travelling in the superior laryngeal nerve (see page 7.38), innervate the laryngopharynx. The sensory innervation of the nasopharynx is supplied by the maxillary (Vb) division of the trigeminal nerve via its pharyngeal branch from the pterygopalatine ganglion.

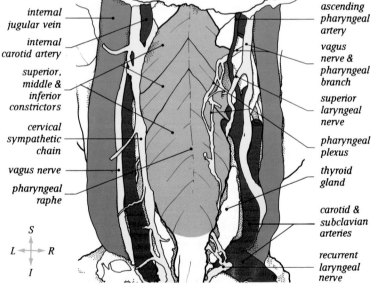

Fig. 7.48 *Posterior view of pharyngeal musculature after removal of cervical vertebral column, posterior part of the skull, right sympathetic trunk and part of the right internal carotid artery.*

PHARYNGOBASILAR FASCIA AND PHARYNGOTYMPANIC TUBE
The inner surface of the pharyngeal musculature is lined by the pharyngobasilar fascia. This fascial sheet completes the wall of the pharynx superiorly and forms a continuous attachment to the base of the skull. Inferiorly the fascia becomes gradually thinner, blending with the epimysium of the pharyngeal muscles.

The pharyngotympanic (Eustachian) tube (see Figs. 7.45–7.47) opens into the nasopharynx above the superior constrictor by piercing the pharyngobasilar fascia. Laterally the pharyngotympanic tube leads into the cavity of the middle ear.

Fig. 7.49 *Oblique view of pharyngeal musculature. Medial pterygoid has been removed to display the whole of the superior constrictor.*

Fig. 7.50 *Posterior view of nasal, oral and laryngeal cavities after opening the pharynx.*

LYMPHOID TISSUE

An incomplete ring of lymphoid tissue (see Fig. 7.45) lies in the wall of the pharynx between the mucosa and the muscles. This tissue is often subject to infection, particularly in children. On each side a palatine tonsil lies between the palatoglossal and palatopharyngeal ridges and has a rich blood supply including its own tonsillar branch from the facial artery. The adenoids, or pharyngeal tonsils, are situated near the roof of the nasopharynx, close to the pharyngotympanic tubes. When enlarged, the adenoids may obstruct one or both tubes, giving rise to middle ear disease. The lingual tonsil lies under the mucosa of the posterior third of the tongue and comprises a diffuse collection of small lymphoid follicles.

BLOOD SUPPLY

The arterial supply to the pharynx is derived from branches of the facial, lingual and maxillary arteries (see page 7.52). The ascending pharyngeal artery (Fig. 7.48) is a direct branch of the external carotid artery and passes upwards medial to the styloid muscles on the lateral surface of the pharynx. Venous blood drains into the pterygoid plexus and the internal jugular vein.

LARYNX

The larynx acts as a sphincter guarding the lower respiratory tract and is responsible for phonation. It lies in the neck and its inlet is continuous above and behind with the laryngopharynx (Figs. 7.51 & 7.52). Inferiorly the larynx is continuous with the trachea. It consists of a framework of cartilages and bone which support the vocal and vestibular folds and the muscles that move them. Anteriorly lie the infrahyoid strap muscles.

SKELETON

The skeleton of the larynx comprises the thyroid, cricoid and arytenoid cartilages, the epiglottis and the hyoid bone.

The thyroid cartilage (see Figs. 7.57 & 7.58) has two flat laminae joined anteriorly to form the midline laryngeal prominence ('Adam's apple'). The posterior margin of each lamina is free and bears a superior and an inferior horn. The tips of the inferior horns articulate by tiny synovial joints with the lateral surfaces of the cricoid cartilage.

The cricoid cartilage (see Figs. 7.57 & 7.61) lies below the thyroid cartilage and is shaped like a signet ring, with a narrow anterior arch and a wide posterior lamina. Its inferior border lies horizontally whilst the superior border slopes upwards posteriorly. Movement at the cricothyroid joints allows the arch of the cricoid to tip upwards whilst the lamina tips backwards.

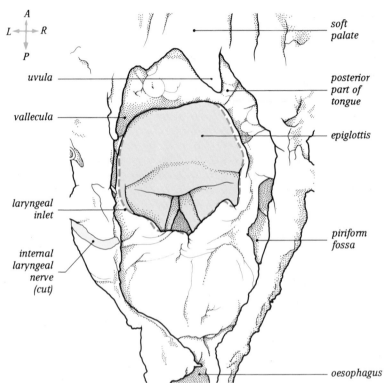

Fig. 7.51 *Posterior view of the larynx, seen through the opened laryngopharynx. The lumen of the larynx is visible through the laryngeal inlet.*

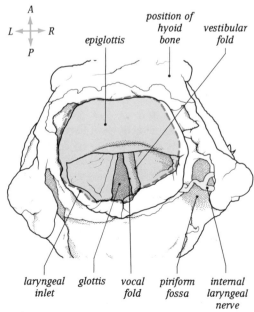

Fig. 7.52 *Superior view into the larynx. The mucosa lining the laryngopharynx has been removed to reveal the internal laryngeal nerve.*

In addition to its articulations with the thyroid cartilage, the upper border of the cricoid lamina bears articular surfaces, one on each side of the midline, for synovial joints with the two arytenoid cartilages. Each arytenoid (Figs. 7.54, 7.57 & 7.61) is pyramidal in shape, with its base on the cricoid lamina and its apex superiorly. It has four surfaces (medial, posterior,

anterolateral and inferior) and two processes. Anteriorly lies the vocal process, to which the vocal fold is attached, whilst its muscular process projects laterally. Each arytenoid is able to rotate around its own vertical axis. In addition, the arytenoids can slide laterally and downwards away from the midline on the slope of the articular surface on the cricoid.

Fig. 7.53 *Some of the intrinsic muscles of the larynx seen after removal of the mucosa of the laryngopharynx.*

Fig. 7.54 *Cricoid and arytenoid cartilages exposed by removal of most of the soft tissues on the left of the larynx.*

7.35

The epiglottis (Figs. 7.54 & 7.57) is attached in the midline to the inner surface of the thyroid cartilage, just below the laryngeal prominence. It extends upwards and backwards behind the tongue. During swallowing, it overlies the laryngeal inlet when the larynx is raised against the tongue.

The hyoid bone (Figs. 7.52 & 7.57) is the uppermost skeletal element of the larynx. It consists of a body bearing greater and lesser pairs of horns.

MEMBRANES AND LIGAMENTS

Several membranes are attached to the laryngeal framework and fill the gaps between the skeletal structures. The cricovocal (cricothyroid) membrane (Fig. 7.56) is elastic and attaches inferiorly to the upper border of the cricoid cartilage. In the midline anteriorly, it reaches the inferior border of the thyroid cartilage, forming the cricothyroid ligament. Posteriorly it is attached to the vocal processes of the arytenoids. The membrane has a free upper border which runs between the arytenoids and the thyroid cartilage and forms the basis of the vocal folds (true vocal cords).

The inelastic aryepiglottic (quadrate) membrane (Fig. 7.56) attaches posteriorly to the body and apex of the arytenoid and anteriorly to the lower part of the lateral edge of the epiglottis. It has a lower free border which forms the vestibular fold (false vocal cord) whilst the upper free edge forms the aryepiglottic fold (part of the laryngeal inlet).

The thyrohyoid membrane (see Fig. 7.58) fills the gap between the thyroid cartilage and the hyoid bone. Its posterior free edges are thickened to form the thyrohyoid ligaments.

Mucous membrane (Fig. 7.55) lines the interior of the larynx. The epithelium is of the respiratory type, except over the vocal and aryepiglottic folds where it is stratified and squamous. A pouch of mucous membrane protrudes laterally between the vocal and vestibular folds, forming the saccule. It contains numerous mucous glands whose secretions moisten the vocal folds.

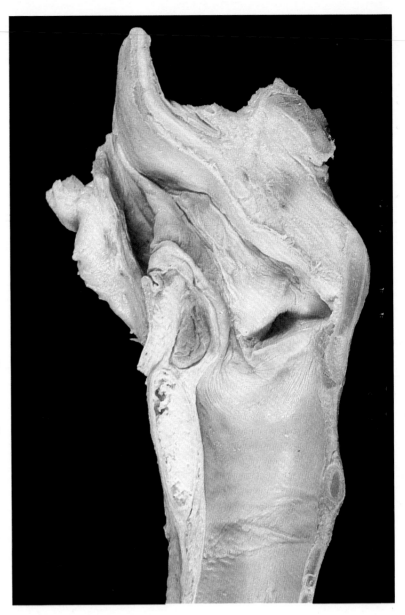

INTRINSIC MUSCLES

The intrinsic laryngeal muscles control the position and tension of the vocal and aryepiglottic folds, therefore modifying the shape of the airway through the larynx, acting both at the glottis (rima glottidis), the gap between the vocal folds, and at the inlet (see Fig. 7.52). During swallowing, the whole airway narrows; but in coughing and phonation, only the glottis narrows. The glottis widens during inspiration, especially when deep. The muscles are symmetrical in their arrangement.

The cricothyroid muscle (see Fig. 7.58) attaches to the anterolateral surface of the cricoid cartilage and to the inferior edge of the thyroid cartilage and adjacent part of the inferior horn. It raises the arch of the cricoid cartilage, tipping the lamina backwards and thereby increasing the tension and length of the vocal folds. This has the effect of raising the pitch of the voice and narrowing the glottis.

The thyroarytenoid muscle (see Fig. 7.60) attaches to the posterior surface of the thyroid cartilage adjacent to the cricovocal membrane. Its fibres pass posteriorly to gain the vocal process and adjacent body of the arytenoid cartilage. The muscle opposes the action of cricothyroid, drawing the arytenoids forwards and relaxing the vocal folds. Part of the muscle (vocalis) lies in the free edge of the vocal fold. The vocalis gives rigidity to the edge of the fold and also modifies tension differentially along its length.

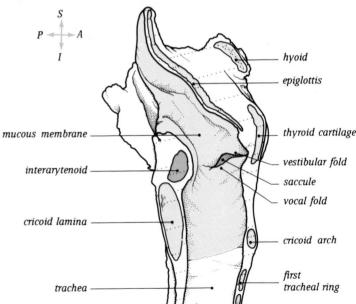

Fig. 7.55 *Median sagittal section showing the lumen and mucous membrane (pink) of the larynx.*

Two muscles attach to the muscular process of each arytenoid. The lateral cricoarytenoid (see Fig. 7.59) attaches to the lateral surface of the cricoid, its fibres passing posterosuperiorly to gain the muscular process of the arytenoid. The muscle rotates the arytenoid around its vertical axis, adducting the vocal folds and thereby closing the glottis. The posterior cricoarytenoid (Figs. 7.53 & 7.59) inclines anterosuperiorly from the lamina of the

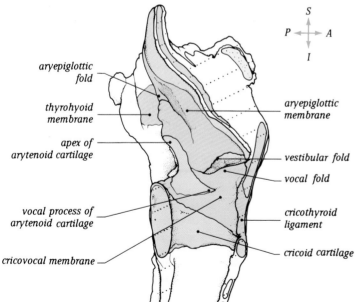

Fig. 7.56 *Membranes and folds of the larynx revealed by removal of the mucosa.*

aryepiglottic fold

thyrohyoid membrane

apex of arytenoid cartilage

vocal process of arytenoid cartilage

cricovocal membrane

aryepiglottic membrane

vestibular fold

vocal fold

cricothyroid ligament

cricoid cartilage

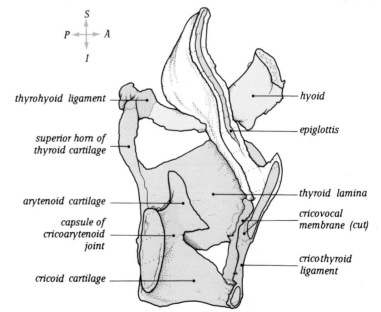

Fig. 7.57 *Bisected skeleton of the larynx revealed by removal of all membranes.*

thyrohyoid ligament

superior horn of thyroid cartilage

arytenoid cartilage

capsule of cricoarytenoid joint

cricoid cartilage

hyoid

epiglottis

thyroid lamina

cricovocal membrane (cut)

cricothyroid ligament

cricoid to the muscular process of the arytenoid. Its action opposes that of the lateral cricoarytenoid, rotating the arytenoid so that the folds are abducted and the glottis opened. Simultaneous contraction of the lateral and posterior cricoarytenoid muscles separates the arytenoids by sliding them down the cricoid lamina.

The interarytenoid muscle (Figs. 7.53 & 7.55) spans the gap between the bodies of the arytenoid cartilages and has transverse and oblique fibres. The muscle approximates the arytenoids, closing the glottis. Some of the interarytenoid fibres continue anterosuperiorly in the aryepiglottic fold to form the aryepiglottic muscle (see Fig. 7.59). These fibres assist in closing the laryngeal inlet and are important during swallowing.

NERVE SUPPLY

The larynx is supplied by the right and left superior and recurrent laryngeal branches of the vagus (X) nerves. Each recurrent laryngeal nerve (Figs. 7.58 & 7.59) ascends from the root of the neck (see page 7.9) in the groove between the trachea and oesophagus. Passing beneath the lower border of the inferior constrictor, the nerve enters the larynx behind the cricothyroid joint.

It supplies motor fibres to all of the intrinsic muscles (except cricothyroid) and carries sensory fibres from all of the structures within the larynx and laryngopharynx below the level of the vocal folds.

The superior laryngeal nerve (Figs. 7.48 & 7.58) arises from the vagus nerve just below the skull and descends to the thyrohyoid membrane where it

Fig. 7.58 *Anterolateral view of the larynx after removal of the pretracheal fascia and the superficial structures of the neck.*

Fig. 7.59 *Deeper intrinsic muscles seen after removal of half of the thyroid cartilage and the hyoid bone.*

divides, forming a motor external laryngeal branch and a sensory internal laryngeal branch. The external laryngeal nerve (Fig. 7.58) descends on the outer surface of the larynx to supply the cricothyroid muscle. The internal laryngeal branch (Figs. 7.52 & 7.58) pierces the thyrohyoid membrane and provides sensory fibres to the larynx and laryngopharynx above the vocal folds.

BLOOD SUPPLY

The laryngeal branches of the superior and inferior thyroid arteries (see Figs. 7.10 & 7.12) supply the larynx whilst venous blood drains via superior and middle thyroid vessels into the internal jugular vein.

Fig. 7.60 *Thyroarytenoid and the arytenoid cartilage after excision of the lateral cricothyroid, interarytenoid and aryepiglottic muscles.*

Fig. 7.61 *Cartilages of the larynx revealed by removal of muscles and membranes on the left side.*

CRANIUM AND CONTENTS

The part of the skull which contains the brain and its immediate relations is called the cranium. Although the detailed anatomy of the central nervous system is outside the scope of this book, there are some important surface features of the brain (Figs 7.62 & 7.63) to which reference should be made when considering the bony features of the interior of the cranium.

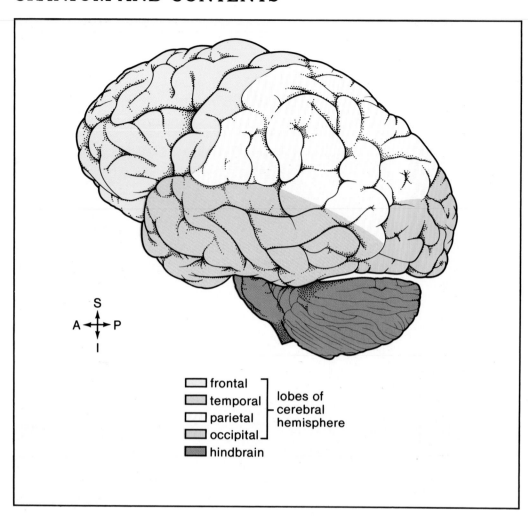

Fig. 7.62 *Lateral view of the brain showing the lobes of the cerebral hemisphere and the hindbrain.*

BONY FEATURES

The vault of the skull consists of four flat bones. Anteriorly is the frontal bone, posteriorly the occipital bone and on each side is a parietal bone (Fig. 7.64). The frontal and parietal bones meet along the coronal suture, and the two parietal bones meet along the midline sagittal suture. Posteriorly the parietal bones meet the occipital bone at the parietooccipital suture. The undersurface of the vault bears a long shallow midline groove for the superior sagittal venous sinus (see below) which terminates at a prominence, the internal occipital protuberance (Fig. 7.65). Below the level of each parietal bone, the greater wing of the sphenoid bone and the squamous part of the temporal bone complete the lateral wall of the vault.

The base of the cranium is characterized by the anterior, middle and posterior fossae, arranged in step-like sequence (Fig. 7.65), the anterior being superior. The anterior fossa, which accommodates the frontal lobes of the brain, is formed by the frontal bone laterally, the cribriform plates and crista galli of the ethmoid bone medially and is completed posteriorly by the lesser wings of the sphenoid bone. The numerous small foramina in the cribriform plates communicate with the nasal cavity (see page 7.28).

The middle fossa, occupied by the temporal lobes of the brain, is formed by the greater wings and body of the sphenoid bone. Posteriorly the fossa is bounded by the petrous part of each temporal bone whilst anteriorly the fossa is completed by the lesser wings of the sphenoid. Each of the lesser wings is perforated by the optic canal which continues forwards into the orbit. Between the lesser and greater wings is the superior orbital fissure which also provides access to the orbit. The greater wing is traversed by the foramen rotundum (opening into the pterygopalatine fossa; see page 7.26) and the foramina ovale and spinosum (both opening into the infratemporal fossa; see page 7.46). Lying in the angle between the greater wing and body of the sphenoid and the apex of the petrous part of the temporal bone is the foramen lacerum, which forms part of the roof of the infratemporal fossa. In the midline, the body of the sphenoid is hollowed, forming the sella turcica. This is limited by the paired anterior and posterior clinoid processes, and accommodates the pituitary gland.

The posterior cranial fossa contains the cerebellum, the pons and the medulla oblongata which is in continuity through the foramen magnum with the spinal cord. The floor of this fossa is formed mostly by the occipital bone, supplemented anteriorly by the body of the sphenoid and the posterior surface of the petrous part of each temporal bone. Anterior to the foramen magnum the occipital and sphenoid bones fuse to form a smooth incline, the clivus, on which the brain stem lies. The internal auditory meatus opens onto the posterior surface of the petrous part of the temporal bone while in the suture between this bone and the occipital bone is the jugular foramen. Running horizontally from the internal occipital protuberance is a groove for the transverse venous sinus (see page 7. 42). An S-shaped groove for the sigmoid sinus (Fig. 7.65) links the groove for the transverse sinus with the jugular foramen. The hypoglossal canal traverses the occipital bone anterolateral to the foramen magnum (see Fig. 7.72).

Fig. 7.63 *Inferior surface of the brain.*

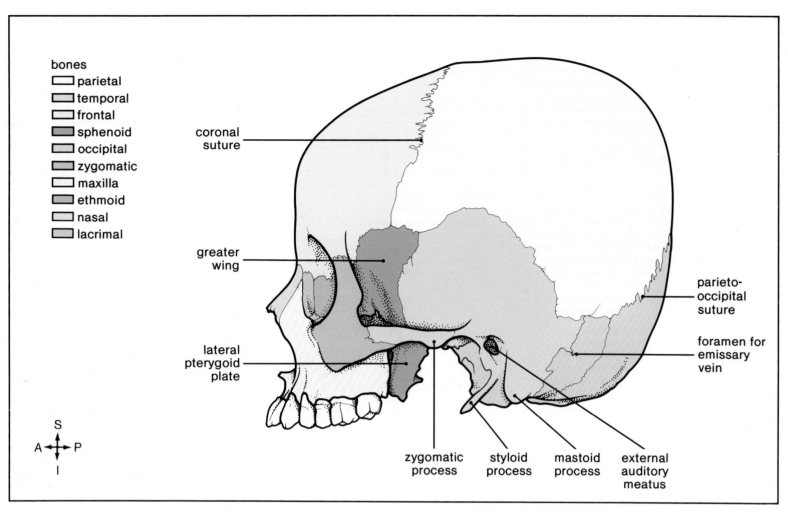

bones
- parietal
- temporal
- frontal
- sphenoid
- occipital
- zygomatic
- maxilla
- ethmoid
- nasal
- lacrimal

coronal suture

greater wing

lateral pterygoid plate

parieto-occipital suture

foramen for emissary vein

zygomatic process

styloid process

mastoid process

external auditory meatus

S
A — P
I

Fig. 7.64 *Lateral view of the skull (without the mandible) showing its bony features.*

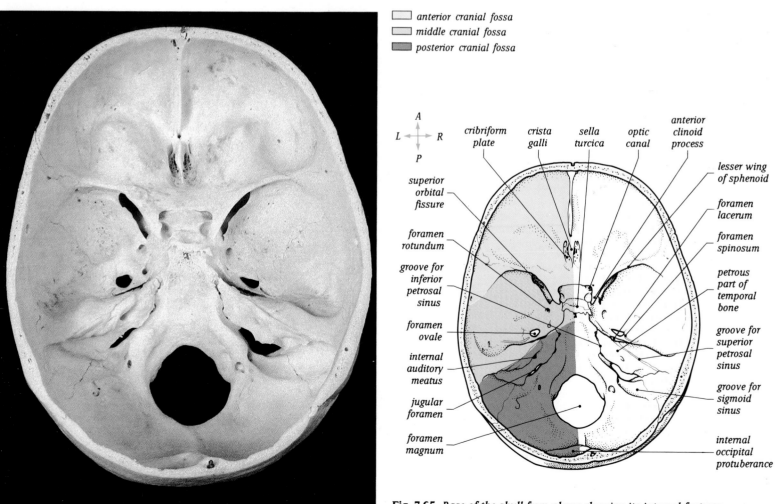

- anterior cranial fossa
- middle cranial fossa
- posterior cranial fossa

A
L — R
P

cribriform plate

crista galli

sella turcica

optic canal

anterior clinoid process

lesser wing of sphenoid

superior orbital fissure

foramen lacerum

foramen rotundum

foramen spinosum

groove for inferior petrosal sinus

petrous part of temporal bone

foramen ovale

groove for superior petrosal sinus

internal auditory meatus

jugular foramen

groove for sigmoid sinus

foramen magnum

internal occipital protuberance

Fig. 7.65 *Base of the skull from above showing its internal features.*

7.41

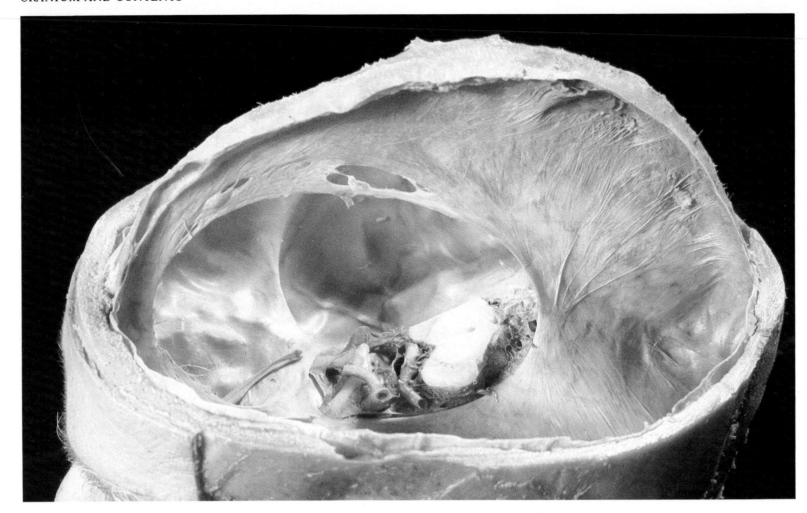

MENINGES

Surrounding the brain are three membranes, the meninges, which comprise the dura mater, arachnoid mater and pia mater.

Dura mater

The dura mater consists of outer periosteal and inner meningeal layers. The periosteal dura attaches to and closely follows the bony contours of the cranial cavity and is continuous through the sutures and foramina with the periosteum on the outer surface of the skull. Although generally bound to the periosteal dura, the meningeal dura is raised in places as a double layer, forming the dural folds.

The largest of these folds is the midline falx cerebri (Figs. 7.66 & 7.67), which projects downwards between the two cerebral hemispheres.

Anteriorly the falx cerebri is attached to the crista galli of the ethmoid bone. It arches over the corpus callosum and gains further attachment to the frontal, parietal and occipital bones. Posteriorly the falx ends by attaching to another dural fold, the tentorium cerebelli (Figs. 7.66 – 7.68). The tentorium forms an incomplete roof over the posterior cranial fossa and separates the occipital lobes of the cerebrum from the cerebellum. Each side of the tentorium slopes upwards towards its midline attachment to the falx cerebri. Anteriorly there is a large aperture in the tentorium through which the brain stem passes. The thickened free edge of the tentorium surrounding this aperture continues forwards to reach the anterior clinoid process. The attached border of the tentorium runs laterally from the internal occipital protuberance along a horizontal groove on the inner surface of the occipital bone, then continues medially along the superior border of the petrous part of the temporal bone to reach the posterior clinoid process. Posteriorly the small falx cerebelli descends vertically from the tentorium and partially separates the two cerebellar hemispheres. The sella turcica in the middle fossa has a roof of dura called the diaphragma sellae, which is attached to the four clinoid processes and has a central aperture for the pituitary stalk.

Fig. 7.66 *Falx cerebri and tentorium cerebelli revealed by removal of the vault of the cranium, associated dura and the cerebral hemispheres.*

Dural venous sinuses

Lying between the two layers of dura are endothelium-lined venous channels (Fig. 7.67). These dural venous sinuses, which often groove the adjacent bones, collect blood from the brain and meninges. They also drain cerebrospinal fluid which has been secreted into the subarachnoid space by the choroid plexuses of the brain. A characteristic of these sinuses is the absence of valves.

The superior sagittal sinus lies in the attached margin of the falx cerebri (Figs. 7.66 & 7.67). The sinus drains posteriorly and has along its length several dilatations called lacunae. These lacunae possess arachnoid granulations through which the reabsorption of cerebrospinal fluid takes place. The sinus also receives numerous cerebral veins. At the internal occipital protuberance the superior sagittal sinus turns laterally, usually to the right, and continues as the transverse sinus in the attached margin of the tentorium cerebelli (Fig. 7.68). Just before reaching the petrous part of the temporal bone, the sinus turns inferiorly to continue as the sigmoid sinus (see Fig. 7.69). This follows an S-shaped course to reach the jugular foramen, through which it is continuous with the internal jugular vein.

S
L ← → R
I

Fig. 7.67 *Coronal section through the posterior cranial fossa showing dural folds and venous sinuses.*

Labels: superior sagittal sinus, dura, falx cerebri, cerebral hemisphere, straight sinus, tentorium cerebelli, transverse sinus, cerebellum

The smaller inferior sagittal sinus lies in the free border of the falx cerebri (Fig. 7.66). The sinus runs posteriorly and at the tentorium cerebelli is joined by the great cerebral vein, which drains the deeper structures of the cerebral hemispheres. The union of these vessels forms the straight sinus

(Figs. 7.66 – 7.68), which continues posteriorly in the attachment of the falx to the tentorium as far as the internal occipital protuberance. Here the straight sinus usually turns to the left to form the transverse sinus, whose course mirrors that on the opposite side.

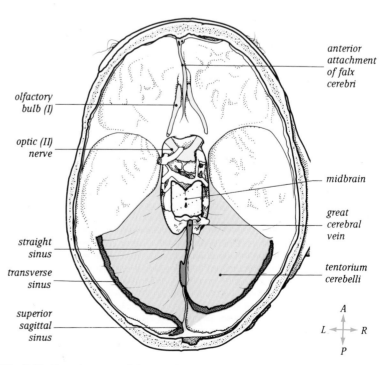

Labels: olfactory bulb (I), optic (II) nerve, straight sinus, transverse sinus, superior sagittal sinus, anterior attachment of falx cerebri, midbrain, great cerebral vein, tentorium cerebelli

A
L ← → R
P

Fig. 7.68 *Superior view of the interior of the cranium after removal of the falx cerebri and cerebral hemispheres. The venous sinuses have been opened. The straight sinus turns to the right and the superior sagittal sinus to the left in this specimen.*

Fig. 7.69 *Interior of cranium after removal of tentorium cerebelli and cerebellum. The venous sinuses have been further opened.*

The cavernous venous sinuses (Figs. 7.69 – 7.71) lie on either side of the pituitary gland and the body of the sphenoid bone. They contain numerous interconnected venous spaces, producing a spongy appearance. The two sinuses communicate with each other and receive blood from the ophthalmic veins of the orbits via the superior orbital fissures. In addition, they receive vessels which pass through the superior and inferior orbital fissures from the pterygoid venous plexuses. Posteriorly each cavernous sinus drains via the superior and inferior petrosal sinuses. The superior petrosal sinus runs along the superior border of the petrous part of the temporal bone to terminate in the junction of the transverse and sigmoid sinuses. The inferior petrosal sinus descends into the posterior cranial fossa and unites with the sigmoid sinus in the jugular foramen to form the internal jugular vein.

Arachnoid mater

The arachnoid mater, the middle of the meningeal layers, is loosely attached to the dura mater, generally following its folds. The arachnoid is separated from the deeper pia mater by the subarachnoid space, which contains cerebrospinal fluid and is traversed by the arteries of the brain and the cranial nerves.

Pia mater

The pia mater is the innermost of the meninges and clings to the surface of the brain, dipping into its numerous grooves or sulci.

Meningeal vessels

Of the many arteries entering the cranium to supply the meninges, one of particular importance is the middle meningeal artery, which arises from the maxillary artery (see page 7.19) and enters through the foramen spinosum. This vessel runs laterally across the floor of the middle cranial fossa, grooving the bone, and divides on the squamous part of the temporal bone into anterior and posterior branches (Fig. 7.69). These branches arch superiorly on the inner surface of the lateral part of the skull and supply the meninges lining most of the vault. Meningeal veins follow the arteries and communicate with the dural venous sinuses and with veins lying outside the skull.

Bleeding from veins or arteries between the meningeal layers can raise intracranial pressure. An extradural haematoma results from extravasation between the dura and the skull. A subdural haematoma is produced by bleeding between the dura and arachnoid layers, where normally no space exists. Blood leaking from the vessels that cross the subarachnoid space will give rise to a subarachnoid haemorrhage, the blood intermingling with cerebrospinal fluid.

ARTERIAL SUPPLY TO BRAIN

The brain receives arterial blood from the vertebral and internal carotid arteries (Fig. 7.70). The vertebral arteries (see page 7.8) enter the posterior cranial fossa through the foramen magnum. Passing upwards and forwards, they unite in the midline on the clivus to form the basilar artery. Branches to the brain stem and cerebellum arise from the vertebral and basilar arteries before the latter divides at the upper border of the pons to form the left and right posterior cerebral arteries. Before supplying the posterior part of the cerebral hemisphere, each of these vessels gives rise to a posterior communicating artery which passes forwards to form part of the circle of Willis by anastomosing with the internal carotid artery.

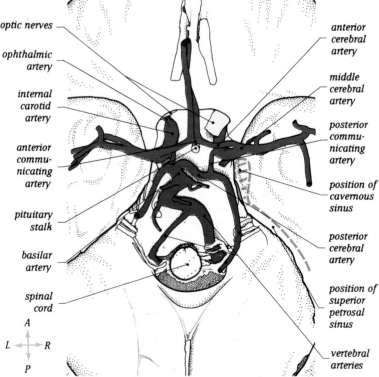

optic nerves

ophthalmic artery

internal carotid artery

anterior commu- nicating artery

pituitary stalk

basilar artery

spinal cord

anterior cerebral artery

middle cerebral artery

posterior commu- nicating artery

position of cavernous sinus

posterior cerebral artery

position of superior petrosal sinus

vertebral arteries

Fig. 7.70 *Superior view of the circle of Willis, exposed by removal of the brain. The basilar and vertebral arteries are asymmetrical in this specimen.*

internal carotid artery

oculomotor (III) nerve

trigeminal (V) nerve

abducens (VI) nerve

facial (VII) & vestibulo- cochlear (VIII) nerves

glosso- pharyngeal (IX), vagus (X) & accessory (XI) nerves

optic chiasma

cavernous sinus

ophthalmic (Va) & maxillary (Vb) divisions

mandibular (Vc) division

trigeminal ganglion

motor root

trochlear (IV) nerve

hypoglossal (XII) nerve

Fig. 7.71 *Cranial nerves revealed by removal of most of the brain. The dura over the right trigeminal ganglion has been excised.*

Fig. 7.72 *Inferior view of the base of the skull showing the principal foramina.*

The internal carotid artery traverses the carotid canal (Fig. 7.72) to enter the middle cranial fossa, emerging from the upper part of the foramen lacerum. The artery turns anteriorly to enter the cavernous sinus, then continues superiorly to leave the sinus through its roof. Here, near the anterior clinoid process, the ophthalmic artery arises and accompanies the optic nerve through the optic canal into the orbit. The internal carotid artery terminates as the anterior and middle cerebral arteries. The middle cerebral artery supplies the lateral portion of the cerebral hemisphere while the anterior cerebral artery ascends between the frontal lobes to supply the medial surface of the hemisphere.

The circle of Willis (cerebral arterial circle) is formed between the branches of the internal carotid and vertebral arteries (see Fig. 7.70). The two anterior cerebral arteries are joined by the anterior communicating artery. On each side an anastomosis, via the posterior communicating artery, between the posterior cerebral branch of the basilar artery and the internal carotid artery completes the circle of Willis.

CRANIAL NERVES
The twelve pairs of cranial nerves enter or leave the skull through various foramina (see Figs. 7.69 & 7.71). The olfactory (I) nerves emerge from the nasal cavity as a number of short branches which traverse the cribriform plates and terminate in the olfactory bulbs.

The optic (II) nerve leaves the orbit via the optic canal and joins the optic chiasma immediately anterior to the pituitary stalk. From the chiasma the optic tracts pass backwards to enter the brain.

Three cranial nerves enter the orbit through the superior orbital fissure. To reach the fissure the oculomotor (III) and trochlear (IV) nerves run forwards in the lateral wall of the cavernous sinus while the abducens (VI) nerve passes through the cavity of the sinus.

The ganglion of the sensory part of the trigeminal (V) nerve lies in a small depression on the apex of the petrous part of the temporal bone. The three divisions of the nerve converge on the anterior surface of the ganglion. From the orbit the ophthalmic (Va) division traverses the superior orbital fissure and continues backwards, embedded in the lateral wall of the cavernous sinus, to reach the ganglion. The maxillary (Vb) division leaves the pterygopalatine fossa via the foramen rotundum and passes backwards along the lower edge of the sinus to the ganglion. The sensory part of the mandibular (Vc) division, accompanied by the motor root of the trigeminal nerve, ascends from the infratemporal fossa through the foramen ovale. The motor root passes beneath and not through the ganglion.

The facial (VII) nerve enters, and the vestibulocochlear (VIII) nerve emerges from, the internal auditory meatus in the petrous part of the temporal bone.

Three nerves leave via the jugular foramen to enter the carotid sheath, namely the glossopharyngeal (IX), vagus (X) and accessory (XI) nerves.

Finally, the hypoglossal (XII) nerve traverses the hypoglossal canal.

ORBIT

The orbit is a pyramidal cavity whose apex is directed posteriorly and base anteriorly. Its bony walls separate it from the anterior cranial fossa above, the ethmoidal air cells and nasal cavity medially, the maxillary air sinus inferiorly and the lateral surface of the face and temporal fossa laterally (Fig. 7.73). Anteriorly the orbit presents a roughly rectangular aperture which is closed by the eyelids. Within the orbit are the eyeball, the extraocular muscles, cranial nerves II, III, IV, V (ophthalmic and maxillary divisions) and VI, and blood vessels, lymphatics and fat.

Fig. 7.73 *Near coronal section, passing through the right orbit more anteriorly than the left, shows the extraocular muscles and relations of the orbits.*

BONY WALLS

The roof of the orbit (Fig. 7.74) comprises the frontal bone, which anteriorly contains the frontal air sinuses. The lateral wall is formed anteriorly by the zygoma and posteriorly by the greater wing of the sphenoid bone. The floor consists of the maxilla anteriorly and the greater wing of the sphenoid posteriorly. From anterior to posterior the medial wall comprises the maxilla, lacrimal, ethmoid and sphenoid bones. The medial walls of the two orbits lie parallel to the median plane while their lateral walls are directed forwards and laterally so that they lie at right angles to one another.

Several foramina and the superior and inferior orbital fissures (Fig. 7.74) allow various structures to enter and leave the orbit. On the medial wall, close to the orbital margin, is a depression called the lacrimal fossa, bounded by the maxilla and the lacrimal bone. The nasolacrimal canal descends from this fossa and opens into the inferior meatus of the nasal cavity. Anterior and posterior ethmoidal foramina perforate the medial wall and allow communication with the lateral wall of the nasal cavity. At the apex of the orbit are the optic canal and the superior and inferior orbital fissures, through which the orbit is in continuity with the middle cranial and pterygopalatine fossae.

FASCIAL LAYERS

Movement of the eyeball is facilitated by its sheath, the fascia bulbi (see Fig. 7.79), which invests it but does not adhere to the sclera and is incomplete anteriorly. The fascia bulbi is attached to the eyeball around the margin of the cornea. Thickenings of the inferior part of the fascia (the suspensory ligament) extend laterally and medially to attach to the orbital walls (check ligaments). The fascia is pierced by the six muscles that move the eyeball. Anteriorly the orbit is closed by the orbital septum, which forms the fibrous layer of the eyelids.

Fig. 7.74 *Bony walls, fissures and foramina of the left orbit.*

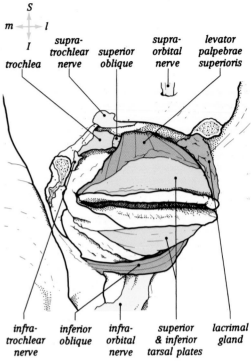

Fig. 7.75 *Contents of the left orbit revealed by removal of the lateral wall and floor of the orbit and parts of the eyelids.*

Fig. 7.76 *Contents of the orbit seen after removal of the lateral wall and floor. The supraorbital nerve lies in a canal in the frontal bone.*

EYELIDS, CONJUNCTIVA AND LACRIMAL APPARATUS

Within each eyelid the orbital septum is thickened to form a tarsal plate (Figs. 7.75 & 7.76) and is perforated between the eyelids by the palpebral fissure. Anterior to the septum lies orbicularis oculi and skin. Levator palpebrae superioris is attached to the upper edge of the superior tarsal plate while a few fibres of inferior rectus are attached to the lower edge of the inferior tarsal plate. Posteriorly each plate has meibomian glands and is covered by conjunctiva. The conjunctival epithelium is reflected onto the surface of the eyeball where it blends with the margin of the cornea. Each eyelid carries a double row of eyelashes together with associated sebaceous glands (which when inflamed form a 'stye'). The lashes on each eyelid extend medially as far as a small elevation containing a central aperture, the lacrimal punctum, leading into the lacrimal canaliculus. The canaliculi carry tear fluid to the lacrimal sac in the lacrimal fossa, and the sac in turn drains via the nasolacrimal duct, in the nasolacrimal canal, into the nasal cavity beneath the inferior concha (see Fig. 7.44).

The lacrimal gland (Figs. 7.75 & 7.76; see also Fig. 7.78) lies in the superolateral angle of the orbit behind the upper eyelid and is deeply indented by the lateral border of the tendon of levator palpebrae superioris. Small ducts open from the deep surface of the gland into the conjunctival sac. Fluid produced by the gland passes medially towards the lacrimal puncta across the surface of the cornea, assisted by blinking of the eyelid. Reflex blinking is initiated if the cornea is touched or becomes dry. Evaporation of the fluid is retarded by the oily secretion of the tarsal glands.

EXTRAOCULAR MUSCLES

Within the orbit most muscles comprise only voluntary fibres, but those that move the eyelids contain smooth fibres as well.

The extraocular muscles are the four recti, the two obliques and one muscle which attaches to the upper eyelids, levator palpebrae superioris (Figs. 7.75–7.77). This is the uppermost muscle in the orbit, and from its attachment to the lesser wing of the sphenoid it passes forwards to form a wide tendon which enters the upper eyelid and blends with the superior tarsal plate.

The medial, lateral, superior and inferior recti (Figs. 7.76 & 7.77; see also Figs. 7.79 & 7.80) attach posteriorly to a fibrotendinous ring which surrounds the optic canal and part of the superior orbital fissure. Passing forwards, these four muscles attach to the eyeball immediately behind the corneoscleral junction in positions corresponding to their names. Collectively they form a cone with its apex at the optic canal and its base around the equator of the eyeball. Nerves and vessels entering the orbit run their course either within or outside this cone of muscle.

The superior oblique (see Fig. 7.78) has a posterior attachment to the lesser wing of the sphenoid adjacent to the fibrotendinous ring. The muscle passes anteriorly along the junction between the medial wall and the roof of the orbit and forms a tendon which traverses a loop of fibrous tissue, the trochlea, which lies at the superomedial angle of the orbital margin and allows the tendon of superior oblique to turn backwards across the upper surface of the eyeball. The tendon lies beneath superior rectus and attaches to the superolateral part of the eyeball behind the equator.

Inferior oblique (Figs. 7.75 & 7.76), lying entirely in the anterior part of the orbit, attaches to the floor of the orbit just lateral to the nasolacrimal canal. The muscle passes posterolaterally below the inferior rectus to attach to the inferolateral part of the eyeball behind the equator.

Three cranial nerves supply these muscles. The abducens (VI) nerve (see Figs. 7.79 & 7.80) innervates lateral rectus while the trochlear (IV) nerve (Fig. 7.77) supplies superior oblique. All the remaining muscles receive motor branches from the oculomotor (III) nerve (see Figs. 7.78 & 7.80).

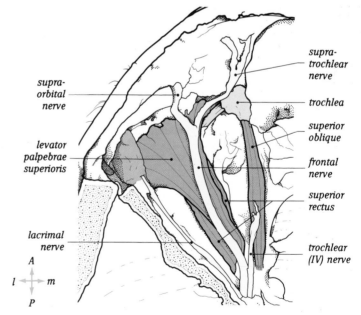

Fig. 7.77 *Contents of the orbit seen from above, after removal of the orbital plate of the frontal bone.*

MOVEMENTS OF EYEBALL AND EYELID

In defining the actions of individual extraocular muscles it is assumed that the eyeball is positioned so that the gaze is directed forwards into the distance. Within its fascial sheath the eyeball is rotated by the extraocular muscles which displace the gaze upwards (elevation), downwards (depression), medially (adduction) and laterally (abduction). Rotation about an anteroposterior axis (torsion) may also occur. Collectively the extraocular muscles also contribute to the stability of the eyeball, the recti tending to pull the globe backwards and the obliques tending to pull it forwards.

The only actions of the medial and lateral recti are adduction and abduction respectively. Superior rectus elevates and adducts whilst inferior rectus depresses and adducts. Both oblique muscles produce abduction, the inferior oblique elevating the gaze and the superior oblique depressing it. Most eye movements involve the coordinated contraction and relaxation of several individual muscles, and elevation and depression are accompanied by movement of the eyelids. Levator palpebrae superioris raises the upper eyelid (opposed by orbicularis oculi) while inferior rectus depresses the lower eyelid.

NERVES

Several nerves reach the orbit from the middle cranial and pterygopalatine fossae. The optic (II) nerve (Fig. 7.78), which conveys visual sensation, traverses the optic canal with the ophthalmic artery. Enveloped by meninges and cerebrospinal fluid, the nerve passes forwards and laterally within the cone of rectus muscles and enters the eyeball just medial to its posterior pole. Other nerves gain the orbit through the orbital fissures.

The oculomotor (III) nerve (Figs. 7.78 & 7.80) enters the cone of muscles via the superior orbital fissure. It has superior and inferior divisions which are often formed before entering the orbit. The superior division supplies the superior rectus and levator palpebrae superioris while the inferior division gives branches to inferior rectus, inferior oblique, medial rectus and the ciliary ganglion. Sympathetic fibres to the smooth muscle in levator palpebrae superioris and inferior rectus enter the oculomotor (III) nerve in the cavernous sinus and travel with its branches to these muscles.

The trochlear (IV) nerve (Fig. 7.78) enters the orbit via the superior orbital fissure, passing above the muscle cone to supply superior oblique.

The abducens (VI) nerve (Figs 7.79 & 7.80) gains the orbit via the superior orbital fissure and passes forwards on the inner surface of lateral rectus, which it supplies.

The ophthalmic (Va) division of the trigeminal nerve divides into lacrimal, frontal and nasociliary nerves, each of which enters the orbit through the superior orbital fissure. The lacrimal nerve (see Fig. 7.77) passes forwards, outside the muscle cone, along the angle between the roof and lateral wall of the orbit. It is joined by parasympathetic secretomotor fibres from the zygomatic nerve (see page 7.26) which are destined for the lacrimal gland. In addition, the lacrimal nerve conveys sensation from the lacrimal gland and the lateral part of the upper eyelid.

The frontal nerve (see Fig. 7.77) lies on the upper surface of levator palpebrae superioris and divides into supraorbital and supratrochlear nerves. The supraorbital nerve (see Figs. 7.75 & 7.77) curves around the upper part of the orbital margin, occupying the supraorbital notch, and conveys sensation from the upper eyelid, forehead, scalp and frontal air sinus. The supratrochlear nerve (see Figs. 7.75 & 7.77) lies more medially, leaving the orbit just above the trochlea to supply sensory fibres to the medial part of the upper eyelid, forehead and scalp.

The nasociliary nerve (Fig. 7.78), lying within the muscle cone, crosses above the optic (II) nerve and continues forwards along the medial wall of the orbit to terminate below the trochlea. Its branches include one to the ciliary ganglion, two long ciliary nerves, posterior and anterior ethmoidal nerves and the infratrochlear nerve. The long ciliary nerves, which carry sympathetic vasoconstrictor fibres that join the nasociliary nerve in the cavernous sinus, pass forwards to supply vessels within the eyeball. The posterior and anterior ethmoidal nerves leave through their respective foramina, supplying ethmoidal air cells. The anterior ethmoidal nerve passes between the frontal and ethmoid bones and emerges on the upper surface of the cribriform plate. Leaving the anterior fossa, the nerve penetrates the plate to run on the inner surface of the nasal bone as the external nasal nerve and eventually reaches the tip of the nose. It conveys sensation from a strip of nasal skin close to the midline and from the nasal septum. The infratrochlear nerve supplies the medial part of the upper eyelid (see Fig. 7.75).

Autonomic nerves

The ciliary ganglion lies just behind the eyeball, lateral to the optic (II) nerve. It receives sensory fibres from the nasociliary nerve, parasympathetic fibres from the oculomotor (III) nerve, and sympathetic fibres from the internal carotid plexus in the cavernous sinus. Only the parasympathetic fibres synapse in the ganglion. From the anterior part of the ganglion, short ciliary nerves (Fig. 7.78) pass forwards into the eyeball, conveying general sensory fibres from the eyeball (including the cornea), parasympathetic fibres to the ciliary muscle and sphincter pupillae, and sympathetic fibres to dilator pupillae.

Vasoconstrictor sympathetic fibres reach the eyeball in the long ciliary branches of the nasociliary nerve. Other intraorbital sympathetic fibres travel in the oculomotor (III) nerve to the smooth muscle component of levator palpebrae superioris and inferior rectus. Parasympathetic fibres reach the lacrimal gland via the lacrimal nerve, which communicates with the zygomatic branch of the maxillary (Vb) division of the trigeminal nerve. The cell bodies of these fibres are located in the pterygopalatine ganglion (see page 7.27).

Fig. 7.78 *Deeper structures of the orbit seen after excision of superior rectus, levator palpebrae superioris and the superior division of the oculomotor nerve along with a quantity of orbital fat.*

VESSELS

The ophthalmic artery (Figs. 7.78 & 7.79), a branch of the internal carotid artery in the middle cranial fossa, enters the orbit through the optic canal inferior to the optic (II) nerve. The artery then accompanies the nasociliary nerve, passing above the optic nerve and continuing forwards along the medial wall of the orbit. Its first branch, the central retinal artery, enters the optic nerve

Fig. 7.79 *Deeper muscles of the orbit seen after removal of the upper eyelid, part of the optic nerve, and superior oblique.*

Fig. 7.80 *Inferior division of the oculomotor nerve revealed by excision of the distal part of the ophthalmic artery and the nasociliary nerve.*

and passes into the eyeball to supply the retina. Occlusion of this artery results in blindness. Other branches of the ophthalmic artery accompany those of the ophthalmic (Va) division of the trigeminal nerve. In addition, there are posterior and anterior ciliary branches to the eyeball, and branches to the extraocular muscles.

Venous blood from the eyeball and adjacent structures drains into inferior and superior ophthalmic veins. The superior ophthalmic vein terminates posteriorly in the cavernous venous sinus while the inferior vein passes through the inferior orbital fissure into the pterygoid venous plexus in the pterygopalatine fossa. Both superior and inferior ophthalmic veins communicate with veins on the face.

CONTENTS OF CAROTID SHEATH

The carotid sheaths form part of the fascial layers of the neck (see pages 7.2 & 7.3) and extend from the base of the skull into the superior mediastinum. Each sheath contains the common, the internal and part of the external carotid arteries, the internal jugular vein and parts of the glossopharyngeal (IX), vagus (X) and accessory (XI) nerves.

CAROTID ARTERIES

The common carotid artery arises on the left from the aortic arch and on the right from the brachiocephalic artery. The vessel ascends within its sheath into the neck and at the upper border of the thyroid cartilage it divides into internal and external carotid arteries (Fig. 7.82). At its origin the internal carotid artery is dilated to form the carotid sinus. The vessel ascends within the carotid sheath without branching and, in company with its sympathetic nerve plexus, enters the carotid canal. In the cranial cavity the internal carotid artery terminates as the anterior and middle cerebral arteries (see page 7.44), having given rise the ophthalmic artery, which supplies the contents of the orbit.

The external carotid artery leaves the carotid sheath, inclines superolaterally and enters the deepest part of the parotid gland where it divides into terminal branches at the level of the neck of the mandible. Separating the external and internal carotid arteries are the styloid process, stylopharyngeus, the glossopharyngeal (IX) nerve and the pharyngeal branch of the vagus (X) nerve.

The external carotid artery has eight branches (Fig. 7.82), supplying much of the extracranial portion of the head and upper part of the neck. The first branch, the ascending pharyngeal artery, arises on the medial aspect of the external carotid artery and ascends on the lateral surface of the pharynx. The next branch, the superior thyroid artery, inclines downwards and forwards from the anterior surface of the external carotid, to supply the thyroid gland and the larynx. The lingual artery passes forwards from the anterior surface of the external carotid artery into the base of the tongue (see page 7.25). The facial artery, another anterior branch, supplies the tonsil and descends under the body of the mandible, grooving the submandibular gland and emerging from beneath the mandible at the anterior border of masseter to supply the face (see Fig. 7.29).

Arising from the posterior surface of the external carotid artery, the occipital artery passes upwards and backwards deep to sternomastoid (Fig. 7.82 & 7.19). The vessel crosses the apex of the posterior triangle of the neck to supply the posterior part of the scalp. The posterior auricular artery arises below the pinna and passes upwards and backwards to supply the pinna and the scalp.

The terminal branches of the external carotid artery arise within the pa   id gland and are named the superficial temporal and maxillary arteries. The former supplies the lateral part of the scalp while the maxillary artery supplies the infratemporal fossa, pterygopalatine fossa and lateral wall of the nose. Postganglionic sympathetic nerve fibres accompany the external carotid artery and its branches.

Fig. 7.81 *Internal jugular vein and some cervical lymph nodes, revealed by removal of sternomastoid and part of the parotid gland.*

parotid gland (cut)
posterior belly of digastric
submandibular nodes
anterior belly of disgastric
submandibular gland
mastoid node
sternomastoid (cut)
jugulodigastric node
deep cervical nodes
internal jugular vein
omohyoid
supraclavicular nodes

INTERNAL JUGULAR VEIN

The internal jugular vein (Figs. 7.81 & 7.82) is formed within the jugular foramen by the union of the sigmoid and inferior petrosal venous sinuses. The vein descends through the neck within the carotid sheath and receives the facial, lingual, pharyngeal, and superior and middle thyroid veins. The internal jugular vein also communicates with the external jugular system via the anterior branch of the retromandibular vein. It terminates by uniting with the subclavian vein to form the brachiocephalic vein.

NERVES

Within the carotid sheath lie the glossopharyngeal (IX), vagus (X) and accessory (XI) nerves, which leave the skull via the jugular foramen. The glossopharyngeal nerve passes inferiorly and leaves the carotid sheath. It winds around the posterolateral surface of stylopharyngeus and enters the posterior third of the tongue. The nerve supplies stylopharyngeus and gives a sensory branch which descends to innervate the carotid sinus (see Fig. 7.25).

The vagus (X) nerve (Fig. 7.82) bears two ganglia, one lying superiorly in the jugular foramen and one below the base of the skull, between which the nerve receives the cranial part of the accessory nerve. The vagus nerve descends in the posterior part of the carotid sheath between the carotid artery and internal jugular vein and gives rise to pharyngeal, superior laryngeal and cardiac branches before traversing the thoracic inlet. The pharyngeal branch passes forwards between the internal and external carotid arteries to gain the outer surface of the pharynx where it contributes to the pharyngeal plexus. The superior laryngeal nerve accompanies the superior thyroid artery and vein supplying the larynx. The cardiac branches of the vagus join those from the sympathetic trunk and descend into the thorax. The right vagus gives a recurrent laryngeal branch in the neck which curves around the right subclavian artery and passes superiorly to reach the larynx (see page 7.9). The left recurrent laryngeal nerve arises from the left vagus nerve in the thorax and passes around the aortic arch before ascending into the neck.

The accessory (XI) nerve (Fig. 7.82) is formed by the fusion of cranial and spinal roots in the posterior cranial fossa. In the jugular foramen the nerve divides into a cranial part joining the vagus nerve and a spinal part which leaves the carotid sheath to supply sternomastoid and trapezius.

LYMPHATICS

Lymphatic vessels from structures in the head and neck accompany the vascular supply and drain into superficial or deep groups of lymph nodes.

Superficial lymph nodes

Several groups of superficial nodes form an incomplete ring around the lower part of the head. The submental nodes lie between the anterior bellies of the two digastric muscles, draining lymph from the tip of the tongue and the mental region. The submandibular group (Fig. 7.81) lies on the superficial surface of the submandibular gland and receives lymph from the submental nodes, from the remainder of the anterior two-thirds of the tongue, from the floor of the mouth including the gums and teeth, and from the nose, face and anterior part of the scalp. The parotid nodes lie on or within the parotid gland, the mastoid group (Fig. 7.81) on the lateral surface of the mastoid process, and the occipital lymph nodes at the apex of the posterior triangle of the neck. The parotid, mastoid and occipital nodes drain the remainder of the face and scalp, including the external ear. Lymph from all the superficial nodes drains into the deep cervical nodes.

Fig. 7.82 *Branches of the external carotid artery and the vagus, accessory and hypoglossal nerves, after removal of part of the internal jugular vein, carotid sheath and posterior belly of digastric.*

Labels: transverse facial artery — maxillary artery — external carotid artery — stylohyoid — facial artery — lingual artery — external carotid artery — superior thyroid artery — superficial temporal artery — internal jugular vein (cut) — sternomastoid (cut) — posterior auricular artery (cut) — occipital artery — accessory nerve — hypoglossal nerve — carotid sinus & internal carotid artery — vagus nerve

Deep cervical lymph nodes

The deep cervical or jugular lymph nodes (Fig. 7.81) form a chain in and around the carotid sheath. Two of the deep cervical nodes are of particular clinical significance. The jugulo-digastric node receives lymph mainly from the tongue and tonsil and the juguloomohyoid node drains the tongue. From the deep cervical nodes lymph drains inferiorly, via the jugular lymphatic trunk, usually into the thoracic duct on the left and into the right lymphatic duct on the right.

CERVICAL VERTEBRAL COLUMN

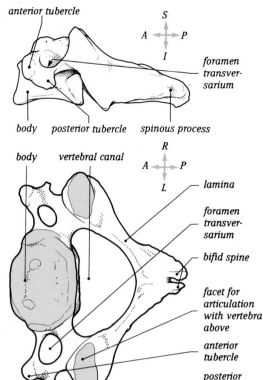

The cervical vertebral column consists of seven cervical vertebrae and their intervertebral discs. It is very mobile and usually has a forward convexity (lordosis). The third, fourth, fifth and sixth vertebrae have a characteristic appearance whereas the first, second and seventh are modified. A typical cervical vertebra (Fig. 7.83), in addition to the features common to vertebrae elsewhere, has two transverse processes, each possessing anterior and posterior tubercles and perforated by a foramen transversarium which transmits the vertebral artery and veins (see page 7.8). The spinous processes are short and bifid and all give attachment to a strong midline fibroelastic ligament, the ligamentum nuchae. This ligament also attaches to the external occipital protuberance and crest.

Fig. 7.83 *Left lateral (upper) and superior (lower) views of a typical (fourth) cervical vertebra.*

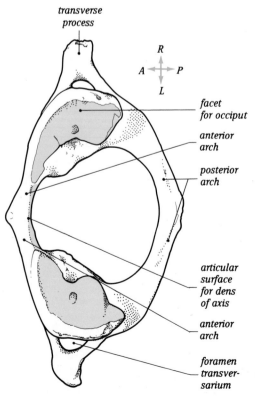

Fig. 7.84 *Left lateral (upper) and superior (lower) views of the first cervical vertebra, the atlas.*

ATLAS
The first cervical vertebra, the atlas (Fig. 7.84), has anterior and posterior arches, relatively large transverse processes and two lateral masses. The atlas has no body and a diminutive spinous process. On its superior surface each lateral mass has a concave facet which articulates with the convex occipital condyle of the skull. At these synovial atlantooccipital joints flexion and extension (nodding movements) take place. The flat inferior surface of each lateral mass articulates with a corresponding facet on the axis.

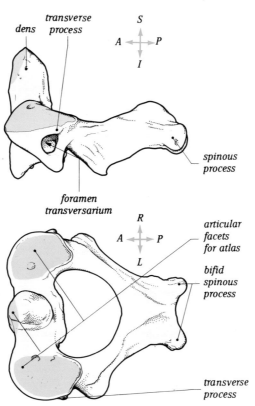

dens

transverse process

S
A ↔ P
I

spinous process

foramen transversarium

R
A ↔ P
L

articular facets for atlas

bifid spinous process

transverse process

Fig. 7.85 *Left lateral (upper) and superior (lower) views of the second cervical vertebra, the axis.*

AXIS

Though the axis (second cervical vertebra; Fig. 7.85) possesses some features of a typical cervical vertebra, it has a unique vertical projection, the odontoid process or dens. This projects superiorly from the upper surface of its body and represents the body of the atlas. The odontoid process articulates by a synovial joint with a facet on the posterior surface of the anterior arch of the atlas (the third component of the atlantoaxial joint), where it is retained by the alar, apical and transverse ligaments (Fig. 7.86; see Fig. 7.87). Movements at the atlantoaxial joint allow rotation of the head as when looking from side to side.

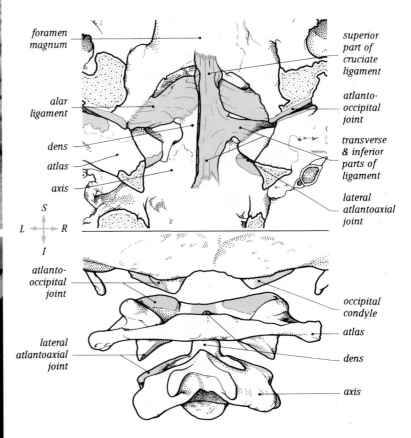

foramen magnum

alar ligament

dens

atlas

axis

S
L ↔ R
I

superior part of cruciate ligament

atlanto-occipital joint

transverse & inferior parts of ligament

lateral atlantoaxial joint

atlanto-occipital joint

lateral atlantoaxial joint

occipital condyle

atlas

dens

axis

Fig. 7.86 *Ligaments of the median atlantoaxial joint revealed by removal of the neural arches of the cervical vertebrae, posterior part of the skull, spinal cord and meninges, and posterior longitudinal ligament. Half of the cruciate ligament has been excised (upper). Base of skull, atlas and axis seen in an expanded posterior view (lower).*

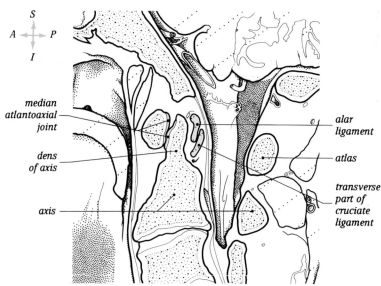

Fig. 7.87 *Near sagittal section through the median atlantoaxial joint.*

In the diagram (Fig. 7.87), labels include: median atlantoaxial joint, dens of axis, axis, alar ligament, atlas, transverse part of cruciate ligament.

SEVENTH CERVICAL VERTEBRA

This vertebra (Fig. 7.88) possesses a long non-bifid spine which provides the inferior attachment for the ligamentum nuchae. This spinous process is easily palpable and hence the vertebra is called the vertebra prominens.

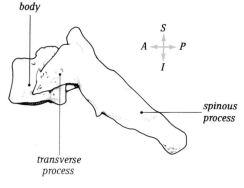

In the diagram: body, spinous process, transverse process.

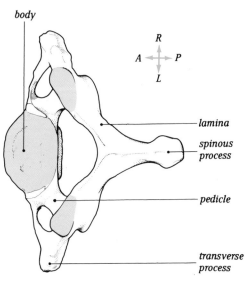

In the diagram: body, lamina, spinous process, pedicle, transverse process.

Fig. 7.88 *Left lateral (upper) and superior (lower) views of the seventh cervical vertebra, the vertebra prominens.*

MOVEMENTS

The joints of the whole cervical column allow movements of flexion, extension, rotation and lateral flexion. These movements are brought about by the prevertebral and postvertebral muscles, assisted by sternomastoid (see page 7.3) and trapezius. The prevertebral muscles flex the cervical spine and comprise the scalene group (see page 7.9) and the longus colli group. The latter passes from the base of the skull down the anterior surface of the vertebral column into the thorax. The postvertebral muscles, also known as erector spinae, occupy the interval between the spinous and transverse processes of the vertebrae. In the neck, erector spinae is supplied segmentally by the posterior rami of the cervical spinal nerves and extends the cervical spine. Lateral flexion is brought about by the unilateral contraction of both pre- and postvertebral muscles.

Injuries to the cervical vertebral column, particularly involving fracture or dislocation of vertebrae, may result in spinal cord injury leading to quadriplegia or death. The atlantoaxial joint is particularly liable to disruption in hyperextension injuries.

Index